I0901262

Stepping Stones and Stepping Stones Plus

Praise for the book

'Stepping Stones is a programme that truly transforms relationships between women and men, older and younger people in communities. As no other guide, it promotes dialogues and understanding between men and women and the different generations: it shows the route to equality. If we can just get this approach fully implemented around the globe, the world would be a better place!'

Doortje Braeken,
Senior Adviser Adolescents,
Gender and Rights,
International Planned Parenthood Federation

'I observed the profound impact of Stepping Stones in a small village in The Gambia. The village consisted of over 30 families, and all but one woman reported spousal violence in the year before Stepping Stones began. In the nine months after the fourteen-week peer-led programme ended, there had been only one incidence of intimate partner violence. The men reported that now they were glad to understand the use of condoms and that they could use them with their wives.'

Susan Paxton, Public health consultant,
author of International Community of Women living with HIV Speakers' Guide

'This manual has been of tremendous benefit and help to stakeholders, middle-level managers and entire health workers in the district. It has increased the knowledge and proficiency of those health workers dedicated to home-based care and counselling of HIV/AIDS patients.'

Frederick Ofosu, Ministry of Health,
Odumase-Krobo, Ghana

'The process was emotionally charged — we were talking about very deep issues. This wouldn't have happened without the Stepping Stones methods. There were young women, widows, mothers with sick children, all taking part. People shared some deep experiences they had never told anyone before.'

Rudo Chikukwa,
Network of Zimbabwean Positive Women

'The girls really love doing the games and drama. Many of them are already involved in unsafe sex; now they're gaining the confidence to say no, or let's use a condom.'

Sarah Tweats, VSO teacher,
Solwesi Technical Secondary School,
Zambia

'I was always scared and ashamed to talk about these things with my husband. He didn't want me to attend these meetings; he used to say that after these meetings, women would rebel against their husbands ... It has been different... I used to live in the darkness...now I am in the light.'

A woman from an indigenous community, Ecuador

'For every worn, rain-splattered copy of Stepping Stones that is in circulation, there are thousands of people that have benefited from it. Communities have been mobilized, lives saved and hope restored.'

Laura van Vuuren,
Medical Teams International,
Seattle, USA

'UNAIDS has included this resource package among the "key documents" recommended for use in innovative community mobilization programmes.'

Noerine Kaleeba,
Community Mobilization Adviser,
UNAIDS

'Stepping Stones has helped ActionAid India to deepen and strengthen our work in the area of HIV and AIDS. ActionAid India has been using Stepping Stones to break the silence about sexuality and HIV among development workers, NGO staff and communities; to create more acceptance of vulnerable groups such as people living with HIV and AIDS, men who have sex with men, and injecting drug users. The changes started by Stepping Stones have created ripples across the country, and the demand for Stepping Stones is growing.'

Christy Abraham, ActionAid India, Bangalore, India

'Here in Latin America and the Caribbean, these materials are some of the most effective tools we have to link the African experience of the AIDS pandemic with the innovative work of local communities.'

Mark Connolly, UNICEF,
Panama City, Panama

Stepping Stones and Stepping Stones Plus

A training package on gender, generation, HIV, communication and relationship skills

Alice Welbourn with Florence Kilonzo,
T.J. Mboya and Shoba Mohamed Liban

PRACTICAL ACTION
Publishing

Practical Action Publishing Ltd
The Schumacher Centre, Bourton on Dunsmore, Rugby, Warwickshire, CV23 9QZ, UK
www.practicalactionpublishing.org

This is a fully revised and updated edition derived from:
Welbourn, Alice (1995) *Stepping Stones*, Strategies for Hope Trust, Oxford, and
Welbourn, A., Kilonzo, F., Mboya, T.J., and Liban, S.M., (2008) *Stepping Stones Plus*, Strategies for Hope Trust, Oxford.

A catalogue record for this book is available from the British Library.
A catalogue record for this book has been requested from the Library of Congress.

ISBN 978-1-85339-891-9 Hardback
ISBN 978-1-85339-8926 Paperback
ISBN 978-1-78044-8916 Library Ebook
ISBN 978-1-78044-892-3 Ebook

Citation: Welbourn, A. (2016) *Stepping Stones and Stepping Stones Plus: A training package on gender, generation, HIV, communication and relationship skills*, Rugby, UK: Practical Action Publishing, <http://dx.doi.org/10.3362//9781780448916>

Since 1974, Practical Action Publishing has published and disseminated books and information in support of international development work throughout the world. Practical Action Publishing is a trading name of Practical Action Publishing Ltd (Company Reg. No. 1159018), the wholly owned publishing company of Practical Action. Practical Action Publishing trades only in support of its parent charity objectives and any profits are covenanted back to Practical Action (Charity Reg. No. 247257, Group VAT Registration No. 880 9924 76).

Cover design: Mercer Design
Illustrations: Petra Röhr-Rouendaal
DVD Production: Jamie Hartzell, Small World Productions
Printed by: Replika Pres Ltd., India

CONTENTS

ACKNOWLEDGEMENTS

First I would like to thank the numerous people who gave us tremendous support in the making of *Stepping Stones* and the accompanying film. They are too numerous to mention all of them by name, but we would like to express our particular thanks to:

The people of Buwenda village, Masaka District, Uganda, where the first workshop based on this manual was organised, and where the film was shot. The Buwenda film crew: Jamie Hartzell, Chris Blokhuis, Zöe Broughton, Tim Muwonge. The Buwenda workshop facilitators: Professor Rose Mbowa, Germine Sebuwufu, Baron Oron and Milton Bakebwa.

Medical Adviser, Dr Nigel Padfield. The authors of the many manuals which have inspired this one.

I am also grateful to the following people for their expert advice on the contents and presentation of the manual and film: Sheena Crawford, Anna Eden, Gill Gordon, Susanna Graham-Jones, Irene Guijt, Okello Hamisi, Vanessa Howe, Margaret Kabanda, David Kabiswa, Sam Kalibala, Emily Katarikawe, Fortunate Kekika, Judith Large, Nicta Lubaale, Sue Lucas, Mary Martin, Mutiba Masereka, Olive Mbogga, Rose Mbowa, Mary-Jane Msungu, Florence Muhangi, Roy Mwilu, John Ngugi, Pat Norrish, Klinton Nyamuryekunge, Baron Oron, Catherine Plewman, Judith Rand, Fiona Robinson, Kirsten Rohme, Germine Sebuwufu, Tina Wallace, and Tina Wiseman.

I would also like to thank those who helped in the preparation of *Stepping Stones Plus*. These include: UNICEF staff member Dr Chris Ouma, Halima Sheikh, Hussein Golicha, Emma Cockburn, Nais Mason, Erika Webi. Also: Elizabeth, Mutinde, and Jamila who are members of OPAHA, Garissa; Marge Berer, Reproductive Health Matters, London; and Amandine Bollinger, Salamander Trust, London.

Other source materials

Thanks to the following for original versions of materials used in this manual:

- TASO (The AIDS Stepping Organization), Uganda, for 'Keeping the Fire Burning'/Bulumbuli diagram (re-drawn for *Stepping Stones* Plus by Julia Whatley) and the 'TASO Game' exercise.
- La Asociación de Hombres Contra la Violencia, Nicaragua, for their 'Join the Circle' exercise which has been adapted to make 'In the spotlight'.
- TJ Mboya, Fridah Musya, Ann Domatob, Susan Govedi, Bonny and Carro Sande, for their exercises about supporting 'prevention of vertical transmission', and involvement of faith-based organisations.
- T.J. Mboya et al for exercises modified from Kidd and Clay (2003) on the following subjects: greater sensitivity of health staff, supporting wider uptake of voluntary counselling and testing, involving neighbours in support of people with HIV and their families, infant feeding, and orphans.[1]

Finally, I would like to thank all who have helped me in the revision and updating of this new edition.

Nell Osborne, Stepping Stones International Community of Practice Coordinator, especially for rewriting all the drawings.

Sophie Dilmitis for revision and update of the *Stepping Stones Plus* references.

Angelina Namiba, who reviewed and updated information in Session E and on breast-feeding in Exercise Q.3.

Aislinn McNamara for preliminary copy-editing. Fiona Hale for further copyediting and valued editorial comments.

Sue Holden and Gill Gordon for all their advice and support, especially in the development of the new sister manual, *Stepping Stones with Children*.

All at Practical Action for the publication of this updated edition.

Especial thanks are due to Glen and Alison Williams of Strategies for Hope Trust who commissioned, published, and distributed this programme worldwide for 20 years until their retirement in 2015.

ENDNOTE

1. Modified by T.J. Mboya et al for exercises modified from Kidd and Clay (2003) on the following subjects: greater sensitivity of health staff, supporting wider uptake of voluntary counselling and testing, involving neighbours in support of people with HIV and their families, infant feeding, and orphans.

REFERENCES

Modified by T.J. Mboya et al for exercises modified from Kidd and Clay (2003) on the following subjects: greater sensitivity of health staff, supporting wider uptake of voluntary counselling and testing, involving neighbours in support of people with HIV and their families, infant feeding, and orphans.

DEDICATIONS

Stepping Stones was dedicated to Mr Mulumba of Buwenda village, Masaka District, Uganda, who died shortly after the shooting of the film which accompanies this manual.

Stepping Stones Plus was dedicated to the honour and memory of my son, Ben, who died suddenly aged 18 whilst this work was in progress.

From you I receive
To you I give
Together we share
By this we live

Stepping Stones and Stepping Stones Plus is dedicated to my own special family, Muna, Ben, Jack and Nigel, who have taught me so much about dying – and living – with all my love and thanks.

Alice Welbourn

PREFACE

The *Stepping Stones* training package has been in use since the first workshop was run in rural Uganda in 1995. It has been used by over 1,000 organisations in over 100 countries and in many different religious and cultural contexts worldwide. Its users find it as useful and relevant as ever in supporting individuals, their peers, and wider community members to prepare for and address the issues that we all face in relation to our sexual and reproductive health and well being, and our relationships.

Over the years, we have seen immense technological advances in the treatment of HIV. It is now possible to live a long, healthy and productive life with HIV, and also to have children born HIV-free, when the right medication is combined with the essential ingredients of care, love, respect, and support.

As the author of *Stepping Stones* I can testify to this. I was diagnosed with HIV in 1992 and I have been on ARV medication since 2000. At the time of writing (November 2015) I have a CD4 count of 970, an undetectable viral load, and I am fit and well.

But medication alone cannot end AIDS.

For those who already have HIV, there is the added possibility that they will experience gender-based violence for the first time, either from intimate partners, other family members, neighbours or work colleagues – or from health care and other institutions.

This is where *Stepping Stones* comes in: it's about timeless issues such as our relationships and the people who create them – amongst peers and across genders and generations. It's only by building long-term, mutually supportive, and respectful relationships that we can overcome the challenges we all face in our lives together. We can keep ourselves and one another safe from fear of violence of any kind (which can often increase vulnerability to HIV) and free of HIV, (other) sexually transmitted infections, and unplanned pregnancies.

How *Stepping Stones* was created – and grew

When I wrote *Stepping Stones* shortly after my own HIV diagnosis, it was a way of trying to make sense of what had happened to me, and so I tried to create a training package for a workshop that might have protected *me* from acquiring HIV. I was supported by many extraordinary people who have helped to shape, produce, and disseminate this programme over the years. Because of the care and support of those around me, I have been able to continue to lead a life fully integrated into my community, and be fully involved in all decision-making about what happens to me. Yet this is very far from the reality for most people with HIV in the world; instead, they are shunned, ostracised, blamed, and excluded from life by their communities, and then die very scared and lonely deaths. Because I was supported so well, I was able to speak out about my experiences, and others have said this has helped them to understand what HIV is – and what it isn't.

Stepping Stones spread around the world largely by word of mouth. There are no big bucks behind it. People say that the best HIV prevention education is for people knowingly to meet someone like themselves who has HIV. However, for those of us with HIV, a supportive environment is critical in order for us to summon the energy to *continue* to speak out and share our experiences and to *keep taking* the daily medication that keeps us healthy. So we hope that this training package will enable us all to understand more clearly how important it is for us *all* to question and challenge our ignorance about HIV, as well as our negative attitudes towards people with HIV, so that we can all learn from each other how very easily HIV can – and does – affect us all.

Stepping Stones Plus

This new edition of *Stepping Stones and Stepping Stones Plus* incorporates both the original *Stepping Stones* programme manual and the supplement, *Stepping Stones Plus*. We designed and published the supplement in response to new scientific advances in healthcare for women with HIV, so that whole communities would support women to have babies safely, when they want to, and to create a new, HIV-free generation. The original manual was designed in 1993–4, a little before antiretroviral therapy (ARVs) had been invented and a long time before it started to become available in most parts of the world. In those days HIV definitely looked as if it *always* meant AIDS and death. For many people with HIV it is still extremely difficult to get hold of ARVs. But this medication can and does make a huge difference to the lives of many people with HIV. WHO[1] now states that ARVs should be offered to an individual, if s/he wants to start them, as soon as they are diagnosed with HIV. So someone who has HIV now may no longer necessarily become sick with AIDS-related illnesses, and may well be able to live a long, healthy, and happy life.

The new exercises and sessions in *Stepping Stones Plus* were designed to supplement the original training package, to provide additional support to communities in understanding how HIV breeds and flourishes on the ongoing root inequities and injustices in our lives, and our collective reluctance to look at or challenge them. The new sessions were designed especially to support women's rights around perinatal care and breastfeeding, to enable us together to have the courage to stamp out many injustices women face in the context of motherhood – and, in doing so, also halt the spread of HIV. Key issues such as supportive health care, support from partners, families, faith leaders and neighbours, and support for other family members are covered. These are all topics that had been highlighted by previous *Stepping Stones* facilitators and trainers as needing more attention. Also, new research has shown[2] that it is from the very people who should be supporting them that women, once diagnosed with HIV, experience gender-based violence (GBV), often for the first time.

Meanwhile, men in many countries seem to fear being tested for HIV but often get sick before their wives or other sexual partners, which suggests that they are likely to have acquired HIV first, especially if their wives are younger. In fact various studies[3] have backed up this observation. In many countries, men are older than their wives or other sexual partners, are expected by their peers to have had several sexual partners before they marry, and to continue to have other sexual partners after they marry. By contrast, women are generally younger than their husbands or other and sexual partners, are expected to be virgins when they first marry, and to be absolutely faithful to their husbands during their marriage. When men get sick, they are nursed and cared for by their wives or daughters. However, they often die prematurely because they haven't had access to the medication that could keep them well. So often men leave their widows and children in a very difficult financial and legal position. Often the man's parents expect the widow to marry the dead man's brother, or to leave the home. But this may not be what she wants to do.

This is why we designed new exercises and sessions for *Stepping Stones Plus* that have now been incorporated in this revised manual to help different sections of the community look more closely at how they feel about people living with HIV, how those of us who have HIV are treated by others, and how the support we receive might be improved.

Ultimately, everyone in the community needs to feel more positive about being tested for HIV, more confident that if they test positive for HIV they will be fully supported by everyone, and more able to keep themselves, and their families, happy, healthy, safe, and alive.

Stepping Stones and Stepping Stones Plus

So, welcome to the 21st anniversary edition! Day by day, the river of life sustains and nurtures each of us in body, mind and spirit. Yet as we cross this great river, we also need to be aware of its strength and power – of its potential dangers and threats – and treat it with respect so that it can best help us to grow and thrive.

These dangers include gender-based violence, especially intimate partner violence, and a virus called HIV, which can bring illness, suffering, and even death and grief, to many.

In this training manual and the accompanying optional DVD, we offer you and your community some 'stepping stones' for overcoming these threats, which often lurk together under the surface as you navigate your way across this river of life. We do not offer any simple solutions, because we believe strongly that communities are capable of developing their own solutions to the particular issues we all face.

We therefore suggest that you each use this training package to help you steer your own way across your own river of life.

HAVE A GREAT JOURNEY!
Alice Welbourn

ENDNOTES

1. WHO (2015a)
2. Orza et al (2015)
3. For instance, one study in Uganda concluded that 'men are the predominant source of new infections in rural villages. Risk factors and preventive behaviors vary with the sex of the infected partner, and seroconversion rates are similar in both sexes.' (Serwadda et al., 1995). See also Abdool Karim (2014).

REFERENCES

Abdool Karim, S. (2014) *State of the Art: Epidemiology and access* Plenary Presentation, AIDS 2014, <http://pag.aids2014.org/PAGMaterial/PPT/1501_2401/final.pptx> [accessed 11 December 2014]

Orza, L. Bewley, S., Chung, C., Crone, E.T., Nagadya, H., Vazquez, M., and Welbourn, A. (2015) '"Violence, Enough Already": findings from a global participatory survey among women living with HIV', *Journal of the International AIDS Society*, 18 (Suppl 5): 20285, <http://dx.doi.org/10.7448/IAS.18.6.20285>

Serwadda, D., Gray, R., Wawer, M., Stallings, R., Sewankambo, N., Konde-Lule Bongs Lainjo, J., et al. (1995) 'The social dynamics of HIV transmission as reflected through discordant couples in rural Uganda', *AIDS* 9 (7): 745–750

WHO (2015a) *Guideline on when to start antiretroviral therapy and on pre-exposure prophylaxis for HIV,* <http://apps.who.int/iris/bitstream/10665/186275/1/9789241509565_eng.pdf> [accessed 15 November 2015]

STEPPING STONES COMMUNITY OF PRACTICE

This 1,200-strong database, which is free to join, links individuals and organisations, large and small, around the world who have used or are using *Stepping Stones* in different contexts and cultures. We have a regular newsletter and you all have so much to share! We are especially keen for you to share with us any evaluations you have undertaken of your work with *Stepping Stones* – you can see others' evaluations on our website. We can also keep you up to date with new ideas and advice about how best to adapt *Stepping Stones* to your context whilst keeping true to the original 'foundation stones', to maximize your chances of using it well. **Do please join us – we ask you this so that we can all support one another to share in our learning journey together**.

Website

If you have internet access, you can learn more about the package and how it works on:
www.steppingstonesfeedback.org

This site also has links to related gender-sensitive participatory approaches to, and articles about, sexual and reproductive health and wellbeing and rights. We also provide information about participatory approaches to monitoring and evaluation, in which community members themselves can be engaged, that complement more formal approaches.

Adaptations

The programme has also been adapted and translated widely across Africa, Asia, Latin America, Eastern Europe, Central Asia and the Pacific, where many similar results from diverse Muslim, Christian, Hindu and other communities have been reported. There may already be a local translation and/or adaptation of *Stepping Stones* **relevant to your needs, and we can help you find** out about these and how to get hold of them.

Vimeo

You can also watch films about *Stepping Stones* on our Vimeo page (https://vimeo.com/salamandertrust) or on your smartphone Vimeo app.

Contact us

You can also email us on:
enquiries@steppingstonesfeedback.org

Alternatively, you can write for the information to:
Stepping Stones International Coordinator
Salamander Trust
Positively UK
345 City Road
London EC1V 1LR, UK

ACRONYMS

ANC	Antenatal care
AIDS	Acquired immune deficiency syndrome
ARV	Antiretroviral
CD4	Cluster of differentiation (a glycoprotein that is used as an indicator to help physicians decide when to offer treatment to people with HIV)
GBV	Gender-Based Violence
HIV	Human immunodeficiency virus
IPPF	International Planned Parenthood Federation
PMTCT	Prevention of mother-to-child transmission
STI	Sexually transmitted infection
WHO	World Health Organization
UNICEF	United Nations Children's Programme
VCT	Voluntary counselling and testing

BEFORE YOU BEGIN ...!

This section presents the following information:
WHAT skills and information are presented in this training manual and DVD package.
FOR WHOM the package was prepared.
WHY the package was prepared.
WITH WHOM to use the package.
WHERE the package could be used.
WHEN the package could be used.
HOW the sessions are structured.
FINAL preparations.

WHAT

What skills and information are to be presented in this manual and DVD?

Some training manuals are like recipe books, which you can dip into to pick and choose different exercises.

Other manuals are like paths across a river, where you should begin at the beginning, and not attempt to jump in mid-way or you risk falling in.

Our manual is of the second kind. It provides you with the details of a training workshop which you could run together with your colleagues in the community where you want to work. The manual describes the sequence of ideas which you can encourage community members to consider and discuss. It suggests appropriate exercises and session timetables for you.

It is important to **follow the sequence of exercises in the sessions as described** and not to jump in and out of exercises in different sessions. Otherwise, the experiences of the earlier exercises will not help participants to cope well with the harder ones that follow. Participants might feel that they have taken on too much and can't cope if they have not been prepared by working through the earlier sessions first.

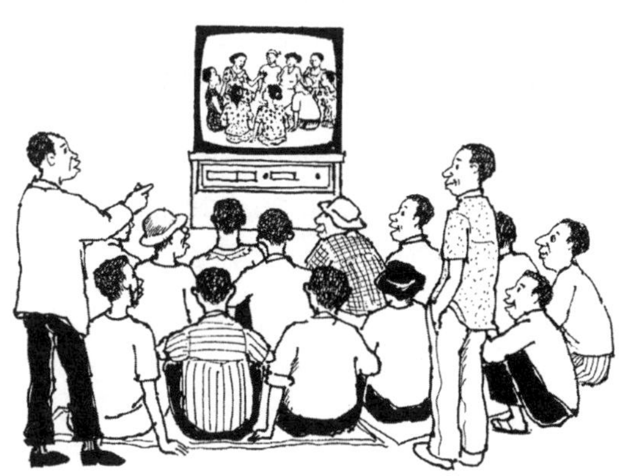

The accompanying DVD[1] provides illustrative material, filmed in Uganda, showing members of a rural community who have discussed and re-enacted their own problems and developed their own solutions. The DVD is divided into fifteen brief clips, each of which provides viewers with a springboard for discussion, enabling them to address their own concerns in a constructive, participatory manner. It shows us how we can learn to behave responsibly towards others as well as to take care of ourselves. **The DVD does not tell a story and only makes sense if each clip is viewed during the appropriate workshop session**. See more about the film in Annex 3.

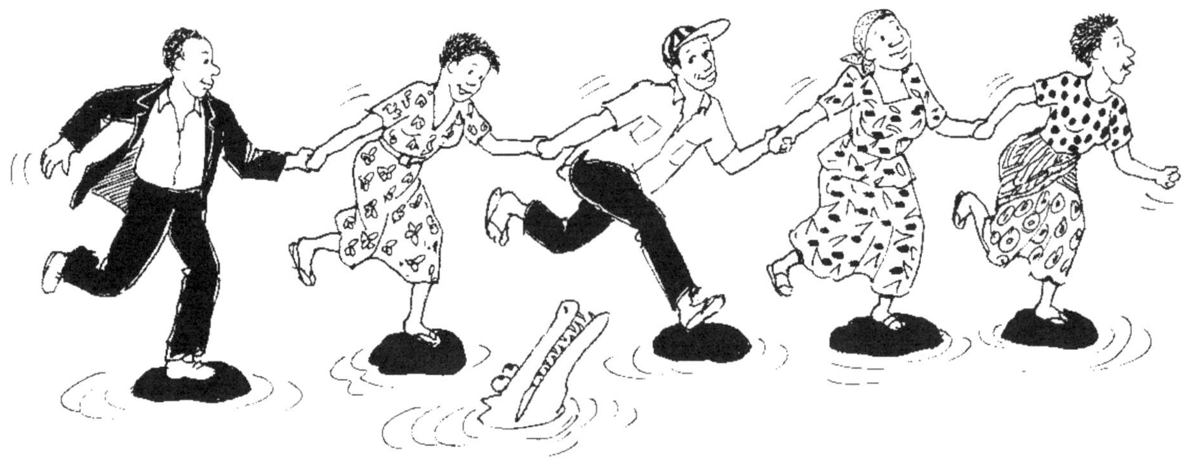

If this training manual and DVD are like a path across a river, the people journeying are the participants, each travelling and discovering him or herself. Each session which the manual describes has a theme, which is captured in the session title. The first sessions (Theme 1: Sessions A–D) focus on exercises which develop group cooperation and which help participants to recognise their own perspectives on life and needs. After two sessions on HIV and safer sex (Theme 2: Sessions E–F), the programme moves on to several sessions which help participants to analyse why we behave in the ways we do (Theme 3: Sessions G–J). A variety of factors, such as alcohol, local traditions, the need for money, social expectations, and our own personalities are considered in some depth. The next sessions (Theme 4: Sessions K–N and second open community meeting) help participants to think about and practise ways in which they can change their behaviour in a manner which allows them both to be more assertive and to take more personal, social, and community-wide responsibility for their actions. There are also *optional* sessions (Theme 5: Sessions O–R and further open community meeting). These support participants and the wider community in moving forward, expanding the network of support across the community, engaging with health settings and faith leaders, and thinking about how best to support both women who are, or wish to be, mothers and the next generation.

The whole workshop aims to enable individuals, their peers, and their communities to change their behaviour, individually and together, through the stepping stones which the sessions provide. To help build understanding across peer groups, during Themes 3 and 4, above, there are two meetings which bring all four peer groups together, in order to share and compare what they have learnt so far. The programme is based on the assumption that community-wide change is best achieved through a personal commitment to change from each of its members. This demands some effort from all those involved and, as we explain below, participants are strongly encouraged to make a commitment to attend all the sessions.

Ideally, there should be four of you working together as facilitators: two men and two women. We explain why on the next page.

FOR WHOM

This manual was written for skilled people who work with local groups in small-scale development settings. You may be professional staff or volunteers. You may be social workers, community leaders, health workers, counsellors, HIV educators, members of support groups of people with HIV, religious leaders or other similar people.

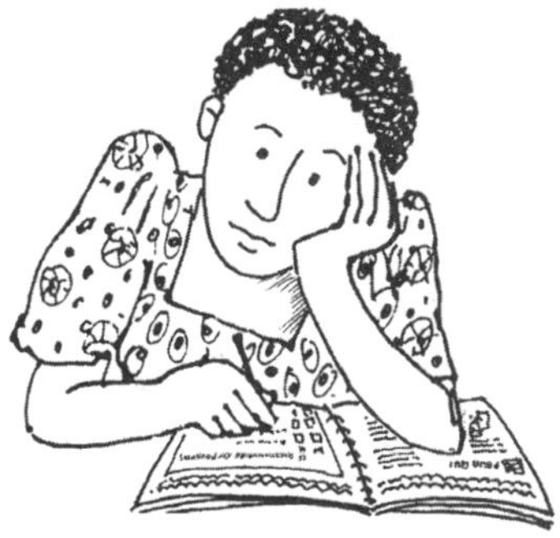

The programme is for use only where there is an ongoing HIV prevention and support programme, or a community health or education programme that includes HIV. **This training package is not for use unless you already have, or plan to have, ongoing HIV work in the community**. The skilled people (you?!) need to have the time to run the workshop in the community over about three or four months. You also need to make a commitment to run follow-up sessions over the course of the following six months or year.

We have designed the manual and its accompanying optional DVD specifically for users in sub-Saharan Africa. The illustrations reflect this part of the world. However, the training programme and exercises described are relevant to many communities elsewhere too.

In order to make best use of this manual, we expect you **ideally** to have the knowledge, qualities, skills, and experience that the quiz below asks about. The quiz below is tough, but maybe it could help you to identify areas where you need training to do your work better. Alternatively, perhaps you could plan to team up with other facilitators who have skills in the areas where you don't. Together you could make a great team! Now have a go at the quiz, ticking the YES or NO boxes according to your particular skills, and see how you score.

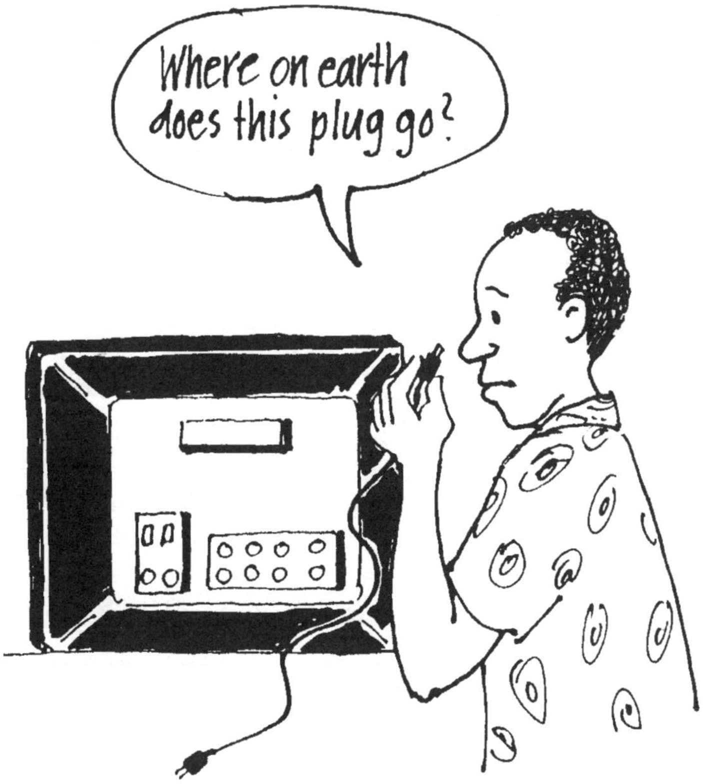

A QUIZ FOR YOU

	YES	NO	
a	☐	☐	Experience with participatory adult learning techniques.
b	☐	☐	Fluency in your community's first language (including the first language of the women in this community).
c	☐	☐	Training in participatory needs assessment.
d	☐	☐	Training in participatory evaluation techniques.
e	☐	☐	A sound knowledge and understanding of gender issues.
f	☐	☐	The trust and respect of a wide variety of people in the community in which you intend to work (old, young, male, female, rich, poor).
g	☐	☐	A basic training in sexuality, including knowledge of your own feelings about sexuality and awareness of your own practices.
h	☐	☐	An ability to discuss sexual matters in public, with a frank, unembarrassed, but sensitive approach.
i	☐	☐	An ability to relate well to people in an understanding, non-judgemental manner.
j	☐	☐	Sound knowledge of basic facts about HIV transmission and prevalence in in the community in which you intend to work.
k	☐	☐	An ability to use humour appropriately.
l	☐	☐	An ability and willingness to be openly self-critical, to be able to say 'I don't know' and 'I'm sorry', and to acknowledge and learn from your mistakes.
m	☐	☐	An understanding of and full respect for confidentiality.
n	☐	☐	A colleague of another gender, who also fulfils all of the above criteria, with whom you can run the training programme jointly (ideally, there should be four of you: two of each sex).
o	☐	☐	A fluent understanding of the language in which this manual is written.
p	☐	☐	Experience in operating a laptop and DVD player and projector.
q	☐	☐	Time in your work-plan to prepare for and run the workshop sessions over about three or four months.
r	☐	☐	Time in your work-plan to hold follow-up sessions over a further six to twelve months.

How did you get on?

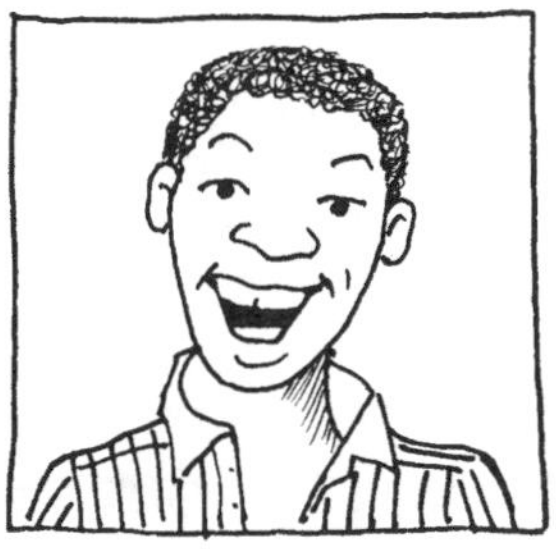

If you have ticked 15 or more of the YES boxes: you are ready to continue study of this training manual and DVD. We suggest that you form a training team with other facilitators who have the skills and experience that you do not have, so that you can share your knowledge with one another. Please see below.

If you have ticked 4 or more of the NO boxes: please have a chat with your supervisor. Perhaps additional training could be arranged for you – or perhaps it would be better for someone else in your organisation to use this manual for training purposes. If you have no supervisor, perhaps you could seek the advice of an organisation which may be able to provide you with appropriate training. It would really help you enormously if you had training or assistance in these areas before you attempt to run this programme. The list of further resources at the back of this manual may also help you. If you don't know anyone who could train you, contact us at **enquiries@steppingstonesfeedback.org**

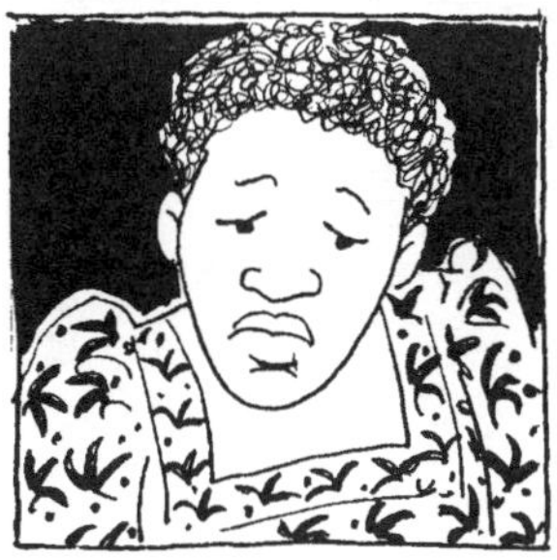

THANK YOU.

If...

If you think this manual is suitable for your use (see above), we strongly recommend the following:

- Work through the whole manual and DVD with a group of colleagues, as if you were participants. You will need ideally two weeks for this.
- Then hold a workshop with the friends or colleagues with whom you plan to use the package for training others. If you know of no one locally, try to meet with others through the help of an interested organisation. We recommend that you run a training of facilitators workshop: practising the whole package on yourselves and completing all the exercises together before facilitating the programme with participants in a community. You will need at least two full weeks for this. Three weeks would be better.

By doing these things you will be able to:

- Become familiar with the material in the package.
- Anticipate and explore areas that are likely to be of particular interest or difficulty in your own communities.
- Gain confidence in handling the subject matter with large and small groups.
- Increase your own understanding of the factors which influence people's ability to cope with HIV.
- Increase your empathy and solidarity with different community groups by understanding that these issues face all of us together – not just them.
- Develop an ongoing support group structure with other facilitators in your area.

Finally ...

This training package is designed to challenge the attitudes and behaviour of people (including us) to themselves and others. You are likely to find this rather frightening. You may also feel rather nervous about things going wrong, or not going according to plan.

Don't worry – there are many other people out there who will feel like you! We warmly encourage you to share your fears and successes with other facilitators in your area, so that you can learn from one another's experiences, suggest alternative options to one another, and so on. We do believe that your efforts to help people better identify their needs and express them to one another more openly will help all of us in our work to address HIV. So please take courage in your skills and ...

NOTE ABOUT FACILITATORS: As people living with HIV have become more supported and respected by their communities, they have felt more able to share their experiences with others and have become powerful peer educators. Can your organisation train and employ people with HIV to be *Stepping Stones* facilitators? If so, they will add a lot to the power of this process in the communities where you work!

GOOD LUCK!

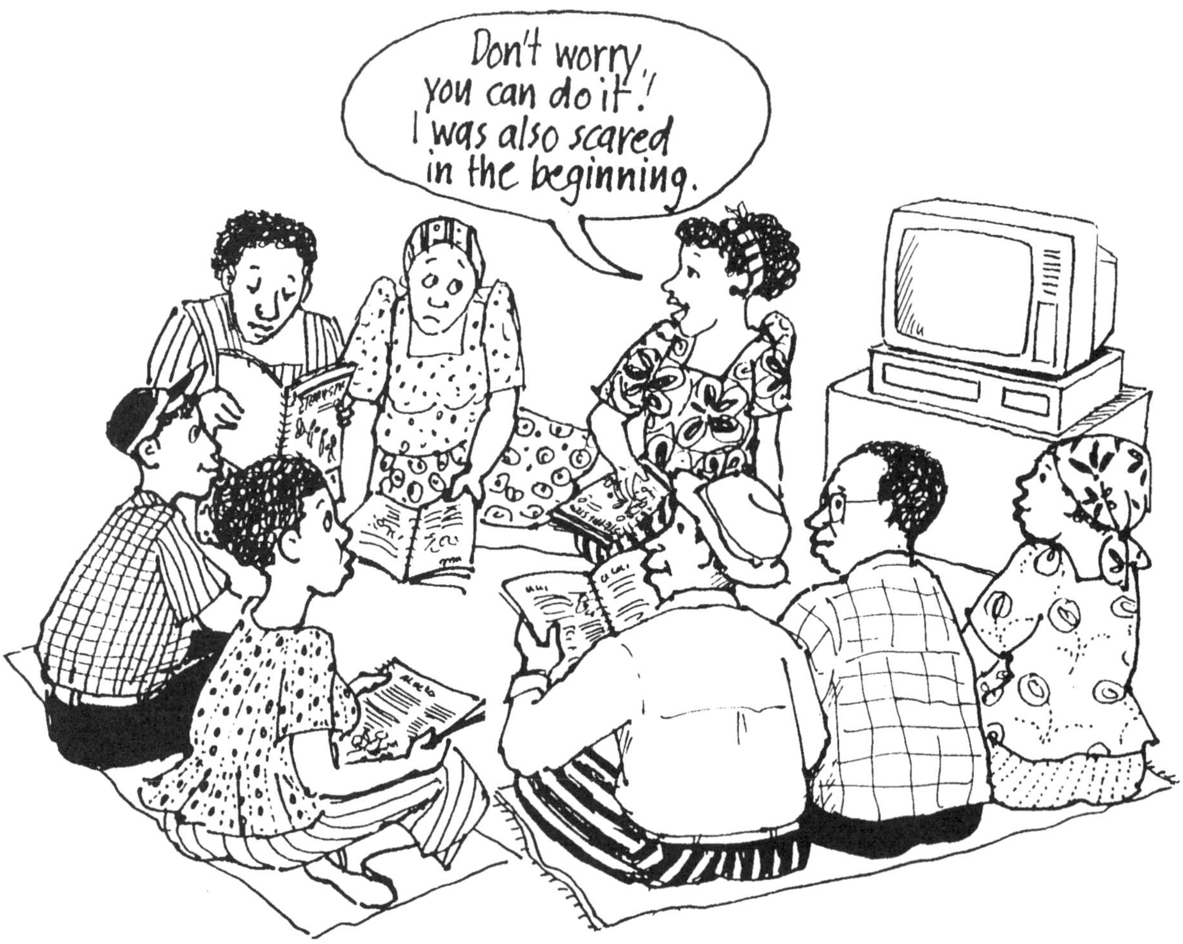
Don't worry, you can do it! I was also scared in the beginning.

WHY

This training manual and the accompanying DVD have been produced in response to a growing need for material to address our communication problems about sexual attitudes and behaviour. We all find it hard to communicate at times, even with our closest friends. Rich people don't understand the needs of the poor; the old often complain about the ways of the young; men and women often argue. Communication presents a challenge to all of us.

We communicate in a huge variety of different ways. Speaking is just one. We communicate to others about ourselves in the way we look at them, in the way we behave, in the way we move our bodies, in the clothes we wear, in the activities we pursue, through the people we mix with, in what we eat and drink, in what we don't say and don't do... so really communication is about the whole of human interaction. And often the message that we think we are communicating is different from the message that someone else has received. We can all think of an example from our own life in the past week where our message has gone wrong. Can you?

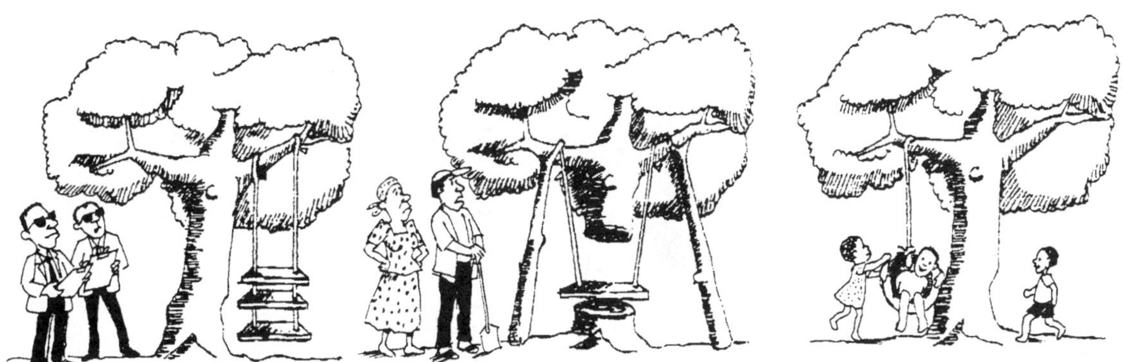

What the experts designed — What the people got — What the people wanted

We find it especially hard to communicate about sex and about death – our expectations, our needs, our hopes, our fears. In almost all societies around the world, sex and death are taboo subjects. People may question our morality if we know or use certain words or perform certain actions related to sex. If we are women, we may fear lack of financial support or mental or physical violence if we talk about sex. We may be thrown out of our homes. If we are men, we may fear teasing and worse from our peers if we are not seen to have a healthy interest in sex, for instance by talking about it frequently or demonstrating our manhood. It's tough! Death too is a subject which prompts great emotion.

Sex is traditionally connected with new life, with birth, with fertility, with blessings and joy. At times, it can also be something threatening or even dangerous. But the main emphasis of sex has always been life-giving.

Yet we know that nowadays, in many parts of the world, there is HIV. And HIV, if untreated, leads to AIDS, so both have close connections with sex and death. Suddenly, in these places, sex is no longer associated with joy and fertility but it is instead connected to death and misery. No wonder many people are scared of AIDS.

The HIV messages we hear all around us are simplified either into an ABC of rules:

	Abstain!
or	**B**e faithful!
or use	**C**ondoms!
(or practise	**N**on-penetrative sex.)

Increasingly, people are encouraged to take pre-exposure prophylaxis (PrEP) or, if they have HIV already, anti-retroviral medication (ARVs), to protect others who might acquire HIV from them.

These rules may sound easy and clear. But they often fail to address our own problems of communication, or our expectations of what Real Sex is. Also medication doesn't protect against unplanned pregnancy or sexually transmitted infections (STIs).

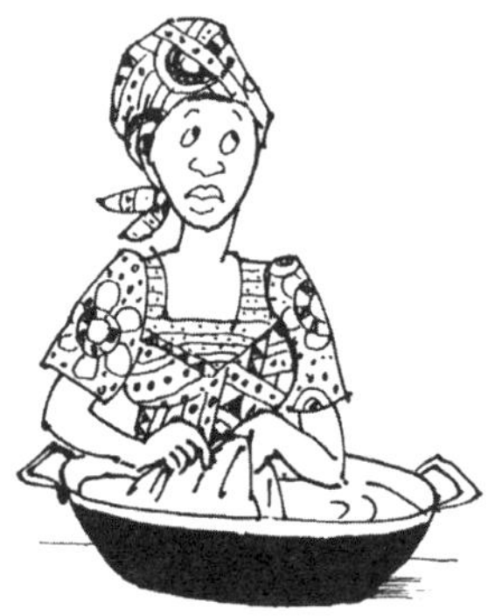

'What does my faithfulness matter if my husband has other sexual partners? Surely his sexual activities put us both at risk? He would throw me out if I suggested we abstain or that he stops seeing other women. And how can I suggest we use condoms when we both want children? What can I do?'

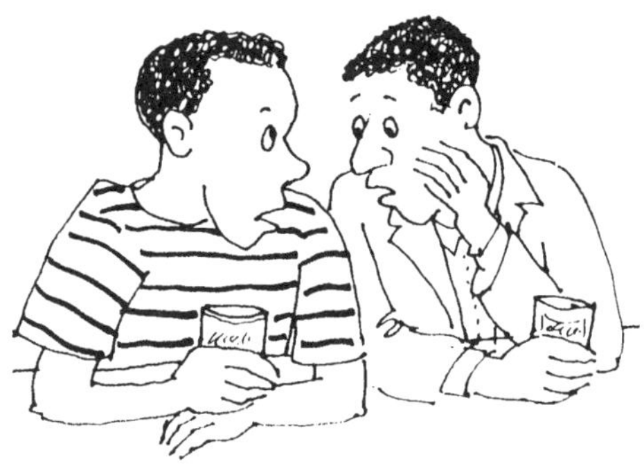

'How can I suddenly suggest to my wife that we start using condoms? I want to be faithful now, but there are times in the past ten years when I haven't been. And I want to protect her from the risk of my past activities. What can I do?'

The whole programme is designed to explore ways in which we can all begin to find a safe way across the river of life. Each session is like one stepping stone, helping us on the way. Instead of being told WHAT to do by outsiders, this programme shows HOW you and your community members can begin to discuss and decide for yourselves what we can all do in our own social contexts, to improve our skills in communication. Through better communication, community members may be helped to achieve something that they want for themselves, their families and their communities: namely, improved care and support for those who are sick and better HIV prevention practices for everyone.

WITH WHOM

Peer Groups

This training manual and the accompanying DVD are designed for use with people in small groups, not for open meetings. This is because it has been shown repeatedly that people share and learn best from talking first with those who are most similar to themselves. If I am an old man, I am most likely to talk openly with other old men. They are my 'peer group'. Similarly if I am a young woman, my peer group will be other young women.

So we recommend strongly that you use this programme with small peer groups only, and not in open meetings. In this way, the discussions will have maximum value for the participants.

There will be times during the sessions when workshop meetings of larger, mixed groups are recommended. But these times will be indicated in the text. For the most part, the sessions are designed for peer groups only.

Selection

So how should these peer groups be selected in the community where you work?

Each community will be different and the relative importance of different divisions in that community will depend upon the issue to be discussed. However, we feel the most important divisions influencing open discussions about sex and sexuality are **gender** and **age,** and/or **marital status**.

We recommend therefore that a minimum of *four* peer groups be encouraged to form amongst your community.

Each community should really decide for themselves how they would like to split up for the sessions.

However, before you go and ask them, please bear the following points in mind.

Particular lines of division which you may find are relevant to people's opinions in a community include:

- gender (male/female)
- age (older/younger adult)
- marital status (married/unmarried/widowed/divorced/separated)
- parental status (parent/non-parent/step-parent)
- religion (e.g. Christian, Muslim, etc.)
- level of formal schooling (e.g. primary leaver, non-literate, secondary leaver)
- socio-economic wellbeing (e.g. well-off, destitute etc.)
- pastoral, agricultural, or urban background
- ethnic group

If your community would also like this workshop to be conducted with older children, be sure to encourage the inclusion of out-of-school children as well as schoolchildren. Some may be old enough to join in with the younger men's and younger women's groups. Alternatively, they may prefer to form their own peer groups. See also our new sister manual, *Stepping Stones with Children*.

For example, in the village of Buwenda *in Uganda, where the DVD was filmed, the people chose to self-select themselves as follows:*

- ***older men***
- ***older women***
- ***younger men***
- ***younger women*** *(including younger single mothers)*

There were some married women in the younger women's group as well as in the older women's group. Their main reasons for choosing which group to join seemed to be age and where they felt most at ease. However, in other communities, women may be much more rigid about dividing themselves on the basis of marital status and whether they have yet given birth or not. How is it in the community where you want to use this training package?

Why are peer groups so important?

Why is dividing up into peer groups so important for this work? Good communication is about good listening and about respecting the views of others. If we want to do this effectively, we need to give everyone the privacy, time, space, and confidence to voice their own views and beliefs in a secure atmosphere.

If you were to run the workshop as an open meeting, the views of young women or young men would rarely be voiced. And if they dared to overcome their shyness and speak

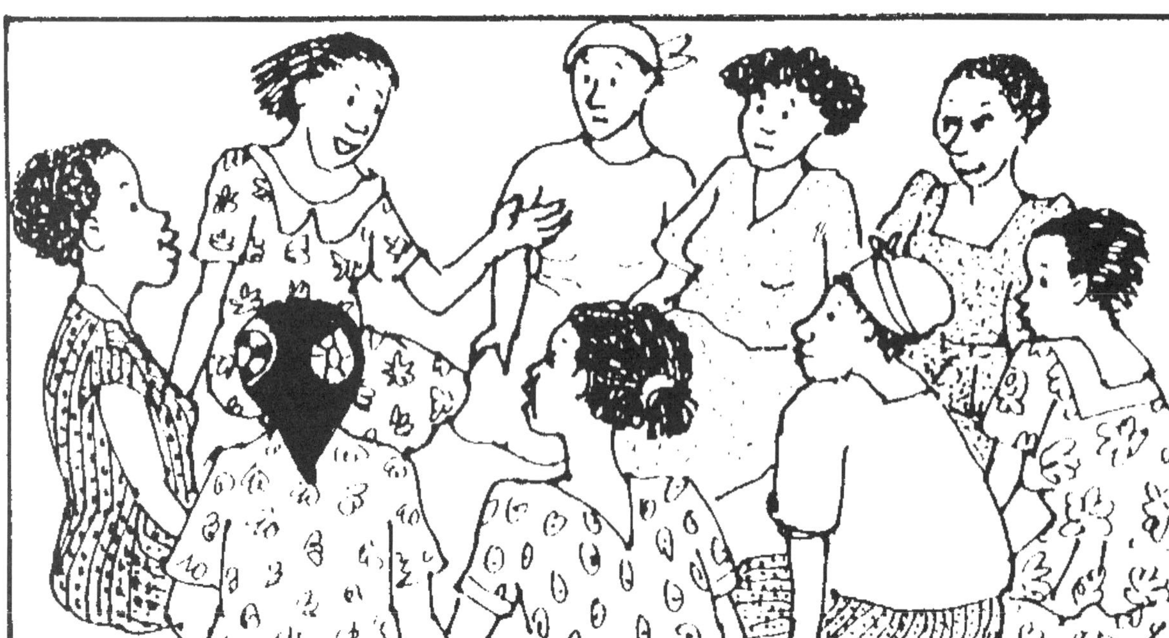

up, their views might be contradicted or laughed at by the older men or women who were present. Then they would have lost the confidence to voice their thoughts in public another time.

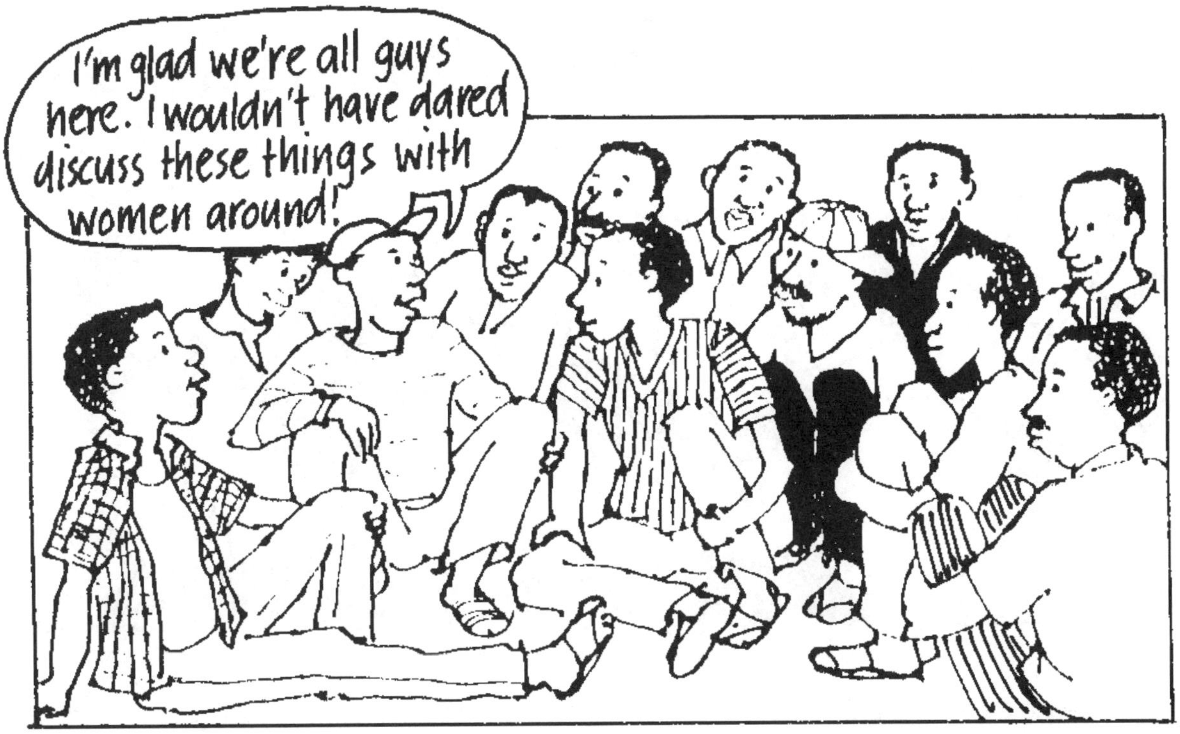
I'm glad we're all guys here. I wouldn't have dared discuss these things with women around!

Think of your own experiences of public meetings. Which people talk most? Which people say nothing? Which people never come to the meetings in the first place? Which people make the decisions for the whole community? Are the decisions made really representative of **everyone's** views and needs?

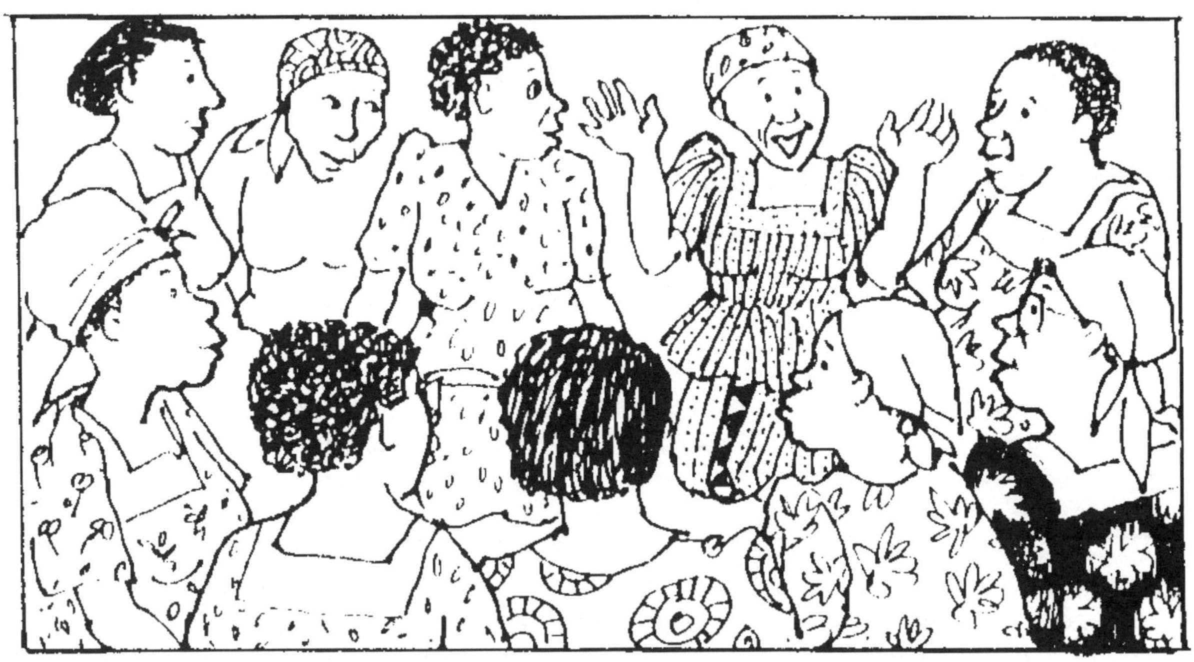

On the other hand, older men also need their own space to talk and learn. Few older men would be happy to examine and ask about a condom, for instance, in front of women or younger men. Their privacy needs to be respected too.

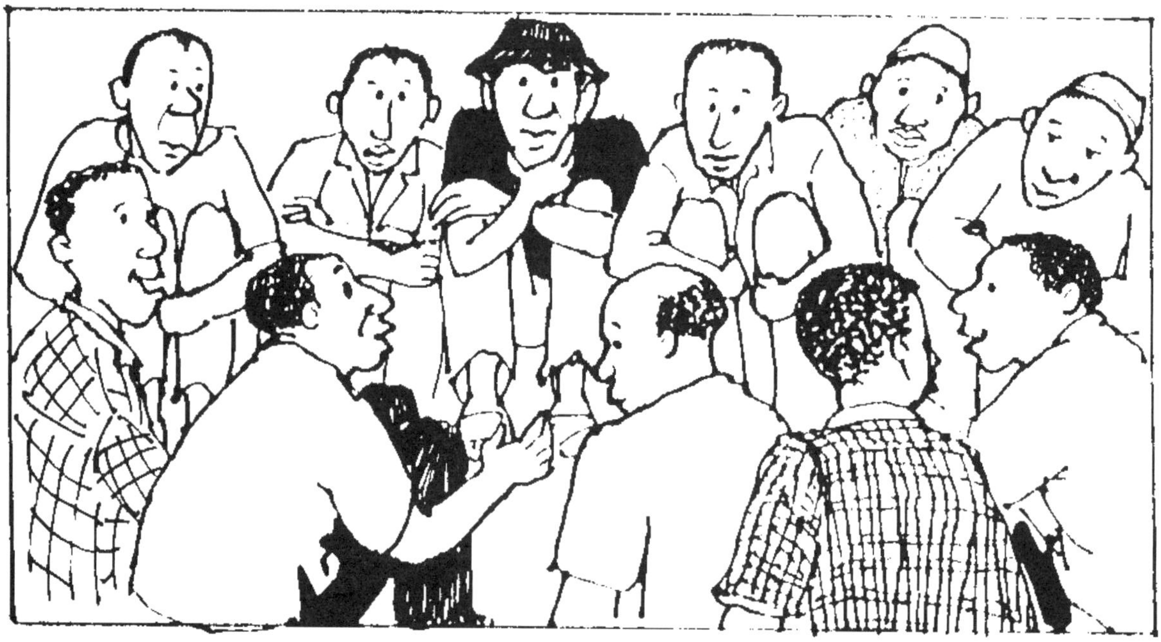

Finally, saying anything in public can be hard enough for a young woman. But talking about her sexuality in a mixed group would usually be impossible. Trust and confidentiality are issues which are extremely important when talking about such private matters. They are much more manageable in a peer group of people of similar gender and age or marital status than they are in a large group.

These are the reasons why we put so much emphasis on working with small peer groups in this programme. Please do try to follow this important recommendation.[2]

People: numbers

Aim for a maximum of twenty and minimum of ten people in each peer group at any one time. This is large enough to allow you to work with quite a few people at one time; and small enough to encourage everyone's individual involvement in the peer groups. (See more about these peer groups above.)

Implications for you the facilitator

This emphasis on peer groups means that it would be best for you the facilitator to work in a team of four: two women and two men. In this way, each of the four peer groups can have their own facilitator, who can guide them through the sessions and in whom they can develop confidence. If it is only possible to have teams of two, it would be best if one of you is male and the other female. Then each of you can run two separate peer group sessions in the community: i.e., the male facilitator can run the sessions with the older men's group and with the young men's group. The female facilitator can work with the young women's group and with the older women's group. Remember that if children want a separate peer group or groups, you may need even more facilitators!

In Buwenda, there were four facilitators: two middle-aged women ran a woman's group each; one young man ran the young men's group; and one older man ran the older men's group. In this way each group felt at home with a facilitator who was most like themselves.

☞ We do recognise that some of you may wish to run a workshop where there are only male members or female members, such as in the army, or with a scout group, with female sex workers, or with the YWCA or YMCA. In these cases, you will not need to divide up along gender lines but you may still have different age groups among your membership, who would best be separated for this workshop. We have written the programme on the assumption that most facilitators would use it in the context of a small community where all different age and gender groups are represented. We believe this formulation has the best chance of lasting success, since it best mirrors the realities of our lives. We have also focused on HIV transmission in heterosexual relationships, because this is widely recognised as the main means of transmission in Africa. We have not addressed in any detail relationships between men or women who have sex with others of their own sex. We have also not addressed issues specifically concerning injecting drug users or sex workers. However, the manual has been successfully adapted for use in different contexts, including these, and we hope that you will also feel able to adapt the text as you go along, in accordance with the visions and needs of your particular participants. Please contact us about adaptations and observe the permissions statement at the start of the manual.

Here is a flow chart which shows you how we recommend that the workshop sessions are structured in a community with four different peer groups.

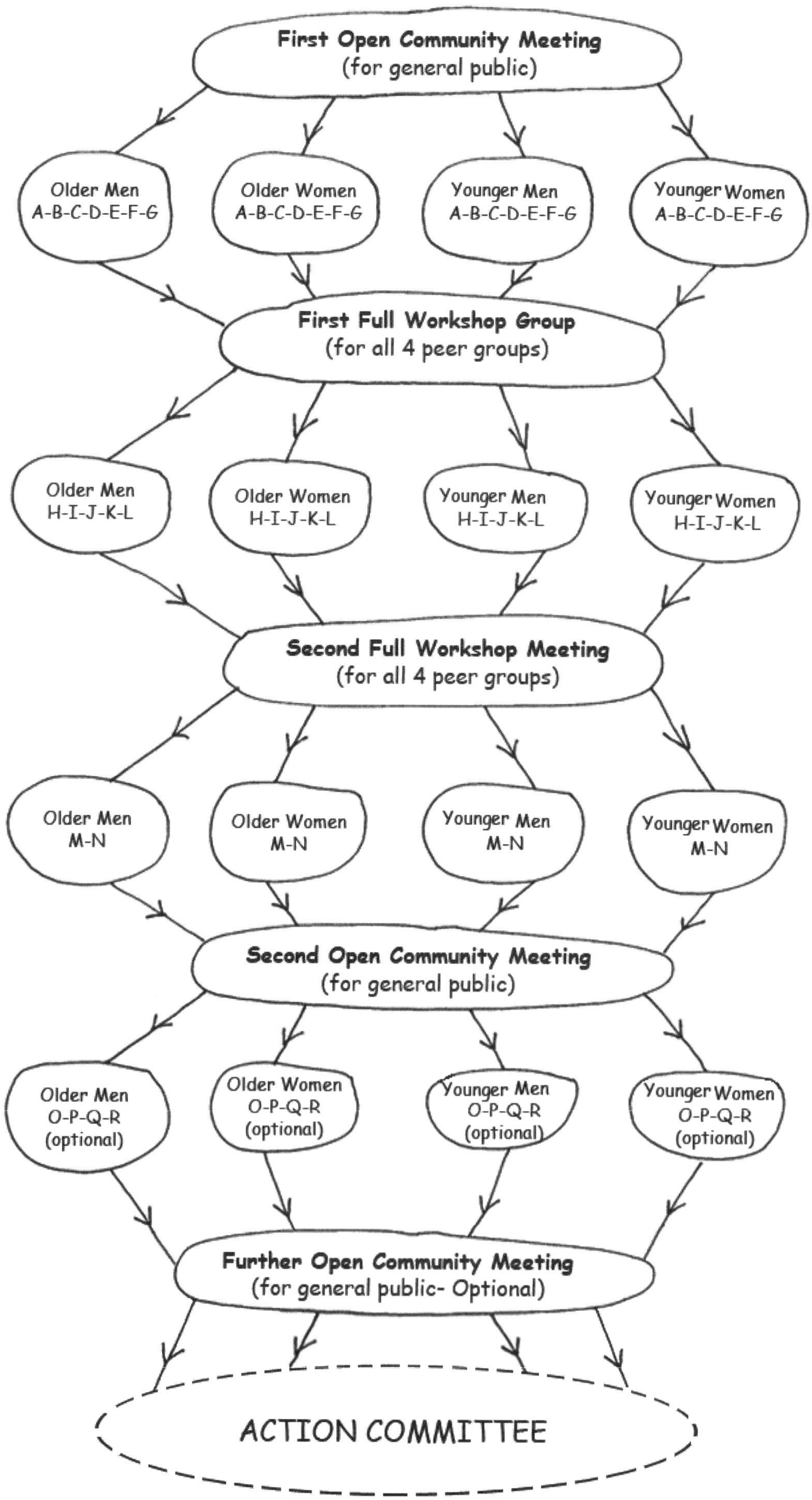
First Open Community Meeting
(for general public)
Older Men
A-B-C-D-E-F-G
Older Women
A-B-C-D-E-F-G
Younger Men
A-B-C-D-E-F-G
Younger Women
A-B-C-D-E-F-G
First Full Workshop Group
(for all 4 peer groups)
Older Men
H-I-J-K-L
Older Women
H-I-J-K-L
Younger Men
H-I-J-K-L
Younger Women
H-I-J-K-L
Second Full Workshop Meeting
(for all 4 peer groups)
Older Men
M-N
Older Women
M-N
Younger Men
M-N
Younger Women
M-N
Second Open Community Meeting
(for general public)
Older Men
O-P-Q-R
(optional)
Older Women
O-P-Q-R
(optional)
Younger Men
O-P-Q-R
(optional)
Younger Women
O-P-Q-R
(optional)
Further Open Community Meeting
(for general public- Optional)
ACTION COMMITTEE

WHERE

Ideal context for the workshop

For many people in Africa, HIV and AIDS are among many problems that they have to face every day. Poverty and the social, economic, and political disadvantages linked to it are constant burdens. Other health problems, such as malaria, TB, diarrhoeal disease, accidents and injuries, and so on also need to be addressed. There are also many other problems to do with sexual health, such as fertility control, infertility, STIs, sexual abuse, and female circumcision, which are rarely adequately addressed.

Many argue that the high prevalence of HIV and the severity of its impact in Africa is closely linked to the lack of health and social service facilities, lack of formal education (especially for women), lack of equality between people in sexual relationships, and sheer general poverty. And, of course, the lack of these things has a great effect on many other aspects of the quality of people's lives, not just on their vulnerability to HIV.

We believe strongly that the issues of communication which are addressed in this training package can influence people in all aspects of their lives, not just in relation to HIV. Therefore we consider that the most effective context for this training workshop would be where other aspects of development work are also in progress. These could be income-generation activities, malaria control, the supply of safe drinking water, adult education programmes, effective immunisation, safe motherhood and child spacing – to name but a few. If activities such as these are already underway in the area (perhaps through good local government services or the work of another development agency), people's basic practical needs are to some extent being addressed. They will therefore be more likely to have some interest in the contents of this workshop. In areas where basic needs are not being addressed, communities will be less ready to address the issues which will challenge them here.

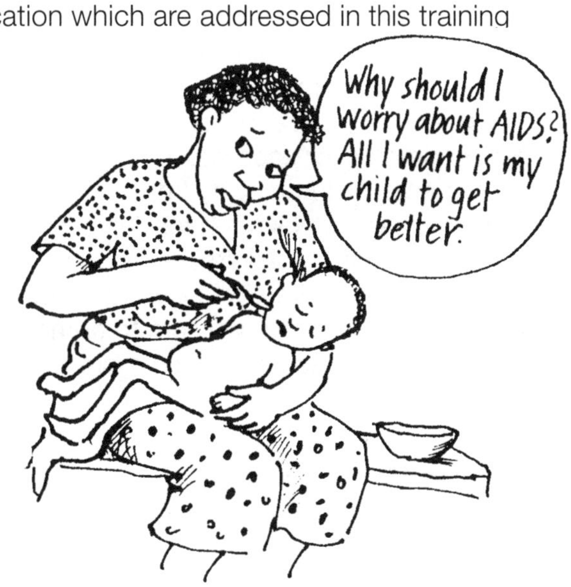
Why should I worry about AIDS? All I want is my child to get better.

Nonetheless, it is clear that many wishing to use this training package will not be working in the context of a broad development approach. We think that sexual health and HIV will still be of enough concern to people for them to be ready to become involved in this workshop. It may well be, as in Buwenda, that this programme could act as a springboard and prompt community groups' interests in other development work.

Finally, those development agencies who are already involved in income-generation and other development activities may find this manual an effective way of introducing the discussion of HIV into their work. **We recommend strongly that income-generation activities be introduced *after the core sessions (A-N)*** (i.e. after the second community meeting, once participants **feel excited about developing future projects together)**. We have seen the success of this approach in Buwenda, Uganda, the original workshop location.[3] This was also found in South Africa by the creators of *Stepping Stones Creating Futures*,[4] a vocational training supplement to the original manual, designed for younger participants.

Community ownership

If community members feel involved in considering and deciding where the workshop should be held, they are more likely to be ready to join in with the project. Therefore we recommend that you discuss locations with some community members first. Make sure that those you consult really represent all the different peer groups with whom you plan to work! Seek their opinions on the best locations. Below are some hints to guide the choice.

Mobile venues: location

Where the package could be used depends on whether or not you have a laptop with DVD player and a projector that have enough battery power, and either a mobile screen or a clear wall space you can use. If you have these, it is a good idea to take equipment to the community, and to conduct the whole workshop within that community's living area, or workplace, or recreation area – whichever seems the most appropriate location.

Mobile venues: privacy

It is a good idea to find quite a **private** place to conduct the workshop since adults are not likely to want to have children around them during the workshop sessions. You may need to think about organising full-time child care for each session, in order to keep children away from discussion areas. Adults often feel inhibited in their discussions if children are around. (Of course, most children in the world know a lot more about sex than we care to admit – and yet they need to know even more to care for themselves!)

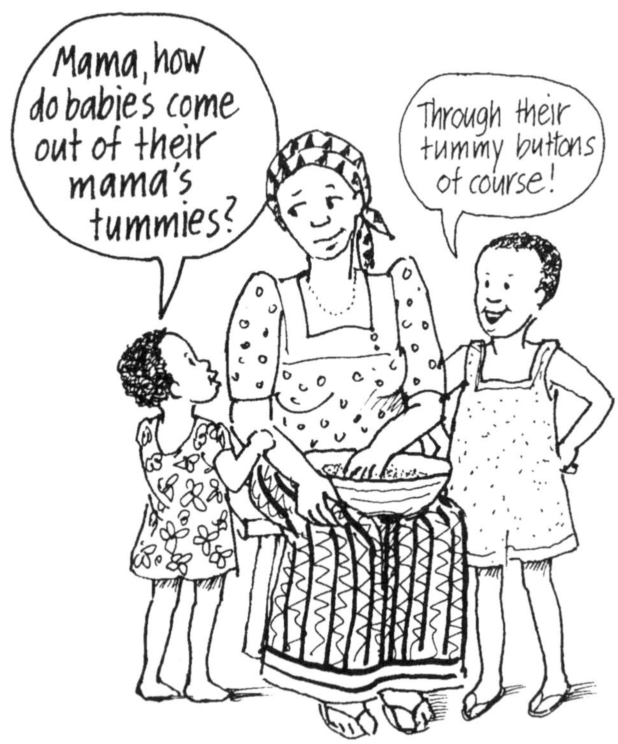
Mama, how do babies come out of their mama's tummies?
Through their tummy buttons of course!

Mobile venues: size

You also need to choose a location where everyone can get to know one another reasonably well and where people feel comfortable. This involves a certain amount of thought about the **size** of your location. For instance, having a meeting of ten people in a huge echoing hall is very difficult. Equally, two hundred people squashed into a class-room designed for thirty is hopeless. (For numbers of people involved, see earlier in this section.)

Fixed venues:

If you do not have mobile DVD equipment and need to bring community members to a fixed venue, again consider location, size, and privacy, as well as transport costs and other difficulties. Try to stick to a maximum of twenty people and minimum of ten in each peer group and, again, try to make sure all the peer group have similar gender and age. (See more about these peer groups earlier in this section.)

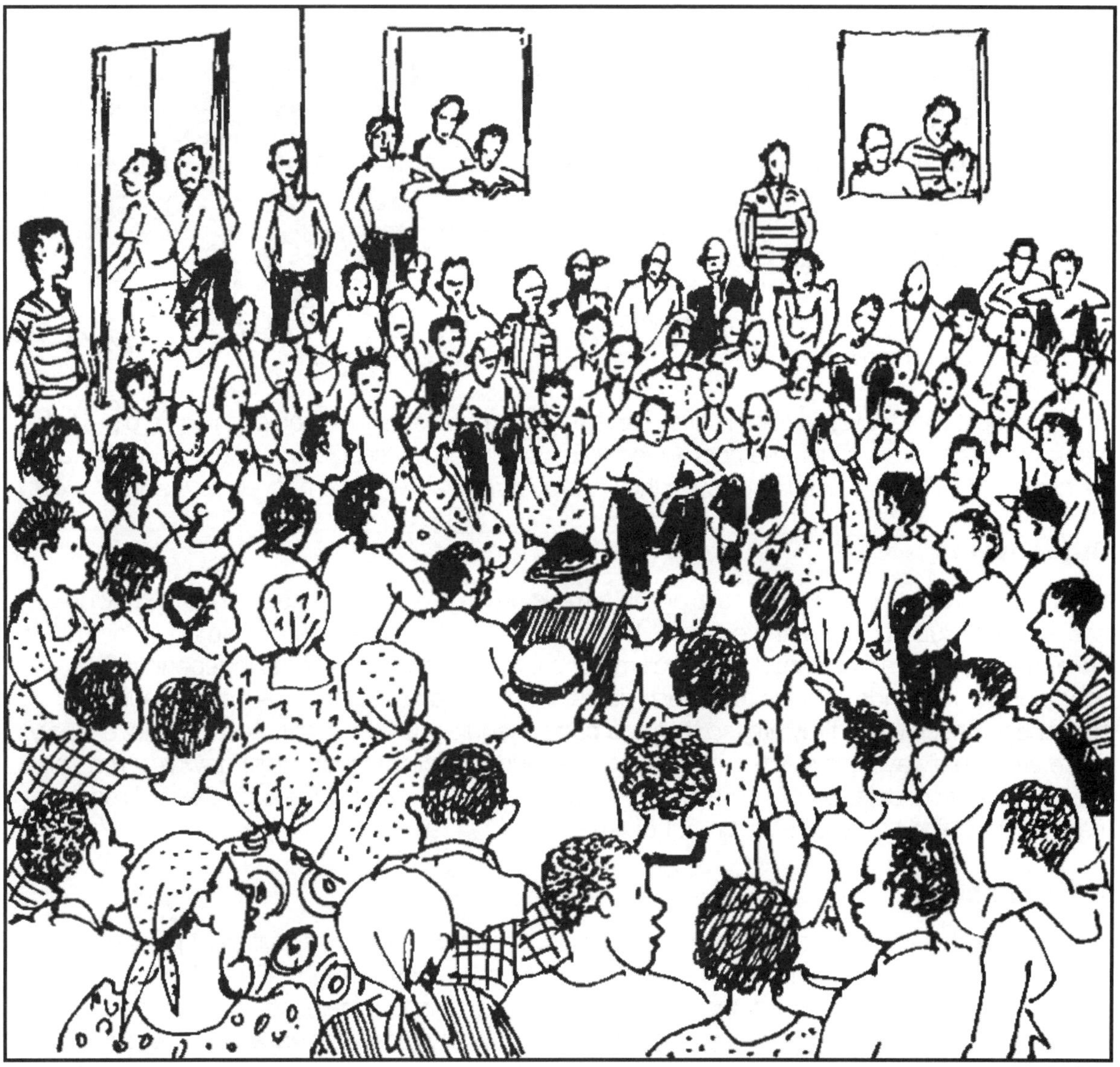

YOUR NOTES ...

WHEN

Time of Year

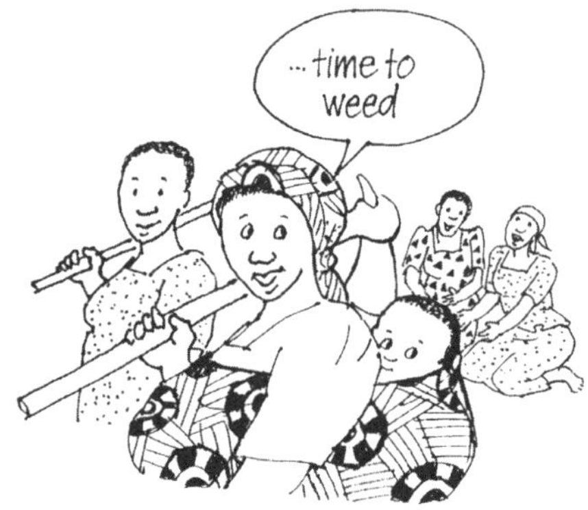

The timing of the workshop should bear the agricultural seasons in mind. Many development projects or workshops fail because we just think about the agency's own planning year and not the local community's. If a workshop clashes with planting time, weeding, or harvesting, attendance is likely to be very low.

Often the best time for workshops is after harvest, when people might be able to relax a bit – both mentally and physically. But remember – women's work in the household doesn't stop just because the harvest is in! You still need to discuss their availability closely with them, even at this time.

Other events

If you plan to run your workshop sessions in a more urban area, the agricultural cycle may be less relevant. But, of course, there are still busy times like Christmas, Easter, Ramadan, or Eid, or there may be other attractions like football matches, market days, elections, Independence Day, or weddings. It sounds obvious that these dates should be avoided. But it is worth planning in advance to check when they are, so that you can schedule your workshop sessions accordingly. There are also always unexpected happenings, like funerals or transport breakdown, which can interrupt your schedule. So it is always a good idea to allow extra time for such possibilities, so that you don't find that you have run out of time.

Time of day

The time of day you meet at can be just as important as where you meet. Different people in a community have different things to do at different times of the **day or night**. For instance, if you arrange a session in the middle of the morning, this may be fine for older men, but may be hopeless for younger men who are away working, or for women who may be fetching water or weeding and so on. The best idea is to ask different peer groups in the community what would be the best times for them to meet with you. You can then arrange session times to fit in with each peer group.

Workshop duration

We suggest that you run the workshop over the course of about three or four months, on a twice-weekly basis. (For a suggested timetable plan, see **opposite**.) We recommend that you do it over this length of time, rather than as an intensive course, so that people can make use of what they learn in their day-to-day lives between each session. This approach has often been seen to be more effective than a short, intensive course.

> Please remember this is only a **suggested** timetable, based on the minimum time of **nine weeks** for the first four themes, with two sessions a week. We expect you may need at least three extra weeks during this time for different peer groups to catch up with one another, or for participants to attend to other commitments. This sort of timetable may be fine for an agricultural community in the post-harvest season, but it may be hopeless for an urban community, or where people have regular hours for paid jobs. **So do plan and write up a timetable with your community, before you begin the workshop!** Remember to include breaks, catch-up time, public holidays, and so on. Remember also that you need at least another four to six weeks for the additional optional sessions (Theme 5); and then at least another six months for follow-up work after the workshop.

A SUGGESTED TIMETABLE

THEME	SESSION	DVD	Wk No.
Introduction	CM1: **First Open Community Meeting**	1. Stepping Stones	1
1. Group Cooperation	A: Let's Communicate B: Our Perceptions C: What is Love? D: Our Prejudices	2. What is Love?	1 1 2 2
2. HIV and Safer Sex	E: HIV F: Condoms	3. The Condom	3 3
3. Why We Behave in the Ways we do	G: Our Options W1: **First Full Workshop Meeting** H: Let's Look Deeper: Part 1 I: Let's Look Deeper: Part 2 J: Let's Support Ourselves	4. Hopes and Fears: The Young Women 5. Hopes and Fears: The Young Men 6. Alcohol 7. Traditions 8. Money 9. Saying 'Yes'?	4 4 5 5 6
4. Ways in Which we can Change	K: Let's Assert Ourselves L: Let's Change Ourselves W2: **Second Full Workshop Meeting** M: Let's Work Together N: Let's Prepare for the Future CM2: **Second Open Community Meeting**	10. Saying 'No'? 11. Coming Home 12. 'I' Statements 13. Trust 14. The Long Journey 15. The Community Challenge	6 7 7 8 8 9
OPTIONAL FURTHER SESSIONS: (you may want a small break before starting these)			
5. Moving Forward Together	O: What Happened Next? P: Nurturing Common Ground: Promoting Care and Support amongst Partners, Families and the Wider Community Q: Supporting Mothers and their Children: Our Community's Future in their Hands R: Accepting HIV within the Family: Supporting Family Members Living with HIV CM3: **Further Open Community Meeting**		10 11 12 13 14

Duration of each session

We suggest that you take between three and four hours for each session, depending on the availability of participants and the level of their interest in the discussions.

In Buwenda, the women's groups discovered that they had so much to talk about that they stayed on, continuing their discussions long after their facilitators had gone home. The sessions opened the floodgates on their thoughts and experiences. Sometimes they would spread the exercises from one session over two meetings, to give themselves more time to talk.

On the other hand, the men's groups tended to complete each session in one meeting. Men, on the whole, find it much harder to talk openly with one another about their experiences, so they tended to prefer to press on to the next exercise, rather than to explore a difficult issue in more depth.

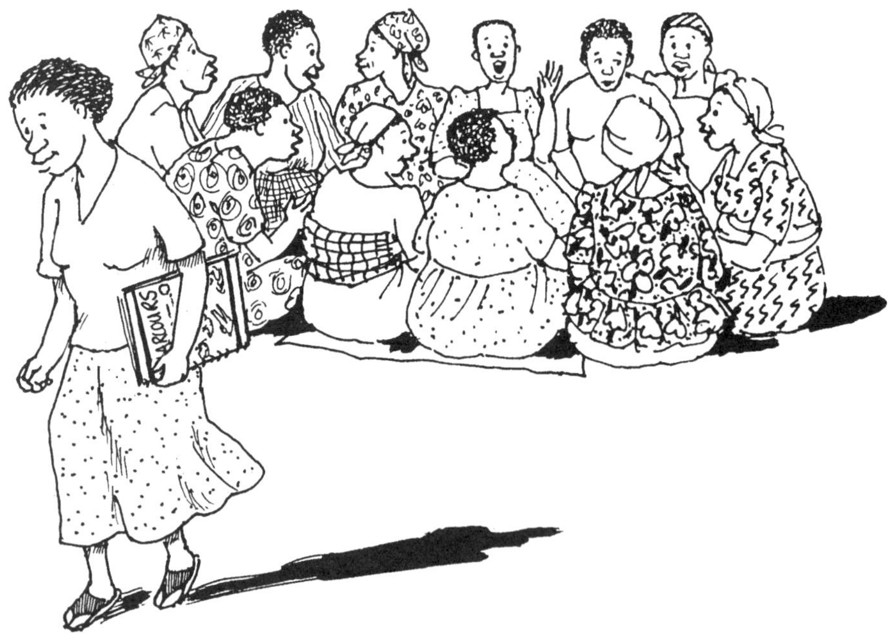

☞ We have deliberately not put individual time recommendations on each exercise. This is because you may find that participants are keen to explore an issue at length. If they do, then it is a pity to break up such a discussion just because this manual says your time's up!

On the whole, therefore, we suggest that in each session you spend around:

30 minutes on the introduction
10 minutes on each of the quick warm-up and wind-down exercises
20–40 minutes on the longer exercises
20–40 minutes on the DVD clips and their discussions.

There are a few major exercises, which may need as much as two hours. These are marked as long exercises in the text.

If you use these recommended times, then most sessions should take 3–4 hours.

We also suggest that, if any of the peer groups feel they need more time, they should have the flexibility to spend more than one meeting on each session. However, it is important that you allow all the peer groups to catch up with one another before each of the first or second full workshop meetings and the second and further open community meetings. **Please discourage the peer groups from thinking of the completion of the sessions as a race!** The more often the men can be encouraged to spend a longer time in discussion the better – for themselves and for everyone else too. (If you do need to split a session into two meetings, see Annex 5, which gives advice on how best to structure any extra session you run.)

Pace

There are several different factors which can affect the speed at which your participants will be able to move through the workshop sessions together. These will include:

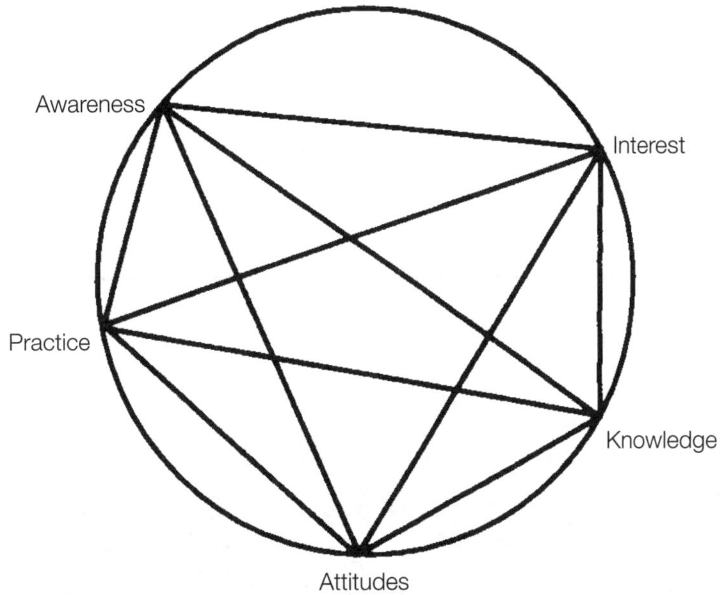

All of these factors – and others – influence one another closely and govern the level of understanding of each peer group. Each peer group will be at a different stage of understanding. (There will also be variations in the understanding of individuals within each peer group.) Do not worry about this: it is inevitable.

We might find, for instance, that older women may want to practise safer sex[5] and already have a good understanding of the issues. But they may be entirely powerless to put what they know into practice, because of their husband's limited understanding of sexual health.

Alternatively, we may find that a young man wants to practise safer sex with his wife because he is unsure of his HIV status. But she may have little understanding of the risks of HIV and may wish to have children, and so be recognised as a woman, as quickly as possible.

Each peer group will therefore have its own starting point and perspective. The important thing is that each peer group is given the time and space to work through the sessions and develop their understanding of all the issues at their own pace. Some peer groups may want to repeat certain exercises or take longer over some of the discussions than the other peer groups. **This is fine – just let it happen.**

Once each peer group has been able to work through all the sessions for itself, **at its own unhurried pace,** there will be a much greater chance of members of different peer groups reaching agreement by the end of the workshop, on the basis of a common understanding of all the issues.

HOW

The rest of this manual describes the eighteen peer group sessions, the three open community meetings, and the two full workshop meetings (the latter are for participants only) which form the programme. In the Annexes you will find additional information to help you run the sessions and ideas for follow-up work.

Here, we run through a few basic principles upon which all the workshop sessions are designed.

EMPHASIS ON WE AND US, NOT THEY AND THEM

We believe strongly that the best way in which people learn is from listening to and talking to others like themselves. This is why we want you to be experienced in participatory adult education techniques before you run this programme. **Lectures on AIDS do not work!**

> *In Buwenda, one of the facilitators said: 'I shared my own secrets with them, so they were encouraged to come up with their own thoughts.'*

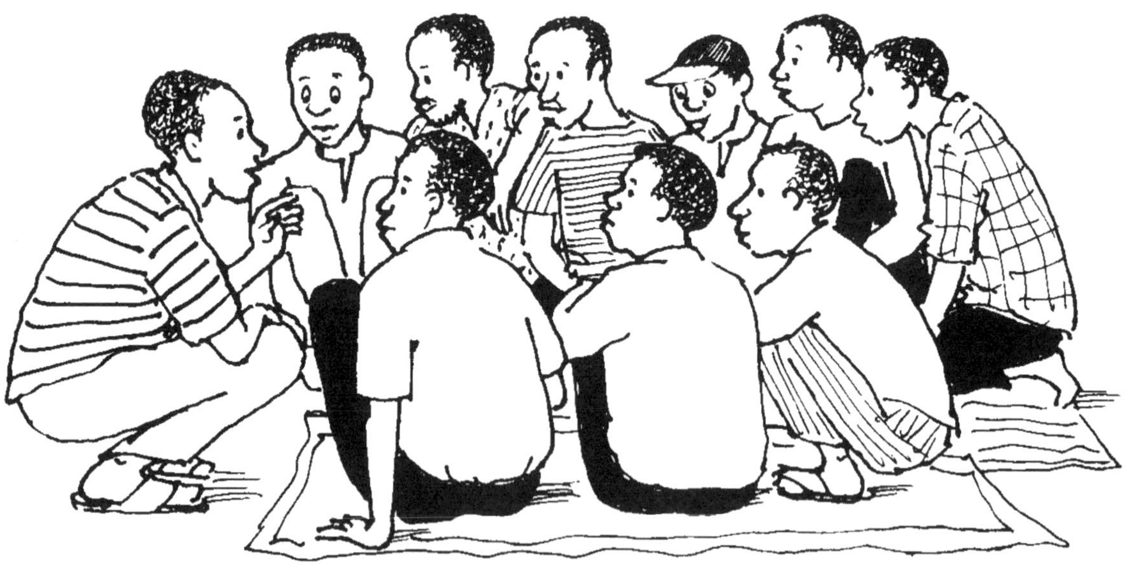

As a part of this principle, throughout the text we have used the words 'we', 'us' and 'our' and have tried to avoid 'they', 'them' and 'their' in talking about issues of concern and dilemmas facing people. We should not pretend to ourselves that we have nothing to learn about better communication and better understanding of ourselves and one another.

If you use the words 'we', 'us', and 'our' during your sessions, you will find that your participants will quickly develop confidence in you as someone who is ready to recognise your own needs alongside theirs.

The work of the group will benefit greatly from this. So do please try to do this.

USING PARTICIPANTS' DRAWINGS

Many people in communities cannot read or write easily, or they only have basic literacy skills. If we depend on written notices or messages in sessions, those who cannot read or write easily will immediately be left out. **They will probably keep quiet about this**, for fear of publicising their lack of skill and being ridiculed. It is therefore very important that you **use no writing** at all in the sessions, **unless you are completely certain that everyone in the group can understand** comfortably what is to be read or is being written.

Luckily, it is easy – and fun – to overcome this difficulty by asking participants to create drawings instead. They can draw on the ground using a stick or chalk, or on flip–chart paper or newsprint using coloured pens. In the DVD, for instance, you will see how the young women made drawings to describe to one another possible life paths for young women in their community. Drawings can be **made and understood by anyone**, whether they can read and write or not. The only thing they may need is some encouragement and praise from you. It does not matter how good or accurate the drawing is: the important thing is that the image means something to the person who has drawn it. When he or she tells others in the group what it means, they will be able to remember what it means also, far more easily than a non-literate person can remember the meaning of a word which they cannot read.

Drawings can be very simple – in fact the simpler they are, the more effective they can be. In a number of exercises in the workshop, the instructions ask you to encourage the participants to draw. So do please have faith that this works – it really does!

In Buwenda, the older women were making up their peer group rules. They chose to draw an ear, which meant that they wanted to encourage one another to listen well. They also drew a watch face, which meant that they wanted to encourage punctuality for meetings. Even though a few women in the group could not read or write, they could all easily understand the drawings of their rules, because they themselves had chosen and drawn them, so no-one felt left out.

NO NOTE-TAKING

Please discourage everyone very strongly from taking notes during the sessions. Nobody needs a pen or paper, except when you provide it for particular drawing sessions (see above). Note-taking by someone can be very unsettling for other members of the group, particularly when people are talking about sensitive or private things. Also, the person who takes notes is not involving him or herself fully in the group's activities.

WORKING WITH OLDER MEN USING GAMES AND EXERCISES

Many of the sessions include games and exercises, which older men often consider rather childish. Great effort is needed from the older men's facilitator to overcome this. We have often heard facilitators say, 'Oh you can't do games with the older men, so we just had a discussion about the issues instead.' Unfortunately, a discussion is rarely as productive as doing and analysing a completed game or an exercise which has a deeper meaning. Facilitators who have been encouraged to be more daring have often realised that it is their own reluctance, rather than the reluctance of the older men (or older women!), which is the main stumbling block.

So do please be more adventurous and encourage the older men to take part in these exercises properly. Encourage the men to think out what the deeper meaning behind the exercise or game might be in relation to their lives. Once they have seen for themselves the benefits of thinking through what they have done, they will feel readier to continue with them in later sessions.

SITTING TOGETHER IN A CIRCLE

We believe strongly that group work like this is far more effective if you all sit in a circle together, at the same level. In this way, no one appears to be more important or less important than the next person. This works best if everyone sits together on the ground on mats. Then no one has a chair in their way when asked to move round the area, and people can feel most relaxed. However, if participants really would feel more comfortable sitting in chairs, and there are enough similar ones for everybody, then you may have to do so. (Even one chair with arms, when the rest have none, makes a difference to the status of the person sitting in it.)

THIS IS NOT A COMPETITION BETWEEN PEER GROUPS

Please remember what was said above: each peer group will need to go through the material at its own pace. In Session D and Session F there is time available to review previous sessions, or for some peer groups to catch up with others if necessary.

FINAL PREPARATIONS

Team contract

You and your co-facilitator(s) need to make a **team contract**. It is crucial to the success of the workshop for you to agree to work together and to help each other as you go along. It may be best for you to choose one of your team as the lead facilitator, or 'workshop coordinator', so that the community leader(s) know whom they can turn to if they have a query about the workshop as a whole.

Other things you are likely to need to agree include:

- A general timetable for the whole workshop.
- Regular preparatory and feedback meetings, before and after each session.
- Who uses the laptop and mobile screen (if needed), and when.
- That there will be advice, support and cooperation – not competition! – between yourselves.
- You may also need to arrange for some kind of external support from someone for yourselves, especially if you find that participants bring a lot of difficult or upsetting problems to the sessions.
- To maintain confidentiality between yourselves regarding specific information about the community.

Before you begin Session F, you need to check whether there is a good, regular, and sustainable supply of male and female condoms available to the community, at a cost which can be afforded by women as well as by men. Session F is likely to create or to increase demand for condoms, so this is very important.

Initial community contact

It is strongly recommended that you meet first with the leader or leaders in your community to explain the purpose and format of this programme to them and to seek their permission to publicise the idea to the rest of the community. Remember to include women's leaders and youth leaders, as well as the older men, religious leaders, political leaders, or leaders of other groups in the community. You may need to conduct several small preparatory meetings, to ensure that you have contacted everyone concerned. The more you have the leaders on your side from the beginning, the more chance you have of conducting a successful workshop. So don't underestimate the importance of this first step! It is especially important, of course, if this is the first involvement that you are going to have with the community.

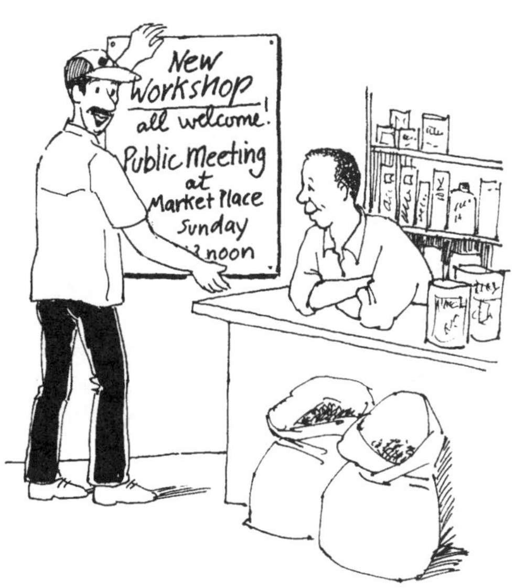
New
Workshop!
all welcome!
Public Meeting
at
Market Place
Sunday

Informal contacts can also help a lot. Go and sit in the bar for a while, if there is one, and chat with whoever is there. Find the headteacher and other teachers at the school, to let them know what is going on and to see if any of them want to attend. If they are old enough, tell the older children around the community about the workshop, to see if they are interested in joining in. Talk to the village shopkeepers or market stallholders. And so on. Let all these people know when the first open community meeting is, invite them to tell others about it, and to come to it with their friends, so they can find out more for themselves.

The optional sessions, (O–R) expect participants to understand many of the issues about attitudes to others covered by the earlier sessions, so we continue to recommend strongly that you use these sessions *only* once the main sessions (A-N and the Second Open Community Meeting) have been completed.

COMPLETE LIST OF MATERIALS NEEDED FOR WORKSHOPS

The exercises in this programme are designed for use by anyone, whether or not they have formal reading or writing skills. They include a lot of active exercises, including role play, movement, and drawing, in order to engage participants more fully in thinking about the issues being discussed.

The following is a list of all the materials which you will need to have available for each peer group to carry out the activities in this manual.

- flip-chart paper
- marker pens
- large ball of string
- long piece of strong rope
- post-it stickers (paper notes which you can stick to flip-chart paper) of different colours
- chalk of different colours
- sticky tape to stick the flip-chart paper together
- blu tack, drawing pins, or something else to stick the flip-chart paper onto walls
- several pairs of scissors
- candles – one for each participant and facilitators; and for all those attending the Further Open Community Meeting and the procession afterwards
- boxes of matches
- a notebook and pen for each facilitator only (not for participants)
- equipment for viewing DVDs listed below (see Annex 2)
- a copy of this *Stepping Stones and Stepping Stones Plus* manual for each facilitator (not for participants)
- photocopies of the body maps from OPAHA, Garissa (Session P.2), or body maps drawn by members of a local support group for people with HIV in your area
- crayons
- index cards
- at least 4 male and 4 female condoms for each participant, as well as one each for facilitators
- item, such as banana, cassava or wooden dildo, to act as a model penis (one for each participant)
- blindfold (a scarf will do)

For community meetings you will also need the items below. The items with question marks are not essential, but would be good to have available if participants would like a general public celebration of the end of the workshop. See more details in Sessions N and R.

- Music instruments? Special clothes for the role plays and for dancing? Refreshments? Food? Candles and matches for everyone.

Three DVDs

The original *Stepping Stones* DVD. This is in this volume.

What can I do? A Strategies for Hope DVD about Canon Gideon Byamagishwa. Available in English, Ki-Swahili, French, Spanish, Portuguese and Russian from Strategies for Hope, www.stratshope.org.

Children First! Stepping Stones with Children in Tanzania A documentary film from the DVD in our sister publication with the same name. It is also available online at https://vimeo.com/125781314.

Please remember also to organise a crèche or other childcare in order to help participants join, stay longer at, and engage fully in the workshop.

ENDNOTES

1. This DVD provides optional films to accompany the sessions. You may prefer not to show the clips to participants. However, it does strengthen the power of the workshop if you use it. We certainly recommend that you watch it whilst preparing to facilitate the sessions so that you can see how each topic was addressed in the original workshop. See Annex 3 for a synopsis of the film clips.
2. See Annex 6 for a discussion about people with particular positions in the community whose involvement it is also important to consider – and whose prior permission it may be vital to obtain!
3. See *Stepping Stones Revisited* (2006) for more on this.
4. *Misselhorn et al.* (2013)
5. For definitions of 'sexual health' and 'safer sex', see Sessions B and E respectively.
6. For details of the DVDs, see list of materials needed on pages 26–27 of this manual.

REFERENCES

Misselhorn, A. Jama-Shai, N. Mushinga, M. and Washington, L.(2014) Creating Futures: Supporting young people in building their 'livelihoods'. HEARD, South African Medical Research Council, Project Empower. Durban http://www.heard.org.za/gender/creating-futures-stepping-stones

Salamander Trust (2015) Children First! Stepping Stones with Children in Tanzania documentary film. Practical Action Publishing. Rugby. Available as part of the *Stepping Stones with Children* package or online at https://vimeo.com/125781314

Salamander Trust *Stepping Stones* Home Page [website], <http://www.steppingstonesfeedback.org> [accessed 11 December 2015]

Salamander Trust Transforming the way we think about HIV [website], <http://www.salamandertrust.net> [accessed 11 December 2015]

The original *Stepping Stones* DVD (optional). This is in this volume.

Strategies for Hope (2006a) What can I do? Strategies for Hope [website and film]. Available in English, Ki-Swahili, French, Spanish, Portuguese and Russian, from: Strategies for Hope www.stratshope.org <http://www.stratshope.org/resources/dvds_item/what-can-i-do> [accessed 11 December 2015]

Strategies for Hope (2006b) *Stepping Stones* Revisited: Stories from the Village of Buwenda, Uganda [film on website] Salamander Trust https://vimeo.com/album/3419245/video/134751173 [accessed 16 November 2015]

Strategies for Hope (2006b) *Stepping Stones* Revisited: Stories from the Village of Buwenda, Uganda. https://vimeo.com/134751173 [accessed 27 January 2016]

Misselhorn. A, Mushinga. M, Jama Shai. N, Washington. L, and Mbatha. M, Stepping Stones Creating Futures: a manual for facilitating livelihoods HEARD, Project Empower and South African Medical Research Council (2013)

Vimeo Salamander Trust on Vimeo [website], <https://vimeo.com/salamandertrust> [accessed 11 December 2015]

FIRST OPEN COMMUNITY MEETING

PURPOSE

To introduce yourselves. To explain the workshop. To find potential participants.

TIME NEEDED: Maximum 1½ hours.

MATERIALS NEEDED: DVD, laptop with DVD player, projector, mobile screen if no wall.

PARTICIPANTS: Anyone from the community who wishes to attend.

SPECIAL INFORMATION

Don't forget to read 'Before You Begin ...!' before using this manual.

AIMS: To announce the purpose of the workshop. To explain how it will be organised. To seek permission of the community elders to run it in this way.

DESCRIPTION: A public meeting of as many adult members of the community as possible, including older and younger men and women. It is probably best to hold it during school time, unless the community are happy for schoolchildren to attend. Of course, if community members are ready to let young people, aged around 12 or more, take part in the workshop too, either in their own groups, or in the younger men's and younger women's groups, then they should be there too. If this is the case, don't forget to encourage out-of-school children as well as schoolchildren to participate. All facilitators should be present.

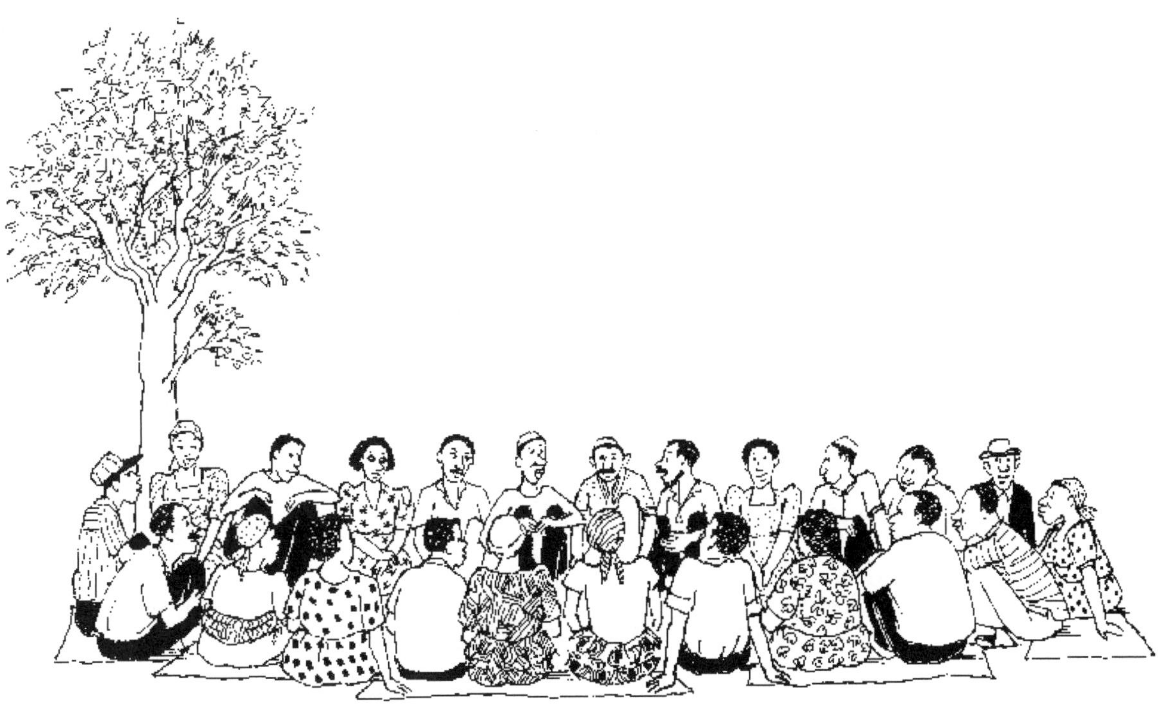

DIRECTIONS

All four facilitators should share the talking. When not actually speaking, any other facilitators present should try as much as possible NOT to be put in chairs at the front of the meeting but instead sit amongst the community members.

1. Thank everyone for sparing the time to come to the meeting.

2. Introduce yourself and let each of your colleagues introduce themselves (so everyone hears a few words from every facilitator).

3. Explain that you are going to tell them about a workshop which they are welcome to join, if they would like.

- (Optional) Say that you will show them a brief DVD which explains a bit about the workshop.[1]
- Then say that you will answer any questions which people may like to ask after the DVD.
- Finally, say that you will finish by asking those who would like to join the workshop to contact the relevant person.

4. Explain that we all find it difficult to talk about sex, but sex is important to all of us as mothers and fathers, husbands, wives, children, grandchildren, grandparents … Explain that the workshop will help us all to explore the good things about sex as well as the bad, and the hopes and the fears that we all have.

It will also help us to learn more about our own needs and expectations of life in general, through talking and listening.

5. Describe how the workshop will last for eighteen sessions, of which this is the first. The last one will be another public meeting for everyone, but most of the others between the first and the last meetings will be meetings just for those who decide to become members of the workshop group. (You can also explain that there will be some further optional sessions afterwards, if people would like them.) You will explain more after the first DVD clip.

6. Then introduce the first DVD clip.[2] Say:

'We would like to show you this so that you can understand better what the workshop is about and what it is hoped that we can achieve during it. The DVD was shot in a village called Buwenda, in Uganda, the first time this workshop was run. There are many different clips which will be shown during the course of the workshop. This introductory clip lasts just a few minutes; please feel free to ask questions afterwards.'

Make sure that everyone can see and hear the DVD clearly.

7. Turn on at '1. Stepping Stones'.

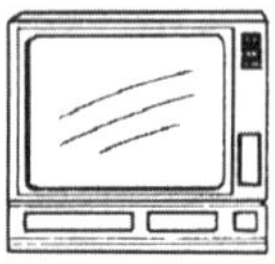

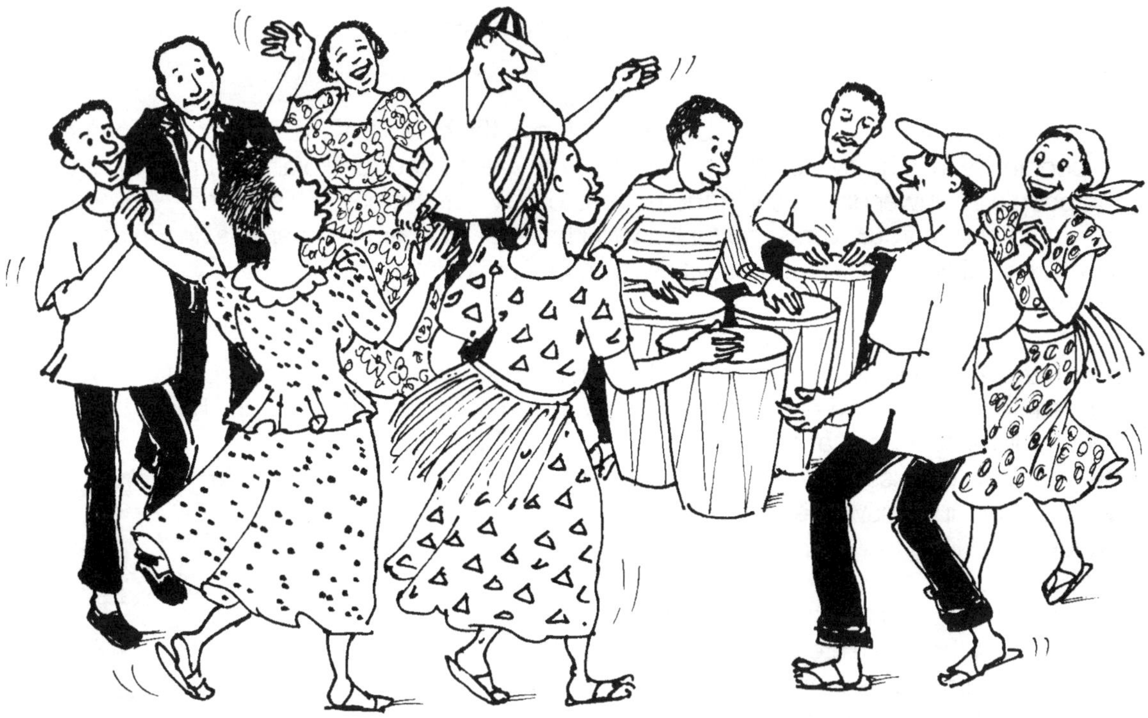

8. Turn off the DVD when it fades to black.

Then explain that, since sex and surrounding issues are so difficult to talk about, much of our work will be conducted in small groups with participants of similar gender and age or marital status.

Explain that this has been found to work well elsewhere, since it reduces embarrassment and encourages us to share our experiences more openly with one another.

Ask them: 'What do you think of this?' and seek their permission to form four separate groups:

- for older men
- for younger men
- for older women
- for younger women.

> ☞ In Ghana, family planning workers found that men and women wanted to talk about sex together and not separately. However, their experience has shown that such discussions are used by individual couples to fight their own particular battles. This is not usually a constructive way forward, either for themselves or for others. So if community members say they don't want to divide into peer groups, explain that there will be opportunities to have joint meetings during the workshop, and afterwards too, but that, to begin with, you would like to ask them to agree to meet separately.

9. Explain again that during the workshop the four smaller groups will meet twice in larger groups, to share their ideas and experiences, but that most of the initial work will happen in the smaller groups.

Explain again that other DVD clips will be shown during the course of the sessions, in order to help people discuss many issues together. You may also need to explain that participants saw the people of Buwenda watching themselves on DVD at the end. This will not, of course, happen at the end of **your** workshop (unless you have a DVD camera available, in which case, maybe you **could** film some of the activities - but beware of letting filming interfere with the workshop).

10. Explain that if someone wants to join in with the workshop, you would ask them to make a real commitment to coming to every one of the twenty three meetings of their group. This is because new things will be discussed at each meeting, which will build on what has been discussed before and so it would be very difficult for the group to have members missing meetings or coming for only one or two.

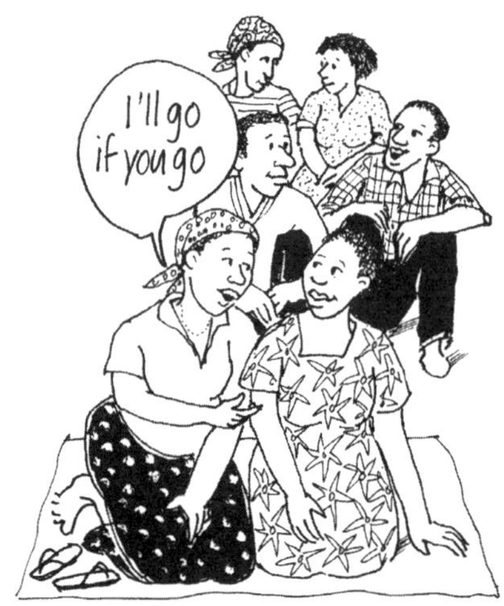

Add that you understand that this sounds like a big commitment, but that there are many things to be discussed as the workshop progresses, and that it deals with a most important aspect of our lives – sex.

11. Ask for any further comments or questions.

12. Thank everyone for coming and participating in the meeting.

Ask those who would like to join the workshop to stay behind for a few minutes after the meeting has closed, so that each facilitator can meet with his/her potential group members in order to find out good meeting times for them and to plan a time for the first meeting of each peer group. Remind the community who each facilitator is, and point out where they will each stand after the meeting.

☞ If more than twenty people want to join any peer group, you and your co-facilitators need to have decided beforehand what you could offer them. You could suggest that an extra peer group be formed straightaway. This might mean that one facilitator would need to run two separate groups of young men, for instance, on two different days of the week. Alternatively, you could ask the extra people to give their names to you so that you can contact them for a repeat of the whole workshop at a later date.

13. Close the meeting.

14. Facilitators each stand in their chosen corner of the public meeting area and arrange a time suitable for their prospective group members to meet.

☞ Facilitators can listen out for conflict development. Don't worry about it. Just take note of the issues and assure the community that these issues will be addressed during the course of the workshop.

FACILITATORS' TEAM FEEDBACK

After the end of the first open community meeting, meet with your co-facilitators to compare notes on how you think the meeting went and the information which you learnt from it. Your co-facilitators could have found useful information that could help you to structure your peer group sessions more effectively.

ENDNOTES

1. This DVD is optional. You may prefer to use no DVD at all or to make your own. Please do contact us for advice on how to do this!
2. There is a synopsis of all the clips in Annex 3. Do not read these out to the participants. They are just to remind you of what happens in each clip. Participants may want to view the clip again. If so, it is usually best for them to have some discussion about it first, then to have a further discussion after the second viewing.

YOUR NOTES ...

THEME 1 – GROUP COOPERATION

SESSION A LET'S COMMUNICATE

PURPOSE

To help a peer group form. To help participants develop skills of listening and the analysis of communication and cooperation.

CONTENTS	TIME NEEDED
Introduction	
A.1	Adjectival Names
A.2	Expectations
A.3	Trust and Confidentiality
A.4	The Straight Line
A.5	Ground Rules
A.6	A Knotty Problem
A.7	Listening Pairs
A.8	Body Language
A.9	Guardian Angels
A.10	Hand in Hand

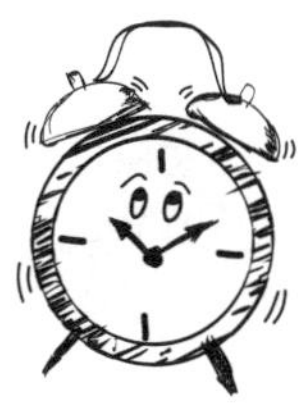

Maximum 3 hours

MATERIALS NEEDED: A roll of flip-chart paper, a scarf for a blindfold, strongly coloured felt-tip marker pens (e.g. three each of red, blue and green).

PARTICIPANTS: Four separate peer groups.

SPECIAL INFORMATION

Don't forget to read 'Before You Begin ...!' before using this manual.

INTRODUCTION

1. Sit in a circle with the group, preferably on the ground. Everyone should be at the same level, including yourself.

2. Introduce yourself, thank everyone for coming and explain that if they want to join in with the workshop, you would ask them to again make a real commitment to coming to every meeting of their group. This is because new things will be discussed at each meeting, which will build on what has been discussed before, so it would be very difficult for the group to have members missing meetings or only coming for one or two.

3. Add that you would particularly like to welcome to the workshop anyone who may have HIV. Reassure everyone that you don't know who may or may not have HIV and that no-one has to identify themselves as living with HIV, or with any other condition, if they don't want to.

EXERCISE A.1: ADJECTIVAL NAMES

AIMS: Icebreaker. For the facilitator to learn the names of participants. For everyone to speak early and to laugh.

DESCRIPTION: Each person introduces her/himself to the rest of the group using an adjective which starts with the same sound as their name: for instance 'Fantastic Florence' or 'Gigantic John'.

DIRECTIONS

1. Explain that you would like to learn everyone's names, since you are going to be working together for several sessions. You would also like to learn something special about each participant.

2. Start off by asking everyone to think of an adjective to describe themselves which begins with the same sound as their own name. Explain that it's not a competition and that, if anyone can't think of one, we could all help. Then ask each participant to think of something special which they like about themselves.

3. Begin the game by introducing yourself: e.g. 'I am radiant Rose and I like my cooking' or 'I am bold Baron and I like my singing'. Cheerful adjectives help everyone to laugh!

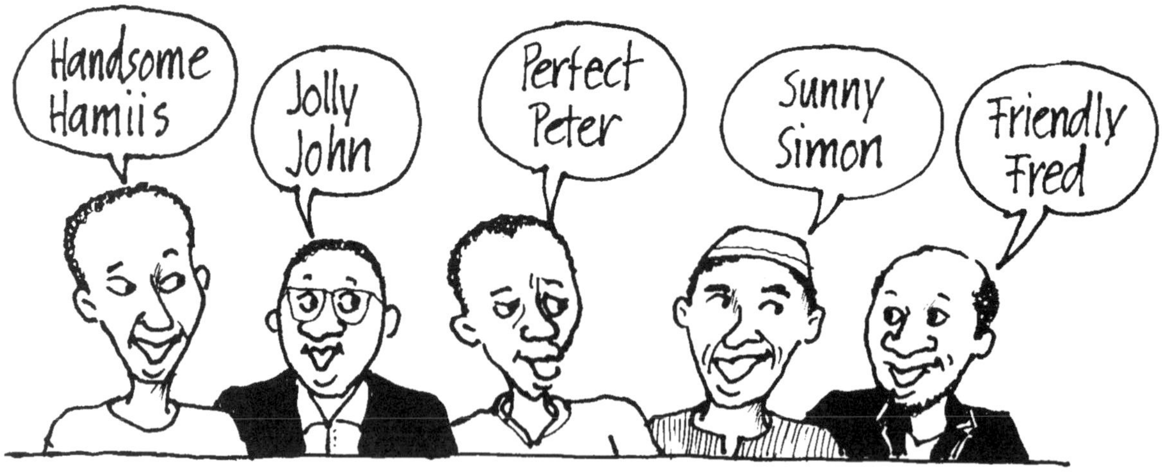

Handsome Hamiis
Jolly John
Perfect Peter
Sunny Simon
Friendly Fred

4. Go round the circle to your right, each group member in turn introducing her/himself to the rest of the group in this way, saying something they like about themselves. Participants may prefer to describe themselves using a clan name or something other than a word whose starting sound matches that of their own name. Whatever works best in your context is fine.

In Buwenda, in the young women's group, one or two women hardly spoke at all to begin with, because they felt so shy. But, later in the workshop, they had built up so much self-confidence that they became much more involved and active.

If someone really can't think of an adjective for him or herself, it may be because they are shy. Bear this in mind, because they may need some help in other exercises. Help now by suggesting a suitable pleasing adjective and encourage others to help too. Some participants may also find it embarrassing to say something they like about themselves. Throughout the workshop, give a lot of praise and encouragement to those who are more shy.

EXERCISE A.2: EXPECTATIONS

AIM: To give each participant a chance to voice their feelings about the workshop. This enables you to gauge their understanding of explanations so far, and to correct any misunderstandings.

DESCRIPTION: Each participant in turn voices one hope and one fear they have about the workshop.

DIRECTIONS

1. Explain to the group that it is always a good idea for a facilitator to find out what a group is thinking.

2. Going round the circle to your left, ask each group member in turn to quickly express one hope and one fear about the workshop. They should be encouraged to say 'I hope that...' and then 'I fear that...'. Finish with your own statements.

3. Do not make any comments about the expectations or fears as you go round the circle.

Feedback and discussion

Once everyone has stated a hope and a fear, you should make some comments. If any hopes are quite beyond the scope of the workshop, you could explain this now. You could also try to reassure people about their fears. Ask everyone to remember their own hope and their own fear, so that at the end of the workshop, you can review them.

EXERCISE A.3: TRUST AND CONFIDENTIALITY

AIM: To define explicitly participants' understandings of these two words in the context of this workshop.

DESCRIPTION: An open discussion about the two words in terms of the effectiveness of the workshop and personal safety.

DIRECTIONS

1. Explain that in this exercise we are going to explore mutual trust between ourselves and our friends, and also confidentiality within the group, since we are going to be talking about some difficult things together.

2. Ask the group to divide into fours and to discuss the following situation amongst themselves for a few minutes. They should imagine that they have some kind of health problem which they feel embarrassed about. They want to seek some advice from a friend or from a health worker. **What qualities** would they look for in the person whose advice they seek? **They should not mention** the name of the person whom they would turn to: they should just concentrate on the **qualities** of that person or those people.

3. Call everyone back into the full circle and ask people to describe the kinds of qualities which have been discussed. **Again, no names** should be mentioned. Point out to everyone that we all seek the same kinds of qualities in people to whom we want to turn when in need. Say that we all have secrets or embarrassing feelings that we would like to share with someone whom we feel could reassure or help us.

4. Finally, explain to the group that confidentiality cannot be guaranteed and that we should all only say what we feel like saying in public. Point out, however, that our greatest source of learning is from our shared experiences. The more that we can show that we care for one another, as well as take care of ourselves, the more we are all likely to learn from one anothers' experiences. So you would like to encourage everyone to think carefully before sharing details of our discussions outside the workshop.

Feedback and discussion

Ask the participants what **they** think of this. **Discourage** them from making any rules about workshop confidentiality, because if someone said something in the workshop which they thought was in confidence and someone inadvertently broke that confidence, it might have bad consequences for the person concerned. However, it is intended that this discussion should raise everybody's awareness of the value to us all of trust and confidentiality.

EXERCISE A.4: THE STRAIGHT LINE

AIM: To help participants experience the value of team support and cooperation.

DESCRIPTION: Participants take it in turn to walk in a straight line blindfold across the meeting area. First they have silence and no guidance. Next they have a lot of encouragement and advice.

DIRECTIONS

1. Provide a blindfold: a scarf would do.

2. Invite a volunteer to come forward to walk slowly in a straight line across the meeting area. Put the blindfold on him/her and turn him/her around several times before s/he sets off in a straight line across the meeting area, aiming to reach an agreed point on the opposite side.

3. Instruct the rest of the group to keep completely silent, giving no encouragement or guidance at all. They should also not touch the volunteer.

4. When the blindfolded person reaches the other side, ask her/him to take off the blindfold. Compare how close s/he is to the point s/he intended to reach.

5. Ask her/him how s/he felt about having no commentary from the others.

6. Ask her/him to replace the blindfold and repeat the exercise, this time with the verbal encouragement of the others. They should still not touch her/him. Then finally, they could repeat the exercise with the participants using their hands to guide the blindfolded person, as well as talking to her/him.

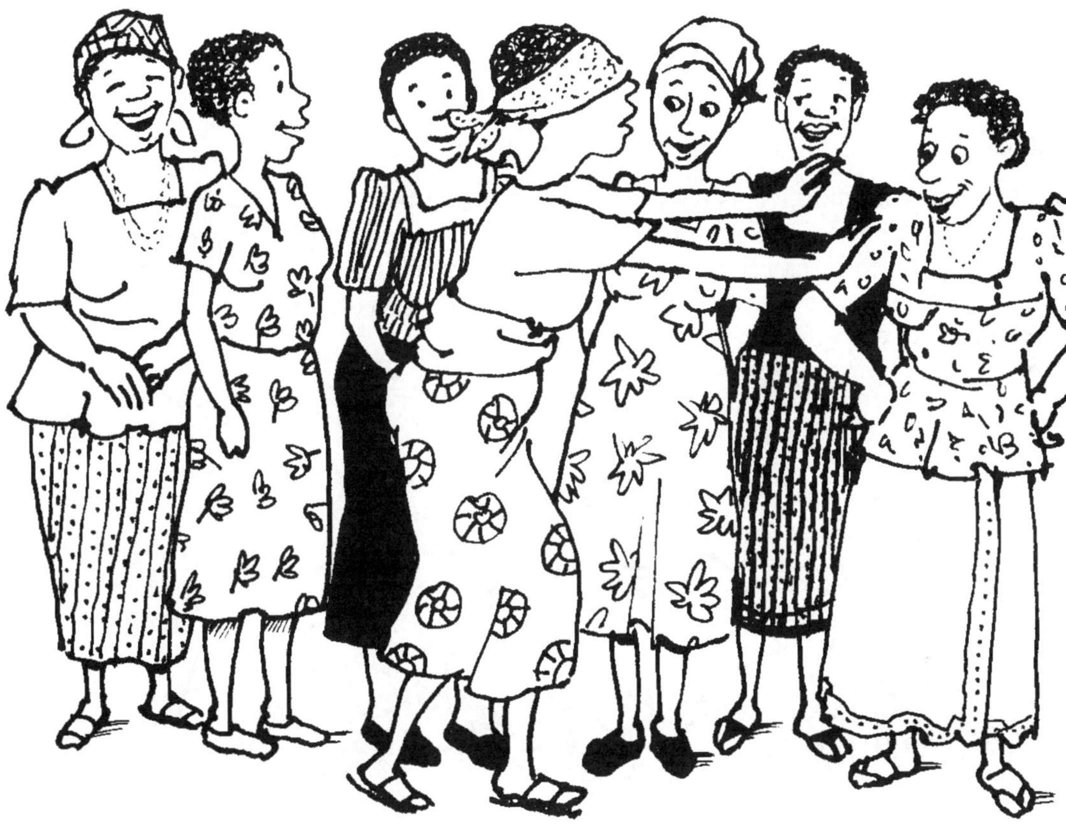

7. On completion, remove the blindfold again and repeat stages four and five above, this time asking how it felt **with** commentary.

8. Repeat the exercise with two or three other volunteers. Explain that this is not a competition, just a game.

Feedback and discussion

Group members are enabled to experience how much safer they feel with the support of their group around them. This exercise emphasises the importance of trust and mutual support in life. Encourage them to talk about these issues, by asking them how their experience in this exercise relates to their real-life experiences.

> ☞ You can explain how this exercise has helped us to explore the advantages of group work over working alone, and how useful listening can be to us!

EXERCISE A.5: GROUND RULES

AIM: To agree on a set of rules for the group during its time working together.

DESCRIPTION: Encourage participants to brainstorm rules which they would like to have for the group.

MATERIALS NEEDED: Flip-chart paper, felt-tip marker pens.

DIRECTIONS

1. Explain to the group that this is their time together and that, in order that they can make the best of this time, it is useful for everyone to agree to some group rules. Suggest certain topics which they may like to include, such as punctuality, respect for other people's views, politeness, being non-judgemental, giving everybody a chance to air their views, not dominating, and so on.

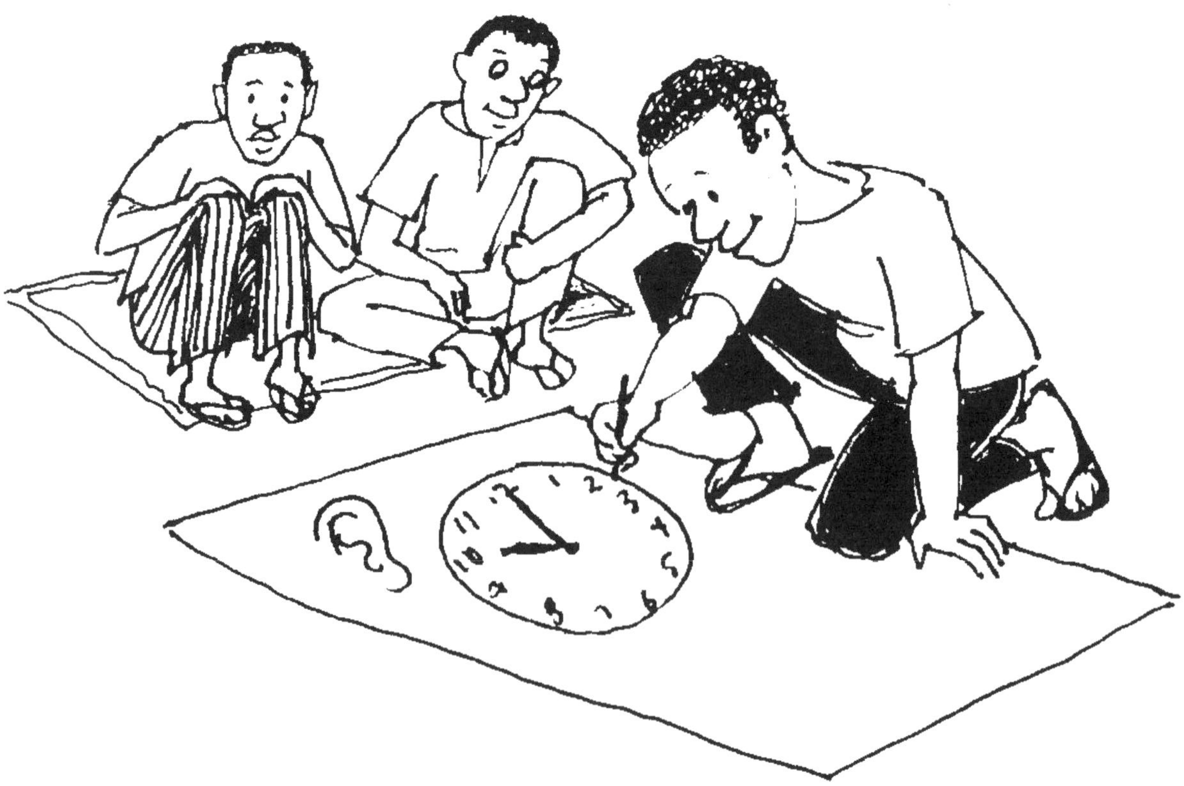

2. Placing a piece of flip chart paper on the floor in the middle of your circle, encourage each group member who has an idea for a ground rule to suggest it. If everyone else agrees to the rule, ask her/him to come into the circle and to draw a symbol of their choice to represent it.

They may need some encouragement to do this initially, but once they are encouraged, they will find it easy to think of an appropriate symbol. You might like to suggest that punctuality, for instance, could be drawn as the sun, or as a clock face. Politeness could be represented by a smiling face, and respect could be shown by the picture of an ear listening. But once you have made some suggestions, **let them choose** what they would like to draw and **let them draw** it. Everyone in the group will remember what it means. (For notes to remind you about why community drawings are important, see 'Using Participants' Drawing' in 'Before You Begin ...!'.)

3. Once all the rules that the group want have been drawn on the flip chart, ask the group to go through them again together so that everyone is clear about them all.

4. Encourage group members to try to stick to these rules, and as a ground rule ask them to remind you and one another if you or any of them appears not to be following them.

5. Ask one group member to take responsibility for the ground rules diagram. Ask her/him to bring it to each of your meetings, so that you always have it on hand to refer to.

> ☞ This acts as a simple introduction to the use of symbols drawn by participants themselves. It is their first joint production. It is helpful to provide a lot of encouragement and praise at this initial stage. It is also useful to emphasise that it doesn't matter if the drawing is not perfect or beautiful: the important thing is that it is a mark on the paper that everyone can recognise and identify with.

EXERCISE A.6: A KNOTTY PROBLEM

AIM: To illustrate in a funny way how the people who can best work out solutions to problems are the ones who have the problems themselves.

DESCRIPTION: Two members of the group try to give directions to the rest of the group about how to disentangle themselves from their problem. This is very hard for them.

DIRECTIONS

1. Ask two people to volunteer to be 'professional health workers' and ask them to go away from the group until called back.

2. Ask the rest of the group to form a big circle by holding hands with the people on each side of them. Then, keeping their hands held tightly, the circle of participants should tie itself into as entangled a knot as possible.

3. Call the 'health workers' back to the group and instruct them to hold their own hands behind their backs.

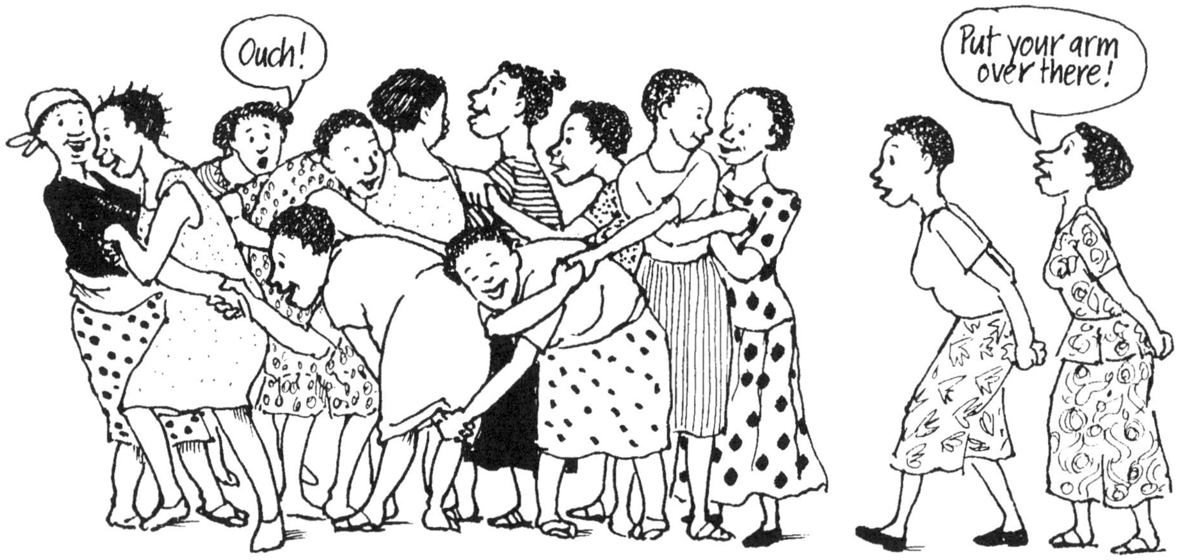

4. Then ask them to unravel the knot of the others, using verbal instructions only, within three minutes. They can move round the knotted circle of people, but cannot touch anyone. Remind the group never to drop their hands and only to follow the instructions of the 'professional health workers' literally, not going out of their way to help them.

5. You will find that the 'health workers' will move around the group and may manage to change the positions of a few of the group slightly, but they will fail to disentangle them! After three minutes, call stop.

6. Now ask the circle members to drop their hands. Then ask them to form a new circle, this time with the 'health workers' and yourself too.

7. Tie yourselves into another knot. Then time your own disentanglement: it should take about 20 seconds.

Feedback and discussion

This exercise shows us and the community how we as managers or outsiders do not have solutions for all problems. Instead the community should have the major role in solving its own problems. Sometimes they only need a little input from outside to make a great advance in their achievements. Encourage the participants to relate this game to their own lives by asking them for examples of when they have experienced this for themselves: e.g. in relation to their parents, school, extension workers, elders, etc.

> ☞ In some societies, it is not considered acceptable to ask men and women to do this exercise together. However we are assuming that the members of your peer group are all of the same gender and similar age: in which case the close contact between participants should not be a problem.

EXERCISE A.7: LISTENING PAIRS

AIM: To help people realise the importance of listening skills to good communication.

DESCRIPTION: Participants work in pairs, taking it in turns to speak. As one speaks, the other first listens carefully to what they say, then stops listening. A plenary session with discussion and summary follows.

DIRECTIONS

1. Describe to participants how we will need to do a lot of listening to one another in this workshop. In this exercise we are going to look together at the skills of good listening.

2. Describe what you want participants to do. They will be asked to divide into pairs, finding someone to work with. Then one of them should start by describing to the other an event in her/his life which made her/him feel very happy. The listener should say nothing, but should just concentrate hard on hearing what is being said. After a couple of minutes, you will ask the listeners to stop listening. At this stage, the speaker should continue to describe her/his happy experience, but the listener should stop listening completely. S/he could yawn, look elsewhere, turn round, whistle, do whatever s/he likes: the important thing is that s/he should no longer listen, although the speaker should continue to tell the story. After another couple of minutes, you will call 'Halt'. At this stage, the speaker and listener should change roles and repeat the two stages of the exercise, with the former listener becoming the speaker and the former speaker becoming the listener.

3. Once you are sure that everyone has understood the instructions, ask everyone to break into pairs. Then call out 'Start', and time each section of the exercise for two minutes. Thus the whole exercise should take eight minutes.

Feedback and discussion

Ask participants first how they felt as speakers, encouraging them to compare telling their story to a willing listener and telling it to a bad listener.

Then ask participants to describe and compare how they felt as good and bad listeners.

Ask participants to describe some of the attributes of good listening and then some of the attributes of bad listening. Ask participants in what other ways we communicate with one another, apart from through language. When someone mentions body language, explain that, by being aware of our own body language, we can often change it in order to communicate a different mood to others around us. This is what we are going to look at next.

EXERCISE A.8: BODY LANGUAGE

AIM: To help participants understand further the role of body language in our relationships.

DESCRIPTION: Through role play, participants are asked to demonstrate how body language can help onlookers understand what is happening without hearing any words.

DIRECTIONS

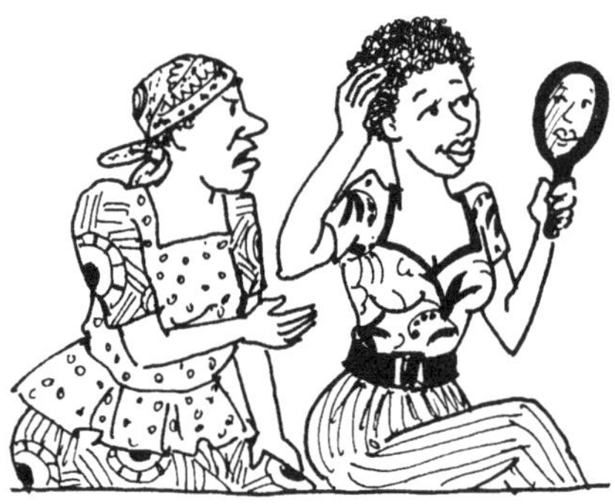

1. Ask participants to divide into pairs, working with someone with whom they have not worked before. Each pair should think of a discussion that one of them has had with someone else which developed into an argument. This could be an argument with their spouse or with a friend. It is up to them to decide. The pair are to create a mime that first establishes the two characters and their relationship, then re-enacts the argument. Throughout the mime they should use no words, only their bodies and faces. They should then re-enact the argument between them also as a mime using no words, only their bodies and faces.

2. Give the pairs a few minutes to work on this. Then ask everyone to return to the circle. Pick out two pairs whose scenes looked particularly clear. Ask the first chosen pair to re-enact their scene in the middle of the circle, so that everyone can see.

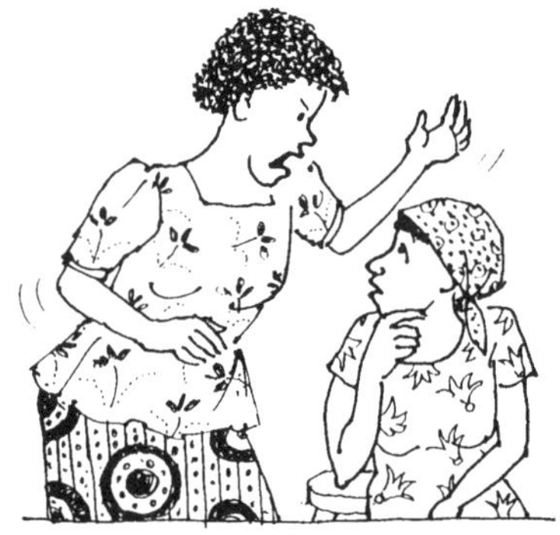

3. Ask members of the audience to tell the story of this pair's argument. It doesn't matter if the audience don't know the details, but point out how easy it can be for us to know what is going on in general through what we do with our bodies.

4. Repeat this viewing exercise with the second pair whom you have picked out.

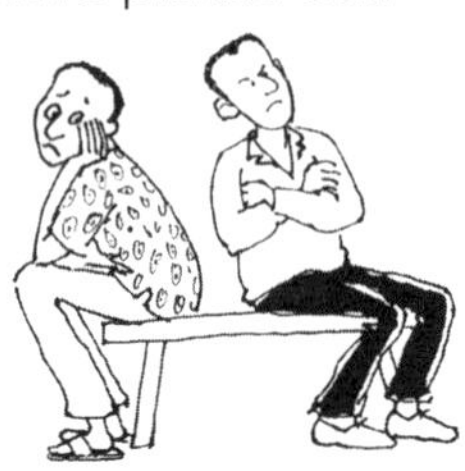

5. Brainstorm with the participants the kinds of emotion which we can communicate with our bodies: pleasure, dejection, anger, submission, strength, weakness, power, and so on. Ask them to add to this list, encouraging them to show different body stances to illustrate each emotion.

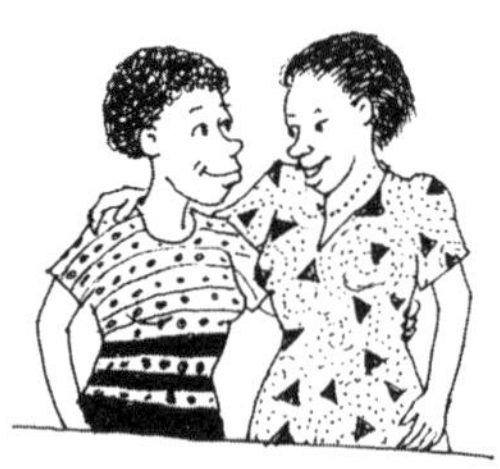

6. Point out also how different eye levels or **relative positions** can make a big difference to communication and to **power** relationships– e.g. teachers standing up, while their pupils are sitting down; elders sitting on chairs, while others stand or sit below them; shopkeepers behind their counters, while customers wait to ask them for goods. Ask participants to give examples of this from their own experience, describing each time whether the person who is higher or lower, behind or in front, has more power and why.

7. Finish by asking participants to start to think about the way that they use their own bodies to say things to one another over the next few days and weeks. Encourage them to think how they might use their bodies differently in various contexts, in order to convey different messages to people.

Feedback and discussion

Encourage participants to be aware that we communicate and listen as much with our bodies as with our words. Explain how some body language can appear very powerful and aggressive, some can appear friendly and warm, whilst other body language can appear very weak and submissive. We say a lot with our bodies!

EXERCISE A.9: GUARDIAN ANGELS

AIM: To make sure each person has support during the whole workshop.

DESCRIPTION: Each person is given the task of looking after someone else in the peer group.

DIRECTIONS

1. Ask everyone to stand up and to join hands in a circle. Stand yourself in the middle of the circle.

2. Then ask everyone to drop their hands and to turn to their right. This will mean that each person in the circle is facing the back of someone else.

3. Next explain that in this kind of workshop, it is always a good idea for participants to look after one another. Therefore you would like to suggest that each participant becomes the 'guardian angel' of the person standing in front of them in the circle. In this way, each person will be looking after somebody and each person will have somebody looking after him or her.

4. Ask everyone to turn back to the centre of the circle. Explain that each of them, as guardian angel, is to keep an eye on the person they are looking after, by asking them at the end of each session, or between sessions, how they are and whether all is going OK for them. This kind of arrangement helps people if they are finding some of the exercises difficult. It also helps people to recognise that **everyone** has something they can offer somebody else. It helps participants to develop bonds of mutual support.

5. Ask if anyone has any questions about this before moving on to the final exercise.

EXERCISE A.10: HAND IN HAND

AIM: Winding-down exercise.

DESCRIPTION: Everyone says something bad and something good about the group.

DIRECTIONS

1. Explain that the time for this session has now run out and that we are going to finish with a closing circle to review this session.

2. Add that in the next session we are going to start to look together at images that we have of the ideal man and the ideal woman in our society. Ask participants to spend a few minutes before the next session thinking about **short** songs they know, or local **short** stories, or proverbs which describe how the perfect man or the perfect woman should behave. Ask them to bring these with them in their minds to share with the group at the next meeting.

3. Everyone stands in a tight circle. Ask the first person to your left to put their right outstretched arm into the middle of the circle and say something they have found difficult about the session then something that they have found good about the session. Ask her/him to use the phrases: 'I didn't like it when …', followed by 'I did like it when …'

4. Ask the second person on your left to repeat this, placing her/his right hand on top of the hand already in the middle, and also saying one thing s/he found difficult and one thing s/he found good about the session.

5. Continue until all the participants have their right hands placed on top of one another in the centre of the circle, and everyone has said something which they found difficult followed by something which they found good about the session.

6. Finish by saying that this tower of hands can represent our strength as a group.

7. Remind everyone of their role as guardian angel.

8. Encourage participants to talk in general about the kinds of issues they have been discussing in these sessions with their friends and neighbours, if they like, but not to share any confidential information from the peer group with others.

9. Ask two or three people to volunteer to stay behind for ten minutes to do a quick assessment of this session. Explain that you will do a similar assessment at the end of every session and that each time you will ask new people to volunteer for this. (For details of how to run the assessment, see Annex 4.)

10. Thank everyone for coming. Fix with them a time and place for the next session which they can all manage. Ask them to remind one another to come on time.

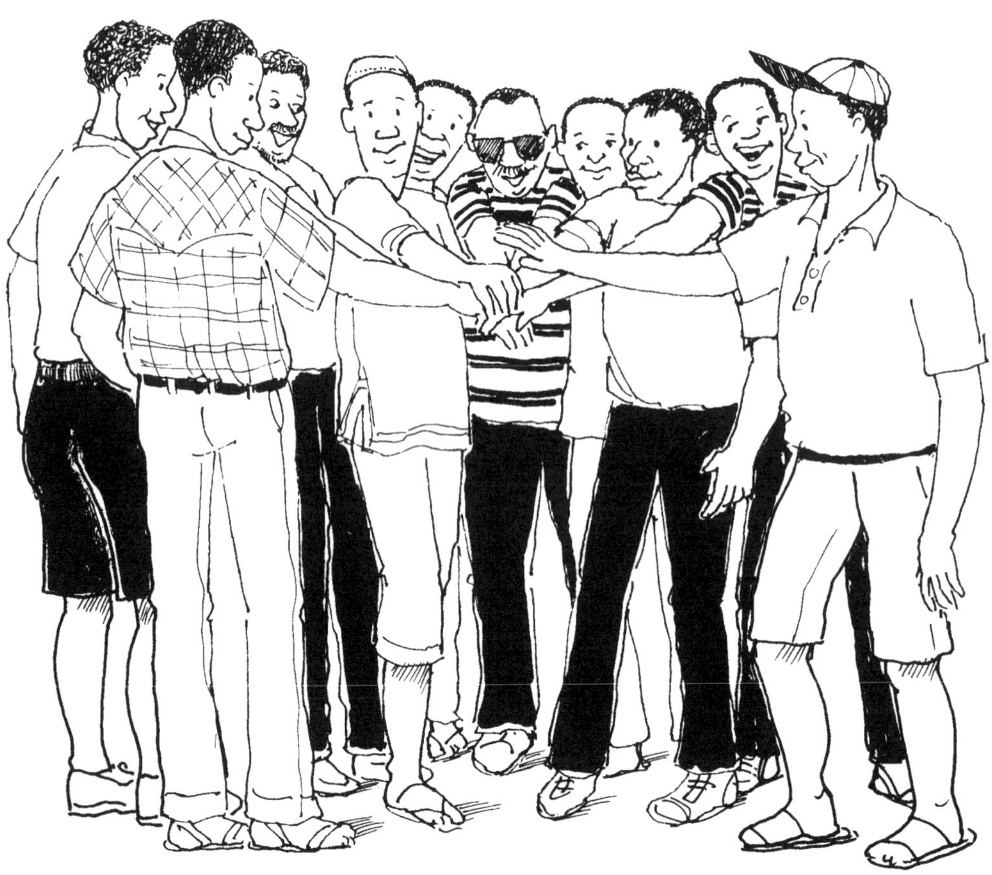

FACILITATORS' TEAM FEEDBACK

After the end of Session A, meet with your co-facilitators to compare notes on how your sessions went and the information which you learnt from them. Your co-facilitators could have found useful information that could help you to structure your next session more effectively. Remember, however, not to share confidentialities between groups. This is the easiest way to ruin the trust that you have begun to build and to wreck the whole workshop!

YOUR NOTES ...

SESSION B OUR PERCEPTIONS

PURPOSE

To help participants recognise how much perceptions influence our judgements of ourselves and others. This includes a first look at images of sex.

CONTENTS	TIME NEEDED
Introduction	
B.1	Mime the Lie
B.2	Fixed Positions
B.3	Ideal Images and Personal Destroyers
B.4	Images of Sex
B.5	Prioritising Problems
B.6	Closing Circle and Local Song

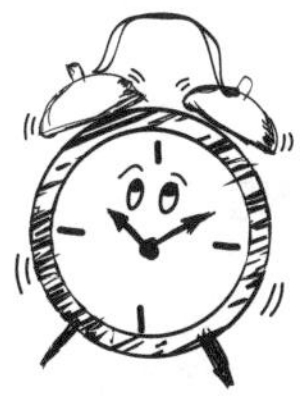

3–4 hours

MATERIALS NEEDED: Pack of 100 small plain index cards (about 12cm x 8cm), 7 small packs of strongly coloured crayons, a roll of flip-chart paper, felt-tip marker pens (4 each of red, green and blue), a roll of sticky tape, scissors, a pack of chalk, a notebook, a pen. (If cards are too expensive, you can use bits of paper, cut to size, but card is a bit stronger and therefore easier to use.)

PARTICIPANTS: Four separate peer groups.

SPECIAL INFORMATION

Don't forget to read 'Before You Begin ...!' before using this section of the manual. If you would like to read up on sexual and reproductive health in preparation for Exercise B.4, see Annex 7 for a list of suggested resources.

INTRODUCTION

1. Sit in a circle with the group, preferably on the ground. Everyone should be at the same level, including yourself.

2. Welcome everyone to the new session. Thank everyone for coming. Enquire about late-comers or non-attendants.

3. Ask everyone to recount very quickly one good thing that has happened to them since the last session.

4. Review the last session. Ask participants to recall what we learnt together at the last session – listening skills, trust, cooperation, body language, finding our own solutions ... Remind them if they have forgotten.

5. Explain that we are going on to discuss other things in this session, but will start with a couple of games.

EXERCISE B.1: MIME THE LIE

AIM: Warm-up game. Shows in a funny, obvious way that what people say they are doing is not necessarily what they are really doing!

DESCRIPTION: Each person in turn mimes an action and, when asked, says s/he is doing something else. The next person has to mime what the previous person said s/he was doing.

DIRECTIONS

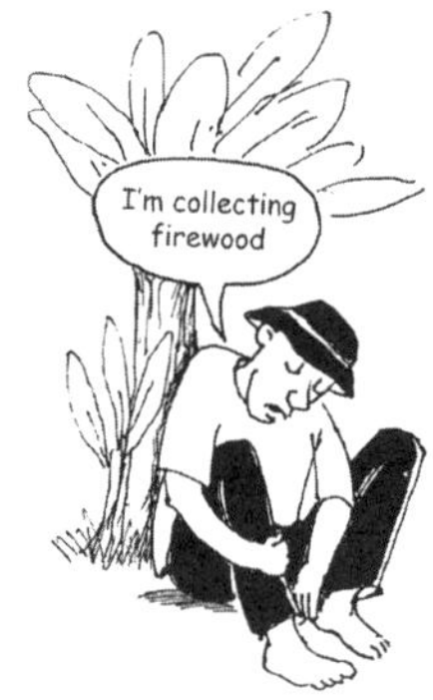
I'm collecting firewood

1. Ask everyone to stand in a circle. You start by going into the middle of the circle and miming an action, such as getting dressed. Ask the person who was next to you in the circle to ask you what you are doing. You reply by saying, for example, 'I am digging the ground!' Everyone will laugh! Next, ask the person who asked you the question to enter the circle instead of you and to mime what you **said** you were doing.

2. When her/his neighbour asks what s/he is doing, s/he also lies, and so the game continues until everyone in the circle has had a go at doing one thing and saying they are doing something else.

> ☞ This is a good warm-up exercise, because it makes everyone laugh and includes everyone. It is also useful to refer back to later in the session: we often say we are doing one thing while in fact we are doing something else. We may lead others into problems if they don't see through our lie.

EXERCISE B.2: FIXED POSITIONS

AIMS: To encourage participants to realise that our perspectives on things are based on who we are and our own experiences. To encourage people to be less judgemental about the actions of others.

DESCRIPTION: Participants stand in a circle and comment about what they see, from different angles, of someone standing in the middle.

DIRECTIONS

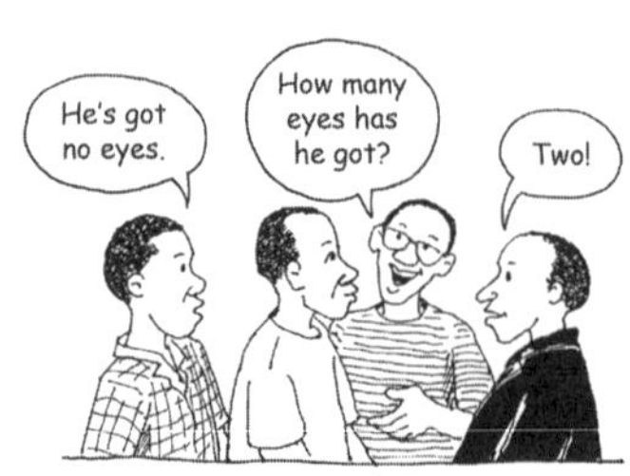
He's got no eyes.
How many eyes has he got?
Two!

1. Form a circle and ask one participant to stand in the middle. Ask her/him to stand still, facing the same way throughout the questions and answers which are to follow.

2. Explain to all participants that you are going to ask some questions. Ask everyone at all times to answer according to what they can actually **see** from their own position, not what they **know** is there.

3. Ask someone standing in front of the person in the middle: 'How many eyes has s/he got?'

4. Ask someone standing behind the person in the middle the same question.

5. Ask someone standing directly to the side of the person in the middle the same question.

6. Then place someone else in the middle and choosing, say, the arms this time, run through the same questions with three different people.

7. Finally, ask one participant to walk round the whole circle, looking at the person in the middle from all angles. Ask the walker to give a running commentary on what s/he is seeing and how her/his vision of the person in the middle changes.

Feedback and discussion

Ask the participants to consider how our perspective on a situation shapes our understanding of it. How can we give ourselves a more complete picture more often? Ask each of the people who were in the middle how it felt to have to keep silent. How would s/he describe him/herself? In what way can we relate this exercise to our everyday experience?

> It is useful to remind participants about this exercise in later sessions. It is often hard for us to remember that there are more, equally valid, views of a situation or a person than our own. We are often quick to judge others without trying to understand more about them first. And we often forget to ask the person him/herself!

EXERCISE B.3: IDEAL IMAGES AND PERSONAL DESTROYERS

AIMS: To explore people's perceptions of the ideal man and the ideal woman, and how these ideal images vary from reality.

DESCRIPTION: Introduction from the facilitator, followed by a drawing exercise and discussions.

DIRECTIONS

1. Remind the participants how in the last session we looked together at verbal communication and at body language, which are two ways in which people relate to one another. We are now moving on to explore how different people in our society are expected to behave.

2. Ask them if they remembered to bring some examples of songs, short stories, or proverbs. Ask five or six people to share them with the rest of the group.

3. After a few general examples, ask participants to break into new groups of three or four and to focus particularly on the ideal image of their own age and gender in their society. Note that, from now on in this exercise, the discussion will focus only on their own age and gender. For example:

- If you are working with the young women, ask them to describe what a young woman is expected to say and do or not say and not do.
- If you are working with the older men, ask them to describe what an older man is expected to say and do or not say and not do.

4. After a few minutes of small-group discussion, ask the participants to re-form a large circle and share with the whole group their ideas on the perfect member of their peer group.

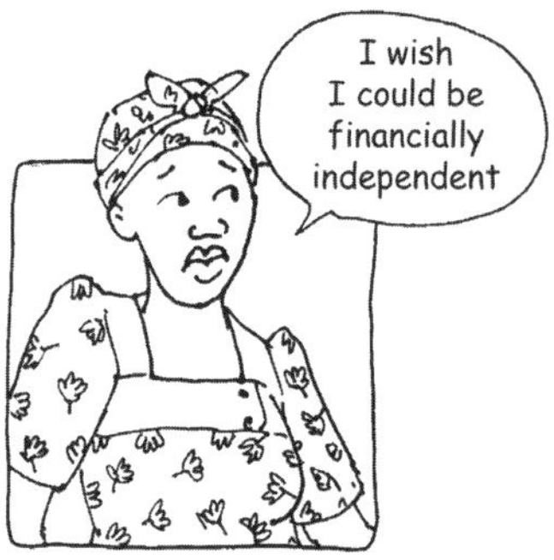
I wish I could be financially independent

5. Next, ask the participants to re-form into the same groups of three or four and discuss how easy they find it actually to live up to the expectations which their society has of them. Encourage the participants to go on to consider what a member of their peer group is most likely to be like.

6. After a few more minutes, ask the groups to re-form a large circle and share with the whole group what their experiences are like in real life.

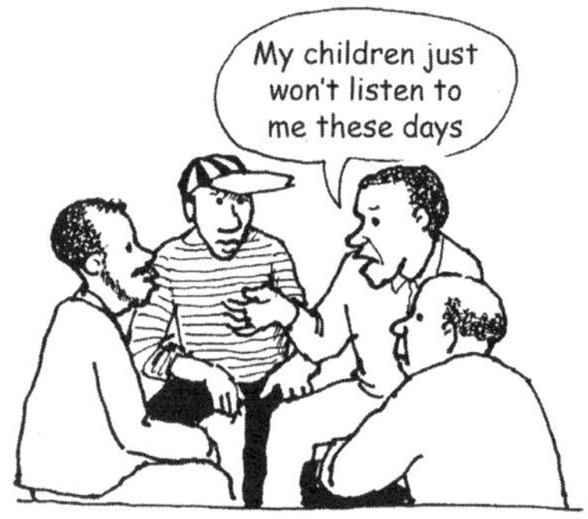
My children just won't listen to me these days

Feedback and discussion

The idea of this exercise is to help people to appreciate that we all have ideal images of how we are supposed to behave and that there is always a gap between our images and reality. We all find our images hard to live up to at times. It can often be reassuring to realise this and to appreciate that we all feel like this.

Sometimes ideal images can actually be **personal destroyers**. For instance, if people believe that 'a woman's place is in the home', this can be used as an excuse to take girls out of school early. Similarly the belief that 'real men drink ten bottles of beer a night' can result in a man drinking far more than he feels happy with, or than is actually good for him. Encourage participants to think about this and to make their own comments about the way some of the examples they have already mentioned can be personal destroyers for them. Finally, ask how would they rather be viewed?

Please emphasise to your group that this is not supposed to be an exercise which reminds them how they should behave! Instead, it is supposed to help us recognise how difficult and limiting some of the labels which our societies put on us are for us to live up to. If your group finds it a bit hard to think of examples to begin with, here are some suggestions which you might make to help them start to express their own ideas. **Do not impose** these ideas on your group: they need to come up with their own descriptions of their lives. But you could say that, in other countries, people have described differences between their ideal and their real lives in this way, before asking participants how it it here, for them.

OLDER MEN – SOME EXAMPLES

IMAGE: leaders and decision-makers with many children, grandchildren, authority, power, money, etc.
REALITY: young don't listen to us, not much authority, too many bills to pay, etc.

YOUNGER MEN

IMAGE: breadwinners, strong, macho, many kids, good income, one wife, etc.
REALITY: many demands on income, unemployment, too many mouths to feed, several girlfriends, etc.

OLDER WOMEN

IMAGE: honoured, looked after by children, respected by all, less work, etc.
REALITY: too much work, grandchildren to look after, no access to cash, etc.

YOUNGER WOMEN

IMAGE: polite, submissive, undemanding, hard-working, obeying father or husband, many kids, etc.

REALITY: too many kids, no money to spend, no personal freedom, etc.

Again, talk **only** about the experiences of the peer group you are working with: e.g. if you are working with younger women, talk **only** about what it is like to be a younger woman in their community!

EXERCISE B.4: IMAGES OF SEX

AIM: To help people to realise that it is no wonder that we have differences between images and realities of sex too.

DESCRIPTION: The peer group will explore different ideas and needs which they have about sex, through drawing them on cards which they will discuss and sort.

MATERIALS NEEDED: Cards, strongly coloured crayons, flip-chart paper, felt-tip marker pens, sticky tape, scissors.

DIRECTIONS

1. Start off by explaining that we have seen how there is a gap between ideal images of ourselves and reality. We are now going to move on to talk about our images of sex in our lives. Explain how sex is something relevant to all of us. As adults we have seen our bodies changing as we grow and, for almost all of us, part of becoming an adult is the expectation that we will have children. Most of us often find sex enjoyable, fun, and rewarding, and almost none of us would have been born if it wasn't for sex! But at the same time, almost all of us at some time in our lives have questions or difficulties related to sex. We may find these questions painful or embarrassing, but we would like some help with them. And help is often very hard to find. This exercise is a way of helping us to share with one another our own understanding of the good things and the difficult things about sex in our own lives. Because we often find it very difficult to talk about sex and our sexual health, we are going to draw about it instead.

If you are doing this with people who are not yet sexually active, you could ask them instead to draw the hopes and fears which they have about sex.

2. Ask participants to divide into groups of three or four. Give each group at least ten index cards and a small pack of crayons. Explain that you would like them to draw one aspect of sex, or something which they feel is connected in some way to sex, on each card and that they can use as many cards as they would like. Explain they can be good or bad, funny, or happy or sad, and the drawings do not have to be skilful – as long as the small group understands the meaning of what has been drawn, that

is good enough. (In the notes later in this exercise, you will find some suggestions of issues that may be of relevance to the peer group with whom you are working.)

> *In Buwenda, by drawing on the cards, the older women's group found themselves able to discuss issues with one another without a sense of personal embarrassment. They gave one another advice on some of the queries and concerns they had. For instance, one woman gave another advice on how to help her husband who took a long time to have an orgasm. Others shared their frustrations about their husbands finishing before the women had had an orgasm. Meanwhile, a common difficulty for the men was that they would like sex to be more exciting.*
>
> *The facilitators said that they felt this kind of discussion in a workshop setting could be very helpful to participants. Normally, if one woman were to behave differently from usual when having sex with her partner, he would accuse her of having had sex with another man and beat her. But since participants in all four peer groups knew this kind of discussion was going on, there would be a general understanding that new ways of behaving had come from suggestions shared in the workshop, rather than through other sexual liaisons.*
>
> *It was agreed by all facilitators that improved sexual relations between partners could only be a good thing for everyone. In particular, they said that men – and women – would be less likely to seek other sexual partners if they felt sexually satisfied in their existing relationships.*

3. Give each small group up to ten minutes, or until they run out of ideas, to draw all the cards they like.

4. While the small groups are busy, lay four pieces of flip-chart paper, long end to long end, on the ground across your circle of participants, anchoring them at the corners with stones, if necessary. Stick the four pieces together with sticky tape.

5. Then call everyone to come back into the big circle, bringing their cards with them. Ask the participants to choose one end of the four sheets as the good end and the other end of the four sheets as the bad end.

6. Once all have agreed on which end is good and which end is bad, ask them to sort through the cards they have drawn and place them nearer to the good end of the four sheets or the bad end, depending on how they feel about them. If they feel that topics on certain cards are similar or are in some way connected, participants should be encouraged to place these cards close to one another.

7. Once all the cards have been placed somewhere on the ground, all participants should move along the four sheets together, starting at the good end. Each card should be viewed by the entire group. The person who drew the card should describe what they have drawn, so that everyone understands what the picture means. Participants should be encouraged to discuss the subject of each card, so that you and they together have a chance to share and learn about the issues raised.

8. Explain that you would like to keep a record of their concerns on the flip charts, if that is OK with them. Ask for two volunteers to help you do this quickly.

- First, ask the volunteers to draw round each card with a marker pen, without removing the cards from the paper, so that the position of each card is recorded.
- Then remove the cards one at a time from the flip chart and, as you remove each card, write a number on the back of it. Write the same number inside the outline of the card on the flip

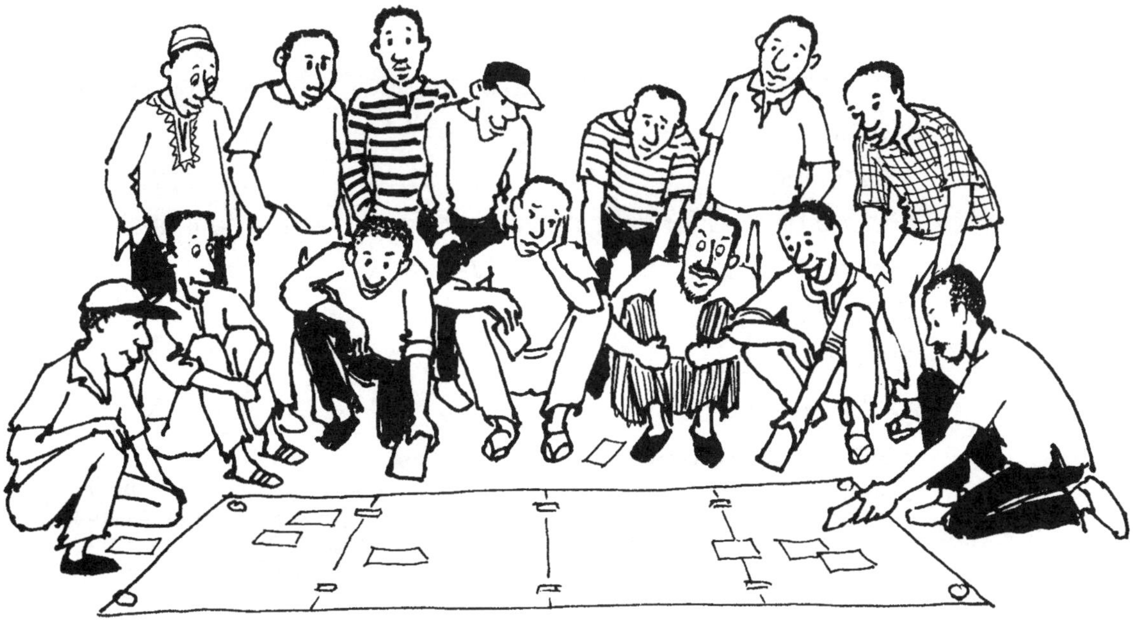

chart. You will then end up with the pile of cards beside you and the four flip charts still lying on the ground, covered with drawings of card outlines, each with a different number inside it.

- Now roll up the flip charts and place them to one side, ready to concentrate on the cards.

Feedback and discussion

This can be a valuable opportunity for participants and you to learn from one another about what this peer group knows about sexual health. If people prefer not to talk about themselves, you can encourage them to talk instead about issues which they have heard about from others. In this way, people often manage to talk about themselves in a way which feels less personal.

Sexual health can be defined as being to do with sex that is pleasurable and free from infection, unplanned pregnancy, and abuse. Each peer group is likely to have its own particular issues which it would like to include in this definition.

People can share their worries with one other and you can learn about problems which people have which are not being addressed. For instance, even though an older man may not publicly show any concern about HIV or AIDS, he may harbour private worries that he fears to express. If we can help him during the workshop to recognise that other older men share similar concerns, we may be able to help him begin to discuss these fears and do something about them. This also gives you an opportunity to learn what priority – if any – participants give to HIV and AIDS compared with other sexual health matters.

> ☞ As with the previous exercise, you may need to make suggestions, talking about 'other people like you elsewhere who have problems such as …' before asking, 'Do you have similar problems here?' to encourage people to start to draw. Here is a list of possible worries for different peer groups. Again **remember not to impose** these ideas on your group: they are intended just as a guide for you to start up the exercise, if needed!

OLDER WOMEN:

Feeling beautiful and attractive
Choice between having children and reduction of risk of contracting STIs
No say in sex
Having fun
Getting blamed for bringing HIV into family when she falls sick first
Getting blamed when child is HIV-positive
Getting beaten by husband
Unwanted sex
Children being hit
Psychological abuse
No orgasm
Being thrown out of home
Expressing love and affection
No financial independence
Cost of condoms
Lack of experience of condoms
Enjoying sexual foreplay
No support when sick
Fear for children's future
Chronic, untreated STIs
Repeated childbirth and too often
Enjoying being massaged
Heavy physical work load
Feeling sexy
Rape
War zone – absent men and physical danger
Commercial sex
Unwanted sex in exchange for money, goods, or favours
Levirate (when a woman is expected to marry her dead husband's brother)
No legal rights of inheritance (or rights not respected by others)
Burden of responsibility for care and support of others
Economic burdens – household, healthcare, school fees
Sex with father of new husband
Being a co-wife
Enjoying orgasm
Enjoying power of sexuality, etc.

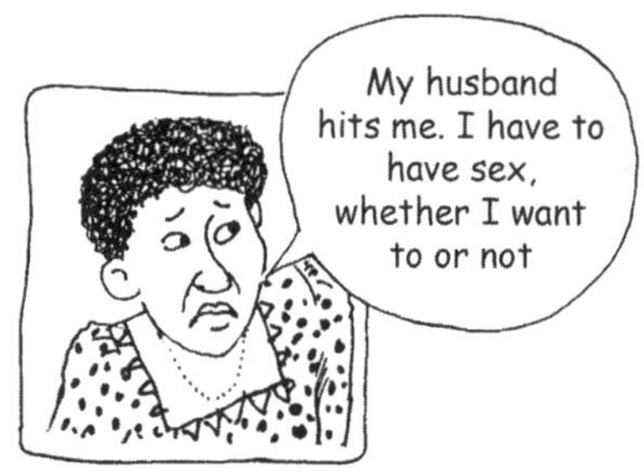
My husband hits me. I have to have sex, whether I want to or not

OLDER MEN: Peer pressure
- authoritarian role
- drinking

- multiple partners
- lack of condom use
- many children

Enjoying power of sexuality
Enjoying being massaged
Where to buy condoms
How to use condoms
Fear of impotence
Feeling sexy
Enjoying sex
Lack of self-confidence in using condoms
Gonorrhoea, syphilis – how to treat, avoid etc.
Personal dilemma of how to mention condom to wife or girlfriend
Expressing love and affection
Enjoying foreplay
Having fun, etc.

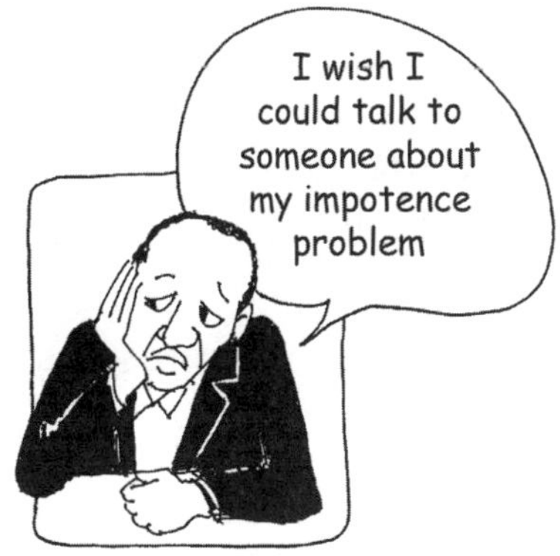
I wish I could talk to someone about my impotence problem

YOUNG MEN: Having fun
Peer pressure

- multiple sex partners
- macho, bravado image
- authoritarian role
- discos, bars
- lack of socially acceptable alternatives
- virility

Enjoying foreplay
Lack of work
Lack of optimism for future prospects
Private dilemmas

- wanting children
- cost of condoms
- lack of self-confidence in using condoms
- how to mention condom to wife or girlfriend

Enjoying orgasm
Lack of education
Migrant labour
Feeling sexy
Circumcision
Away at war
STIs – how to get rid of them, avoid them
Where to get and how to use condoms

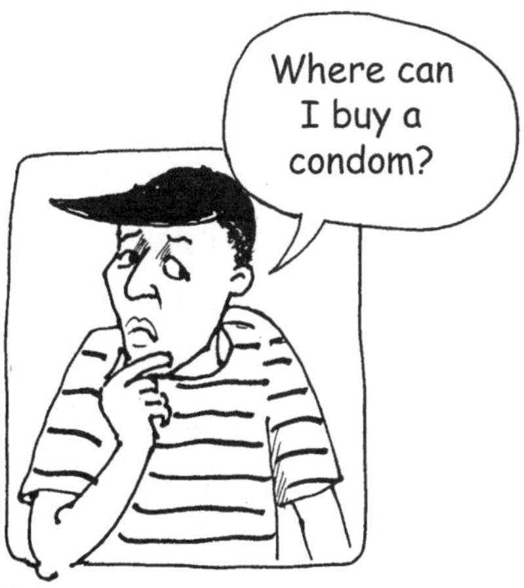
Where can I buy a condom?

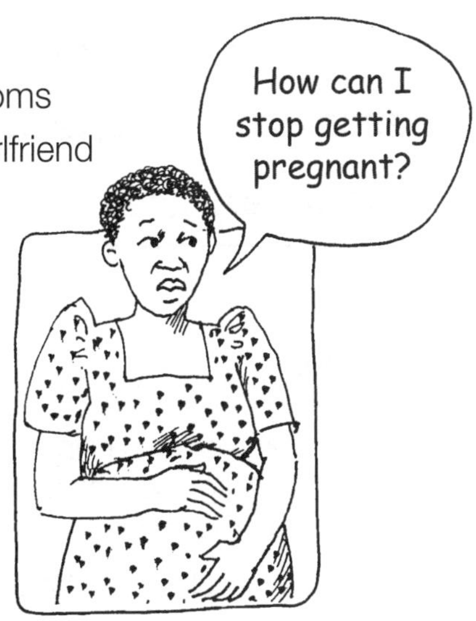
How can I stop getting pregnant?

Expressing love and affection
Enjoying power of sexuality, etc.

YOUNG WOMEN:

Enjoying power of sexuality
Feeling beautiful and attractive
Pressure from parents to have rich boyfriend
Idea that motherhood means being grown up
Peer pressure
- clothes, etc.
- money
- having rich boyfriend

Having fun
Fear of condom getting stuck or worse
Fear of infertility from condom use
Cost of condoms
Fear of infertility if sex delayed
Lack of education
Lack of work with secure income
Lack of independence – submissive role
Feeling sexy
Sex work
Transactional sex
Rape
How to avoid or cope with teenage pregnancy
Expressing love and affection, etc.

EXERCISE B.5: PRIORITISING PROBLEMS

AIM: To enable participants to prioritise their own concerns about sex and related issues.

DESCRIPTION: Participants are asked to sort cards according to their perceived urgency.

MATERIALS NEEDED: The cards drawn above, chalk, notebook and pen for you.

DIRECTIONS

1. Explain that it is often helpful for people to think about which problems or concerns they find most pressing and which less so. Suggest that the participants could now divide up the problem cards into different categories, such as:

- issues they would like to be dealt with NOW

- issues they would like to be dealt with SOON
- issues they would like to be dealt with LATER

2. Suggest that the participants form the cards into four different parallel lines on the ground in the middle, one for each category above and one for all the cards which present good aspects of sex. They should decide for themselves which line is which. Lines could be marked out with a stick if the ground is soft, or with chalk if it is hard.

3. Once everyone has agreed which line represents which category, hand out the cards to groups of participants, so that everyone becomes involved in distributing them between the four piles. Listen to the discussions which they have about the distribution, especially any disputes over which line to place a card in. This will help you to understand a lot about people's perceptions and priorities.

In Buwenda, the women spoke of various gynaecological problems, including several related to untreated STIs. As a result, arrangements were made with the Ministry of Health in the district capital for extra training of local health staff in diagnosis and treatment of STIs. This will greatly improve the service available to women – and men – in the area and address their immediate problems, as well as being likely to help reduce the rates of HIV transmission in the area.

4. Record in a notebook the numbers of the cards placed in each line, for future reference.

5. Explain that you have now learnt a lot together about their needs and concerns – as well as what they enjoy about sex! Suggest that, if they wanted to, they could together present their concerns about their health problems to local development agency staff, or hospital and health-clinic staff, or teachers, or whoever is concerned in the area. This information could help these staff to provide a better service to community members. Suggest that there could perhaps also be issues which they might like to discuss at a wider community meeting. Perhaps participants could together identify someone with whom they could take up their immediate concerns, and decide who should go to speak with this person.

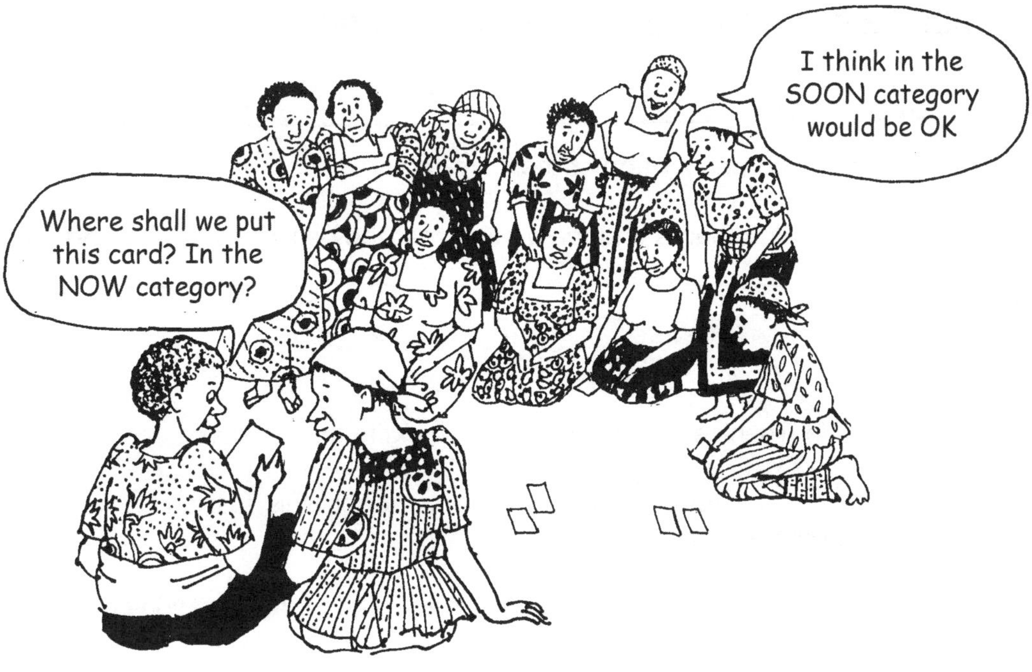
Where shall we put this card? In the NOW category?
I think in the SOON category would be OK

Some communities may want you to liaise on their behalf with local health staff. But it is not a good idea to offer to do this unless you really think they would like you to.

6. Finally, say that it is now time to close this session, but that at your next meeting you will be going on to explore what love means in our lives.

Feedback and discussion

There will really be discussion and feedback throughout this exercise. It is likely that some of the things which the participants discuss will never have been aired openly before. Now is an ideal time for you to learn, by listening to their discussions as they sort the cards. If there are any disputes about where to place a card which cannot be resolved, agree to let the card's number be recorded in both (or more!) columns to reflect the disagreement. Participants are also likely to find this exercise a very valuable way of sharing experiences amongst themselves.

Don't forget to take a note of the card numbers and which lines they have been placed in at the end of this exercise. This information is very important and you should use it when planning the next sessions.

- If HIV has not been placed as a priority, it is important to recognise this and also for you to think about what can be done to help people address the concerns which they **have** prioritised. Once **their** prioritised concerns have begun to be addressed – by you or by other relevant bodies – their readiness to respond to **your** HIV concerns is likely to increase. Often the other sexual health concerns they have will have an impact on HIV anyway.
- If concerns about HIV **have** been prioritised, this is encouraging because it may make the following sessions easier to run. On the other hand, it is important still to note what else people have prioritised. For instance, just because people are concerned about HIV does not mean that their worries about infertility, or teenage pregnancy, or impotence are less valid!

EXERCISE B.6: CLOSING CIRCLE AND LOCAL SONG

AIM: To finish the session on a happy note.

DESCRIPTION: The participants choose a song that they all know to sing together.

DIRECTIONS

1. Sit together in a circle. Thank everyone again for coming to this session.

2. Ask each person to say one thing which they have learnt from this session and one thing they are looking forward to before the next session.

3. Arrange a mutually suitable time and place for the next session. Ask everyone to remind one another about it.

4. Encourage participants to talk in general about the kinds of issues they have been discussing in these sessions with their friends and neighbours, if they like, but not to share any confidential information from the peer group with others.

5. Remind everyone of their role as guardian angel.

6. Remember to ask for three new volunteers to stay behind for ten minutes afterwards for a quick review of this session. (See Annex 4 for details).

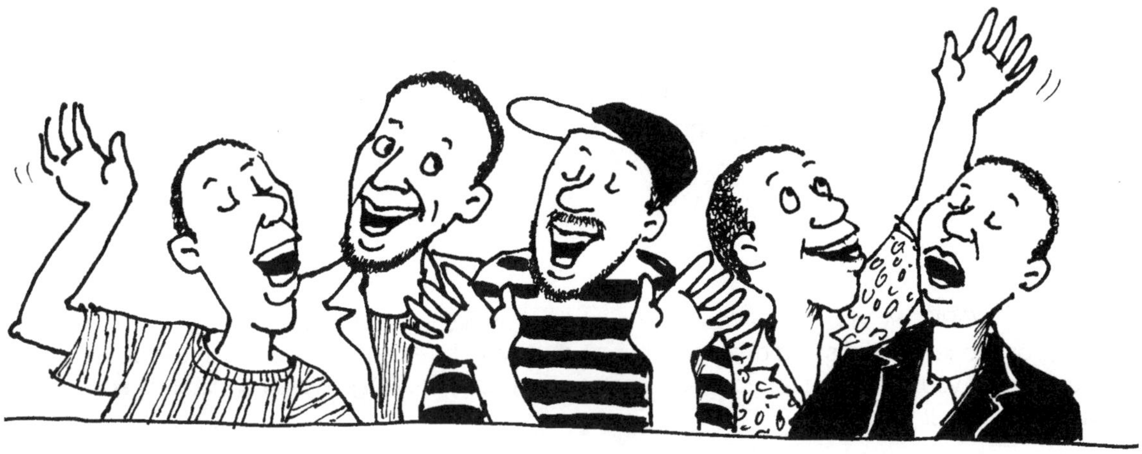

7. Ask all participants to think of a happy song which they all know that they would like to sing together now, to finish off the session.

8. Try to join in with it, especially if it includes dancing!

FACILITATORS' TEAM FEEDBACK

After the end of Session B, meet again with your co-facilitators to compare notes on how your sessions went and the information which you learnt from them. Your co-facilitators could have found useful information that could help you to structure your next session more effectively. Remember, however, not to share individual confidentialities between groups. This is the easiest way to ruin the trust that you have begun to build and to wreck the whole workshop!

At this stage, you also need to **think very carefully about how you run the rest of the workshop**. If people have put high priority on HIV and AIDS, then the workshop can be run as they are presented here. However, if participants are more concerned about STIs or teenage pregnancy, for instance, you may want to modify the following sessions to take more account of these local concerns.

Alternatively, you may feel the need to link their concerns with HIV and help them to reach a realisation that all these issues are inter-connected. In order to do this, you may want to spend some more time at this stage in addressing participants' own perceived needs and desires before moving on to further sessions in this manual.

Whichever route you choose, there is no doubt that the exercises on assessment of vulnerability, better communication and mutual planning and support are of general benefit to everyone, whatever their priorities.

NOW IS THE TIME TO PLAN YOUR WORKSHOP IN THE WAY WHICH BEST SUITS YOUR OWN COMMUNITY![1] GOOD LUCK!

NB: At this stage, you also need to be aware that some people may wish to come and ask your advice about their own situation. You need to either refer them to someone who can give them the right help, in confidence, or decide with your co-facilitators and others what role – if any – you want to play in personal counselling. On the whole, as a facilitator it is better not to become involved in giving personal advice to individual participants. This is because your relationship with the person and with the rest of the group will change as soon as you become drawn into individual participants' personal issues. Also, the role of counsellor is a skilled one. Trained counsellors, for instance, do **not**, in general, give advice. Instead they enable their clients to decide what to do for themselves, through asking them relevant questions and giving them appropriate information. This is very hard to do successfully unless you have been trained properly. But you need to make the best decision for yourselves and your participants, depending on your own community and situation.

ENDNOTE

1. Thanks to ACORD, we also have adaptation guidelines available which highlight which are the 'foundation stone' sessions and exercises that must stay in the adaption, and which are optional exercises, that you can adapt for your own community (ACORD 2007). Please contact us so we can advise you on this!

REFERENCE

ACORD (2007) *Implementing Stepping Stones* ACORD, London. http://www.steppingstonesfeedback.org/resources/5/SS_ACORD_Implementing_Stepping_Stones_2007.pdf

YOUR NOTES …

SESSION C WHAT IS LOVE?

PURPOSE

To explore what we look for and expect to give in love.

CONTENTS	**TIME NEEDED**
Introduction	
C.1	Fruit Salad
C.2	What is Love?
C.3	**DVD Clip 2**: 'What is Love?'
C.4	Sitting on Knees
C.5	Closing Circle

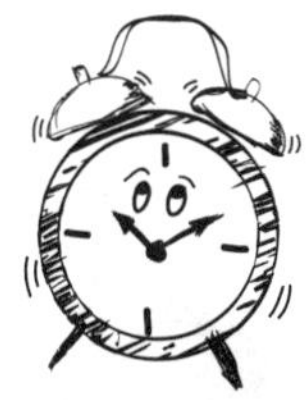

3–4 hours

MATERIALS NEEDED: DVD, laptop with DVD player, projector, mobile screen.

PARTICIPANTS: Four separate peer groups.

SPECIAL INFORMATION

Don't forget to read 'Before You Begin ...!' before using this section of the manual.

INTRODUCTION

1. Sit in a circle with the group, preferably on the ground. Everyone should be at the same level, including yourself.

2. Welcome everyone back to the new session. Thank everyone for coming. Enquire about late-comers or non-attenders.

3. Ask each participant to recount quickly something good which has happened to them since the last session.

4. Review the last session. Ask participants to remind us what we learnt about then – images and reality, our views on sex, prioritising our own concerns ... Remind them if they have forgotten.

5. Explain that we are going on to discuss other things in this session, but will start with a game.

EXERCISE C.1: FRUIT SALAD

AIM: Energiser.

DESCRIPTION: Person in middle of sitting circle calls out and others have to change place.

DIRECTIONS

1. Stand in the middle of the sitting circle. Everyone but you needs to have an established place to sit. For instance, if participants are sitting on mats, agree how many should be sharing each mat before the game begins.

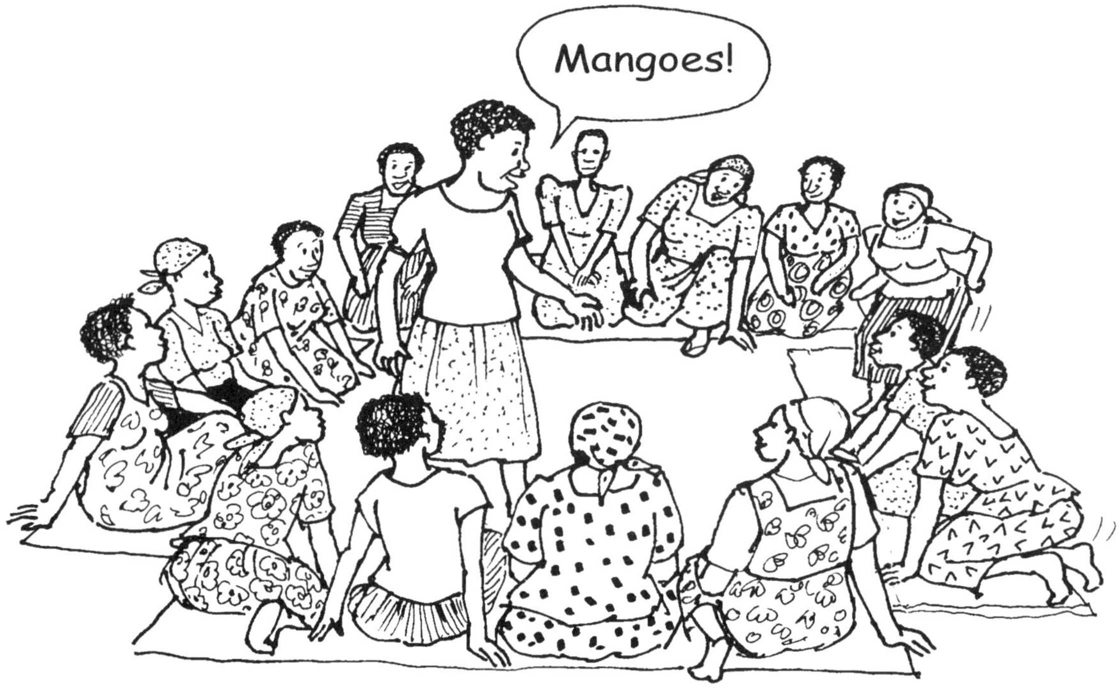

2. Ask the participants to name three different fruits. Then go round the circle, giving each participant in turn one of these names. For instance, the first person could be a mango, the next a banana, the third an orange. The fourth would then be another mango. Go round the whole circle until everyone, including yourself, has one of the three fruit names.

3. Next explain that you are going to call out one of the fruit names. Everyone with that name has to jump up and find somewhere else to sit. You are also going to find a place to sit. The person who doesn't find a new place will be left in the middle and will have to call out the next fruit.

4. Add that if someone calls out 'fruit salad!', then everyone has to jump up and find another place to sit!

> This game is good at making people laugh and waking them up. To end the game, finish up in the middle again yourself, by being slow to move. Then say it is time to move on to the next exercise.

EXERCISE C.2: WHAT IS LOVE?

AIM: To explore what we mean by 'love'.

DESCRIPTION: Pair work, followed by group discussion

DIRECTIONS

1. Ask participants whether they can give you a word or words which mean 'love'. Is everyone agreed upon this word or expression? Is this a word or an expression which applies to the love someone has for their partner (i.e. their husband, wife, or recognised partner) alone, or can it also be used to describe feelings between boyfriends and girlfriends, or between lovers who are not publicly recognised as a couple, or between brothers and sisters? If other words or expressions are used to describe **those** relationships, ask everyone to agree on those also.

2. Once everyone has agreed upon one or two words or expressions meaning love between partners (and, if necessary, other words meaning love between boyfriends and girlfriends, lovers, or sisters and brothers), ask everyone to divide into pairs, preferably with someone whom they have not worked with before.

3. **Love between friends or family members with no sex involved**. Ask each pair to take it in turns to describe to each other three qualities which they show to a close brother or sister or friend whom they particularly love; and then three qualities which they expect from the same brother or sister who loves them. If someone has no brother or sister, perhaps they could think of a cousin or a close friend instead.

4. Call everyone back to the full circle. Ask participants to share their thoughts, firstly on qualities they show to this person and then on qualities they expect from him or her. If there is general agreement, move on. If not, encourage participants to discuss the different views further in the whole group. Finally, do participants believe that the person they were thinking of would agree with the qualities they have chosen? In what ways might their views differ?

5. **Love between partners who have a publicly recognised relationship and where they have sex**. Next, ask each pair to take it in turns to describe to each other three qualities which they would show to a partner (i.e. a husband or wife or publicly recognised partner) whom they love, and then three qualities which they expect from a partner who loves them. If the participants are not currently in a relationship, they can describe an imaginary relationship instead. Discourage participants from talking about lovers whose relationship is not publicly recognised. Qualities of love between lovers will be discussed later. (Splitting the discussion is not supposed to suggest that we are making a moral statement about the rights or wrongs of one or other! Instead, the point is to try to help people explore how public recognition affects a sexual relationship in their own culture.)

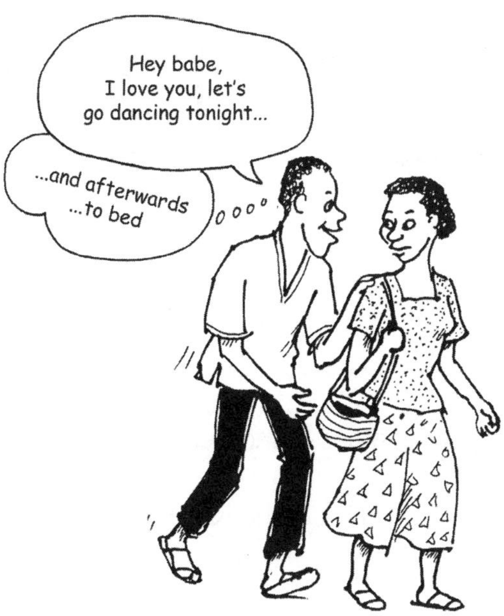
Hey babe,
I love you, let's
go dancing tonight...
...and afterwards
...to bed

6. Call everyone back to the full circle. Ask them to share their thoughts again, firstly on qualities which they would show to a partner (i.e. a husband or wife) whom they love, and then on qualities which they expect from a partner who loves them. Again, if there is not agreement, encourage participants to discuss the different views further in the big group. Do participants believe that the qualities they have chosen would be agreed by their wife or husband? In what ways might their views differ?

7. Finally, if there are some clear differences in the qualities of love described between partners and those described for sisters and brothers or friends, point these out to participants.
Ask them to define these differences more clearly. Encourage them to try to explain why these differences exist.

- What differences, for instance, do the existence of sex, or of formal contracts, or public recognition of a liaison have on the qualities of the relationships?
- Does love = sex, or does love = marriage? Do they automatically go together?
- If love does not equal marriage, what are the minimum levels of respect which they think each member of the couple should show each other?

> This exercise is designed to prepare participants for the DVD clip by getting them to share some of their own ideas. Encourage participants to focus on their own perspectives first and on their partner's perspective only when asked to. It is likely that issues such as trust, sharing, responsibility, sex, money, and so on will all be mentioned. Love is a complicated thing! **NB:** If polygamous marriage is common in your area, encourage participants to talk about the qualities of this kind of relationship also.

EXERCISE C.3: DVD CLIP 2: 'WHAT IS LOVE?'

AIM: To explore further what we mean by 'love'.

DESCRIPTION: Watching DVD, followed by pair work and group discussion.

MATERIALS NEEDED: DVD, laptop with DVD player, projector, mobile screen.

DIRECTIONS

1. Explain to participants that we are now going to watch a DVD clip about two married couples. Ask them to stand up, have a good stretch, and move round to a new position so that they can all see the DVD screen.

2. Say that, while they are watching the clip, you would like them to think about the relationships of these two couples in the light of the qualities which they have just been describing. Explain that they will have a chance to discuss what they think about the couples' relationships after watching the DVD together.

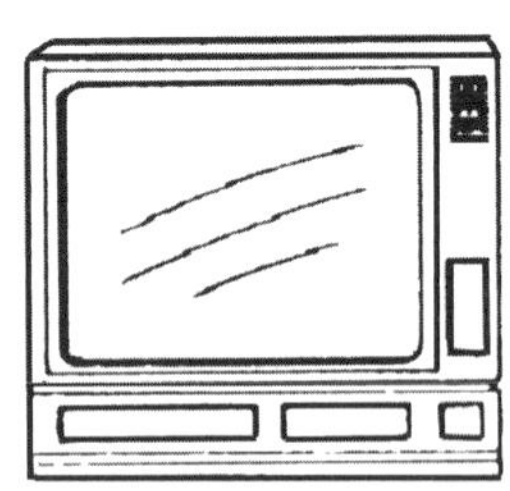

Make sure that everyone can see and hear the DVD clearly.

3. Turn on the DVD at the point where it says '2. What is Love?'.

4. Turn off the DVD at the point where the screen goes black.[1]

5. Ask participants to form pairs again and discuss the following points:

- What did they think were the better and more challenging qualities of the Senyondos' relationship?
- What did they think were the better and more challenging qualities of the Kaumas' relationship?
- What advice, if any, would they like to give to whom?

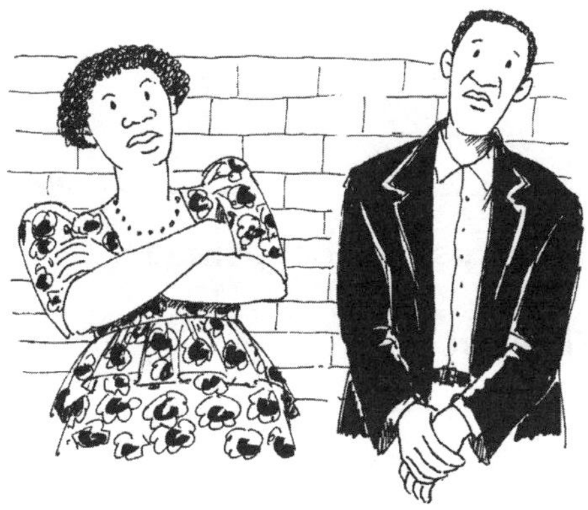

6. Bring the pairs back to the full circle. Ask for feedback on each of the three questions. If there are differences, encourage the group to explore them.

7. Next ask participants to form new pairs. Ask the pairs to talk about the difference between qualities of love between people in a married relationship and lovers (i.e. people who are not married to each other). Do the people involved give and expect the same qualities in the relationship as would a married couple, or different ones? In what ways would the relationships be different?

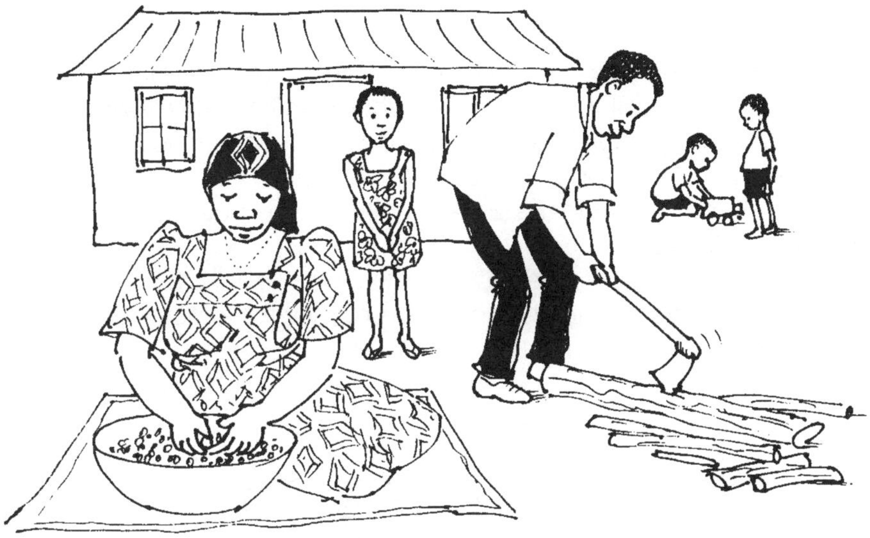

8. Ask participants to form a large group again. Encourage them to tell the whole group what they have discussed. If there is general agreement, draw out the main points. If there are different opinions, explore these further.

9. Finally, ask participants whether the DVD has in any way altered or strengthened the views they held before on the qualities which they look for in their own relationships.

It may help participants to understand that it is normal in this part of Uganda for women and children to eat on the floor while their husbands sit at table. It is also expected that women and children kneel in front of their husbands, other men, or older people. However, it is very unusual for a man to work together with a woman and help her with her tasks. Even in poor families it is the children who normally do the wood-chopping and digging work – not the husband. Therefore Mr Kauma's actions are not because of poverty but because of his respect for his wife.

Try to ensure that everyone has a chance to air their views in their discussions, but do not encourage an argument to develop! This is a chance for people to respect and listen to one another, without having to agree with everything which is said by others. There may well be some people who are feeling upset by these exercises. You need to be sensitive to their needs. The next exercise is designed to give them some support from the group.

EXERCISE C.4: SITTING ON KNEES

AIM: Fun exercise to bring group together and encourage trust and cooperation.

DESCRIPTION: Everyone sits on one another's knees in a circle.

DIRECTIONS

1. Explain that you are all going to stand closely in a circle, yourself included, then everyone is to turn to their right, so that each person is facing the back of someone else.

2. Ask everyone to put their hands on the shoulders of the person in front of them. Explain that you are going to call out '1,2,3, SIT!' and that they should call out slowly with you. On the word 'sit', everyone should carefully sit down on the lap of the person behind them, still holding on to the shoulders of the person in front. This really works, but takes care! If your group is really brave, you can try to shuffle around in the circle together in this position! This is a fun exercise and gives everyone a good feeling

3. Afterwards, ask participants how it felt to do this. Did they think they were going to be able to? How does the exercise relate to real-life experiences?

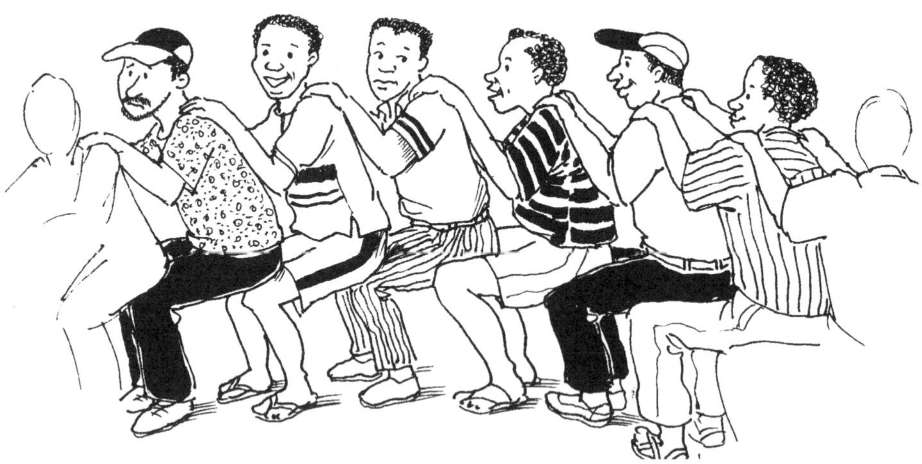

If your participants are too elderly to do this, perhaps you could substitute another, less active, exercise which also illustrates trust and cooperation. For instance 'Cross the Circle'. This is also a fun exercise. Participants stand and form a big circle, facing inwards. Each participant identifies someone standing opposite her/him. When you say 'go', each participant must close his/her eyes, walk across the circle and stand in the place of the person opposite her/him. All participants do this at the same time and they mustn't peep! People get in a muddle but sort themselves out eventually. Afterwards, ask participants how it felt to do this with their eyes shut and how the exercise relates to real-life experiences.

EXERCISE C.5: CLOSING CIRCLE

1. Thank everyone again for coming. Ask each member of the group in turn to mention one thing that they have learnt today and one thing that they are looking forward to doing before the next meeting.

2. Ask if there are any more questions about today's session.

3. Encourage participants to talk in general about the kinds of issues they have been discussing in these sessions with their friends and neighbours, if they like, but not to share any confidential information from the peer group with others.

4. Remind everyone of their role as guardian angel.

5. Remember to ask three new volunteers to stay behind for ten minutes to review this session with you. (See Annex 4 for details.)

6. Remind everyone of the time and place for the next meeting and say you look forward to seeing them all again there.

FACILITATORS' TEAM FEEDBACK

After the end of Session C, meet again with your co-facilitators, to compare notes on how your sessions went and the information which you learnt from them. Your co-facilitators could have found useful information that could help you to structure your next session more effectively. Remember however not to share individual confidentialities between groups. This is the easiest way to ruin the trust that you have begun to build and to wreck the whole workshop!

ENDNOTE

1. Remember the synopsis of the optional film clips in Annex 3. Do not read out the synopsis to the participants; is just for your benefit. Participants may want to view the film clip again. If so, it is usually best for them to have some discussion about it first, then to have more discussion after the second viewing.

YOUR NOTES ...

SESSION D OUR PREJUDICES

PURPOSE

To challenge the judgements which we make about one another.

CONTENTS	**TIME NEEDED**
Introduction	
D.1	Pass the Picture
D.2	Taking Risks
D.3	Who's Labelling Whom?
D.4	In the Spotlight
D.5	Catch-up Time (optional)
D.6	Closing Circle

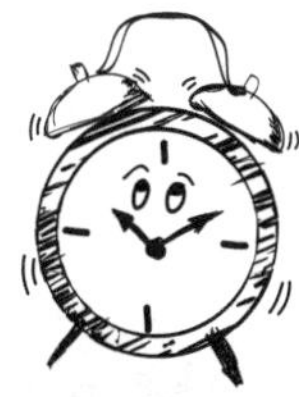

Maximum 3.5 hours

MATERIALS NEEDED: Roll of flip-chart paper, 4 felt-tip marker pens, 20 small index cards about 12 cm x 8 cm, about 40 strongly coloured crayons, sticky tape, scissors. (If cards are too expensive, you can use bits of paper, cut to size, but card is a bit stronger and therefore easier to use.)

PARTICIPANTS: Four separate peer groups.

SPECIAL INFORMATION:

Don't forget to read 'Before You Begin ...!' before using this section of the manual.

INTRODUCTION

1. Sit in a circle with the group, preferably on the ground. Everyone should be at the same level, including yourself.

2. Welcome everyone to the new session. Thank everyone for coming. Enquire about late-comers or non-attenders.

3. Ask each participant to recount quickly something good which has happened to them since the last session.

4. Review the last session. Ask participants to remind us what we learnt then - thoughts about love and what it means to us ... Remind them if they have forgotten.

5. Explain that we are going on to discuss other things in this session, but will start with a game.

EXERCISE D.1: PASS THE PICTURE

AIMS: Fun warm-up game to illustrate different people's perceptions of what they hear.

DESCRIPTION: A picture is drawn and described in words to others who try to reproduce it.

DIRECTIONS

1. Ask for five volunteers to leave the training area for a few minutes.

2. Bring out a piece of flip-chart paper, ask the remaining people to agree on a picture, and for two or three people to draw it. It could include, say, a person, a house, a tree, and some animals. Do not make it too complicated.

3. Then hide the picture and ask someone to call the five volunteers back to the group.

4. One volunteer is shown the picture. This volunteer must then describe the picture in words to the second volunteer, who in turn describes it to the third volunteer, and so on.

5. When the fifth volunteer has heard a description of the picture, s/he should be handed a new piece of flip-chart paper and some marker pens. S/he should then try to draw the picture as s/he understands it to look from the description. S/he should receive no help from the rest of the group.

6. When s/he has finished the picture, compare it with the original. There should be some interesting differences!

7. Thank the five volunteers for their willingness to help. Point out that it is often much harder than we suppose for us all to understand things in the same way.

EXERCISE D.2: TAKING RISKS

AIM: To help participants to reflect on their own behaviour with regard to risk-taking in life in general.

DESCRIPTION: Individual reflection, followed by paired listening.

DIRECTIONS

1. Explain to participants that when people have problems, or seem confused or scared, they like to have clear, simple answers to things. However, we have seen how our lives are full of

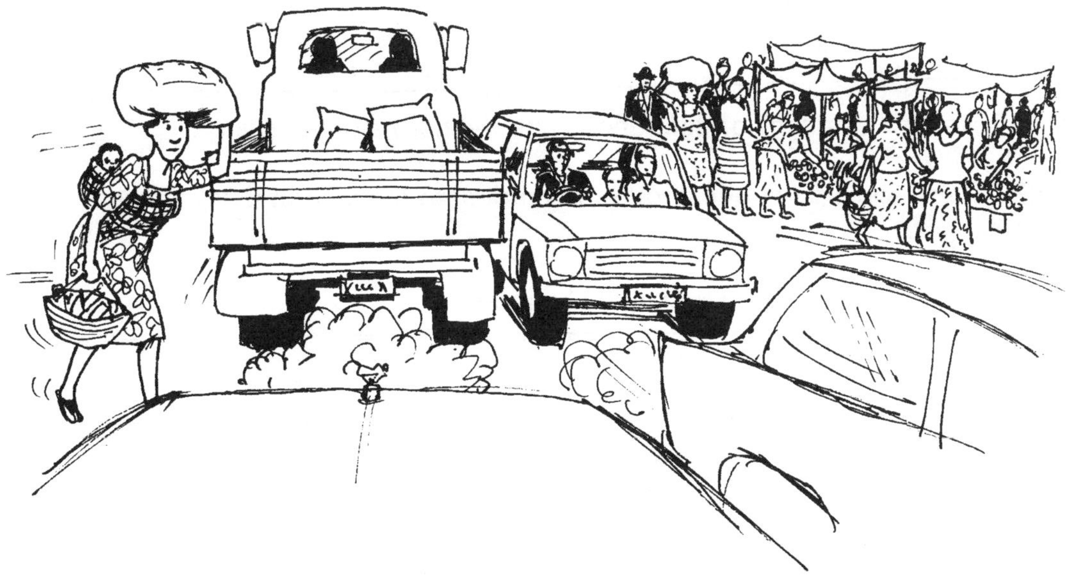

uncertainty and that easy solutions are rarely available. Explain that we are now going to do an exercise which will help us to think about how we handle risk in our own lives.

2. Ask participants to work alone first of all and consider the following for a few minutes:

Think back over your life and identify any occasion when you took a risk. It may have been something quite trivial or it may have had great significance.

- What factors influenced your decision to take a risk?
- What were your feelings at the time?
- What was the outcome of taking that risk? Was it positive or negative?
- Are you generally a risk-taker?
- How do you view risk-taking in others?
- What implication does this have for your attitudes towards HIV and AIDS?

3. After a few minutes, ask participants to choose a partner and share what they want of their situation. Encourage them to do this as a listening exercise – each person taking a turn to talk and a turn to listen. Give them a few minutes each.

4. Call everyone back into the full circle. Encourage them to draw out any general observations on risk-taking behaviour and any ways in which it may affect our responses to HIV and AIDS.

> ☞ We often tend to feel that it is OK to take risks: if they turn out well we might be praised for our courage! But we tend to blame others if they take risks and things go wrong. We are also much less harsh in judging ourselves, on the whole, than we are in judging others. Participants can be encouraged to recognise how judgemental we often are about the problems of others. It is also worth pointing out that we are all taking risks all the time: when we walk through a field (snakes or scorpions); when we cross a road in the town (traffic); when we give birth to a baby; when we cut something with a knife; and so on. Life without risk-taking would be very difficult!

EXERCISE D.3: WHO'S LABELLING WHOM?

AIMS: To develop awareness of differences and the harms of 'labelling'.

DESCRIPTION: People greet one another according to the kind of label that is being worn.

MATERIALS NEEDED: Cards, crayons, sticky tape.

The idea of this exercise is to help people to experience in some way the misery that people with HIV feel when faced with the prejudice of others. Just because someone has HIV does not mean that they suddenly become unhuman or evil. **Just as with lying or stealing, HIV can happen to anyone. Moreover many people acquire HIV without having any intention to, and without realising that they may be putting themselves at risk of HIV. So it is often not fair to say that what they have done is wrong! Yet people's attitudes to them can change radically once it is known that they are HIV-positive. Is this fair? This exercise seeks to explore this**.

DIRECTIONS

1. For this exercise, you need as many cards as there are people in the group, including one for yourself. Distribute the cards, so that each person has one. Pass round the crayons too. Identify the person sitting opposite you. Those on your left, as far round as that person, are to draw on their card a face representing a good quality that someone may have. You could give suggestions, such as a generous person, someone who has been kind and caring, someone who is a good listener, someone who is always cheerful, and helpful, and kind, and so on. **Remind people that all of us have these qualities in us.**

2. Meanwhile, everyone on your right, up to and including the person opposite you, is to draw a picture of someone who has a challenging quality. For instance, their picture could be of someone who has lied, stolen, been selfish, or done something else which is not respected.

- **Before they start, remind people that we have *all* also done something which we have later regretted.** We may have done it in the heat of the moment and then regretted it. Sometimes it can take longer for us to regret an action. Either way it does *not* mean we are a bad person – just that we have done something we realise later was not wise. *Does anyone want to share an example of this?*
- **Sometimes we have little or no control over what we do.** For instance we may be part of a group of friends who steal mangoes or bananas from someone else's tree, we may lie to protect a friend who has done something wrong and got into trouble, we might have done something because an older person has told us to and we felt we had to ... *not* doing something unwise or wrong is often hard! *Does anyone want to share an example of this?*
- **Say there is often a reason behind why we have done something we have later regretted and this programme will help us to think of other ways round this behaviour in future.** Often showing our concern helps the person to get through this problem, instead of showing any anger. *Does anyone want to share an example of when someone has shown them concern instead of anger?*

- **Explain that in this game by showing our concern to someone when they behave in a way they may later regret, we can support each other not to use this kind of behaviour in future.**

3. When everyone has drawn their card, ask each person to hold up their card in turn and show it to the rest of the group, explaining the image they have drawn.

4. Then ask everyone to pass their cards to you and shuffle them so that they are all mixed up.

5. Next, leaving the cards in a pile, ask everyone to stand up and to move round the circle, greeting ten or so others warmly, as they normally would.

6. Then, ask each person to come to you in turn. You should then take a card from the pile and stick it with sticky tape to the back of the first person, without letting him/her see what is drawn on it and then ask them to return to their seat. **Tell everyone not to tell one another what the picture on their back shows.**

7. Continue this with the rest of the cards, not letting them be seen by the others, until you have stuck one on everyone's back.

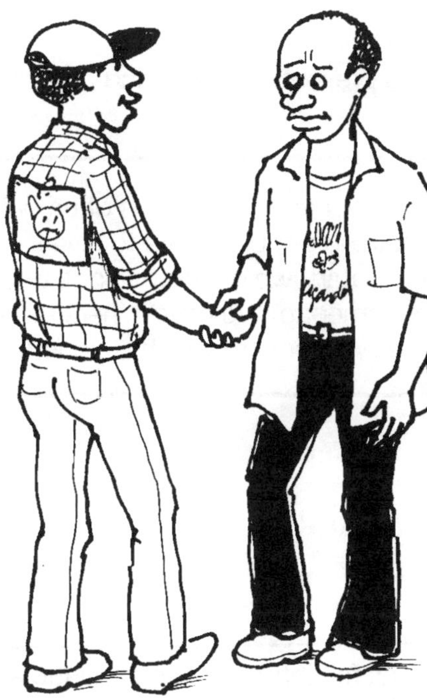

8. Ask someone else to stick the last card on your own back: try to leave a card showing a negative quality for yourself, if you can!

9. Ask participants to stand and move around again, greeting one another. This time, however, the style of their greeting should depend on their reaction to the label which they see on the back of the person they are greeting. So if, for instance, they are greeting someone with a 'stealing' picture on their back, they should use their face and movements to show concern for that person as they greet them. If they meet other people whom they feel less concerned about, they can greet them and smile at them freely. If they can't remember what the picture on the back of someone means, then they should treat that person with concern.

10. After everyone has greeted one another again, ask them to come and sit in a circle, leaving their labels on.

11. Then ask the group the following questions:

- How did you feel during the first meeting with your friends?
- How did you feel during the second meeting?
- Did **others** treat **you** differently? How?
- How did that make **you** feel?
- Was it easier or harder to show concern instead of anger?
- How can we support one another to show more concern for others in future?

12. Next, ask everyone to reach round to their labels and take them off, so that they can see how they have been labelled. Clear up any uncertainties that people may have about the meaning of their labels. **Remind everyone this is only a game and that we all have done things in our lives that we later regret. This programme is here to help us all support each other by showing concern, so that we can all feel supported to behave in ways we prefer in life in future.**

13. Then ask:

- What have we learnt from this exercise?
- How can we relate this lesson to HIV in our community?
- Why is this exercise so relevant to prevention of HIV and care for people with AIDS?

Remember to emphasise that acquiring HIV is often out of people's control and that it is *very rarely* something people intend to give to someone else. Just like the examples we thought of at the start, we often do things we later regret with a friend, as part of a group, or to protect someone. We need others around us to show *concern*, instead of anger, to help us find a way forward which is constructive.

EXERCISE D.4: IN THE SPOTLIGHT

AIMS: To illustrate how we have all felt left out or stigmatised at times for many reasons, how quick we can be to judge others without understanding things from their point of view, and how miserable this can make us feel if we are the ones being judged.

DESCRIPTION: Participants and the facilitator stand holding hands in a circle and follow the facilitator's instructions.

DIRECTIONS

1. Explain how we are going to look further into how it feels to be 'different'. Ask participants to join hands in a circle and not to talk during the exercise but just to do as you ask them. Then ask them to think back through their lives to when they were children, as well as more recent years. Ask participants to 'be stared at' if they have ever been laughed at, told off, felt left out because of something they have said or done, or for some felt different in some way from

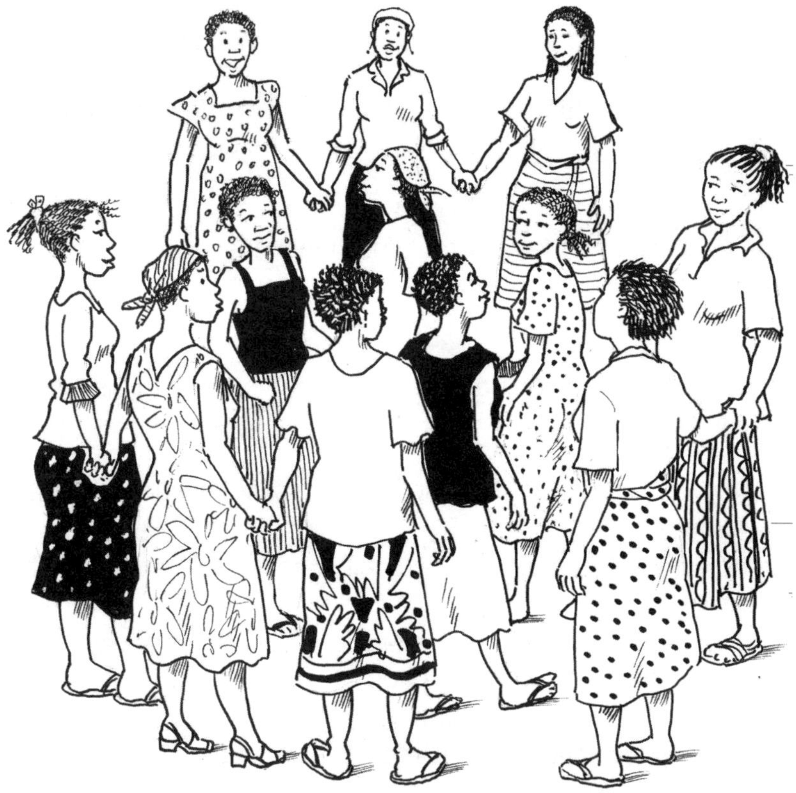

others around them. It is a good idea to start off with some examples which have happened to you. Here are some examples, but you can use your own:

'Be stared at if you have ever felt left out because of your eyesight.' Anyone to whom this has happened then needs to move into the centre of the circle of participants, and walk slowly around inside the circle, looking at all the others who are still holding hands, and making eye contact with each of them in turn. They should also make eye contact also with each of the others inside the circle. When they have walked around the complete circle, and made eye contact with everyone, they rejoin the circle, in their original place or a different one, and hold hands again.

'Be stared at if you have felt left out because you were too young.' Again, anyone to whom this has happened needs to move into the centre and walk around the circle slowly, making eye contact with each of those who haven't left the circle in turn, as well as each of those who have, before rejoining the circle and again holding hands with their neighbours.

Other examples that you might like to use:

BE STARED AT if you have ever felt left out for being too small, too tall, too fat, too thin or because of your skin colour; for being a girl, a boy, a woman, a man, too poor, too rich, too slow, too fast; for not being able to read, for being too educated, for being out of work …
BE STARED AT if you have ever been told off for telling a lie, telling the truth, stealing something, giving something away, hurting someone, helping someone, breaking something, hitting someone, gossiping about someone, eating too much …

2. Encourage participants to think up their own examples and to suggest these to the group themselves, after four or five of your suggestions.

3. After a few rounds, bring in some examples such as: if you have ever done something which you later wished you hadn't; if you have ever not done something which you later wished you had; if you have ever been told off for something you didn't do; if you have ever felt unfairly

treated for doing something which others were doing too; if you have ever felt unfairly punished; if you have ever felt guilty because someone else was punished instead of you.

4. By this time all the participants should have been stared at a few times. Try to make sure that everyone has joined the group at least three or four times before asking the group to sit down for a discussion.

5. Ask participants how it felt to remember the times when they felt singled out, put in the spotlight and stared at. Ask several participants to describe their own feelings about the exercise and what it has shown them.

Here are some of the points which you can encourage participants to discuss if they don't mention them themselves:

- Different people can feel 'stared at' for completely opposite reasons (e.g. being too tall or being too small).
- Participants can be surprised that others have felt stared at for something they hadn't realised was an issue.
- Some participants may feel stared at for something which others always thought was an asset (e.g. being tall, or pretty, or good at school).
- There may be participants in the group with disabilities such as poor eyesight or a limp, or someone who wants children and can't have any. Women can be stared at for wearing jeans or short dresses, and can be seen as 'bad women' for wearing these clothes. Language barriers, wealth, having something new or old, having something unique, being ignorant about something, holding a belief different from others: all of these can produce negative reactions in others. Participants may be more aware of their feelings – but then they may also not be. Ask participants how fair or unfair they think it is for people to be stared at or feel left out for any reason, and especially because of having a medical condition.
- Encourage participants to identify other forms of reaction – i.e. not just staring, but whispering about people, being pointed at, being excluded from a job, a school, a discussion, a club, a place of worship ... What else?
- Encourage participants to discuss how it feels to be stared at. Some of the issues mentioned may not feel too big, but others may feel very big to those participants who may feel upset at being treated unfairly by others. Help participants to realise that we often judge and condemn others unfairly, without perhaps realising how strong an effect our words or actions can have on them.
- Have participants ever 'stared' at someone negatively just to go along with the views of their friends when, in fact, they have perhaps felt this treatment to be unfair? How did they feel about that?

6. Ask participants what they think this exercise has taught them about themselves and about others around them.

7. Explain how, in other countries, people have realised that, if there are some people in a community who stare at others and judge or pick on them a lot for being different from themselves, this can often be because they have somehow been judged themselves when they were growing up: they are now treating others unfairly because they have felt unfairly treated themselves. Ask participants whether there may be similar issues in their community. Ask participants also whether it is fair to judge others for being different from yourself just because you have felt unfairly treated.

8. Finally, ask all the participants to stand up again, join hands in a circle once more. All of you are going to to ***smile*** together at each person in turn, and to use a word or two to ***praise*** her

or him for all his or her great qualities – whether tall or short, with or without glasses, fat, thin, whatever – encourage all the participants to celebrate diversity in all its forms. Spend just 15 seconds or so focusing on each person as you move round the circle, *smiling* all together at each person in turn. Point out that it is our diversity which makes us all so special and which singles us out in the world. It is something which we should be celebrating, not criticising all the time. Encourage everyone to feel positive about their uniqueness and feel good about being ***smiled*** at for a change!

> This exercise can raise strong emotions for some participants, either because they have felt stared at, or bullied, or because they recognise themselves doing this to others and feel either guilty or defensive about it – or both. Please be aware of this, especially if some participants become defensive, or go very quiet, or maybe even cry. If this happens, you could repeat the 'Hand in Hand' exercise from Session A and remind participants that we can all work to support one other in these exercises.

EXERCISE D.5: CATCH-UP TIME (optional)

AIM: Time for peer groups to catch up with sessions so far, if they have fallen behind other groups, or to review work which they have already covered.

DESCRIPTION: Continuation of exercises not yet completed, or free time for the peer group to structure as it would like.

DIRECTIONS

1. If you still have exercises to cover, please continue with them.

2. If you have kept up with the suggested schedule, your group may wish to spend some time discussing further some of the issues which have been raised in previous exercises. Do try to avoid pushing ahead onto later sessions, because participants need time to digest what they have already learnt. Alternatively, they may be ready to go home early for a change!

EXERCISE D.6: CLOSING CIRCLE

1. Thank everyone again for coming. Ask each member of the group in turn to mention one thing that they have learnt today and one thing that they are looking forward to doing before the next meeting.

2. Ask if there are any more questions about today's session.

3. Encourage participants to talk in general about the kinds of issues they have been discussing in these sessions with their friends and neighbours, if they like, but not to share any confidential information from the peer group with others.

4. Remind everyone of their role as guardian angel.

5. Ask for three new volunteers to stay behind for ten minutes, to do a quick review of this session. (See Annex 4 for details).

6. Remind everyone of the time and place for the next meeting and say you look forward to seeing them all again there.

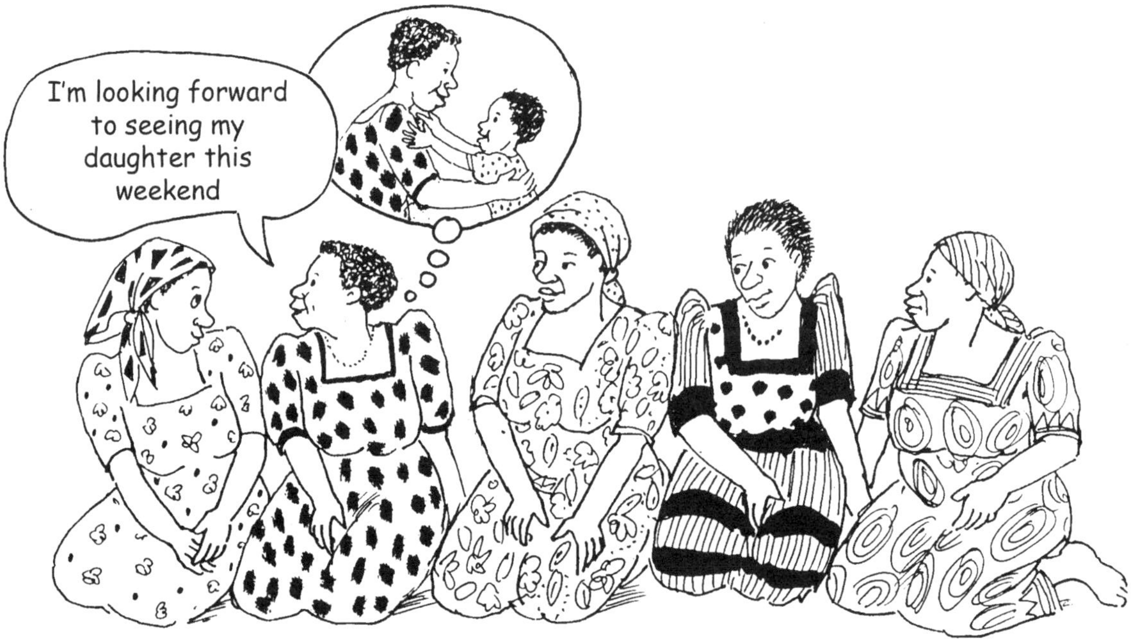

FACILITATORS' TEAM FEEDBACK

After the end of Session D, meet again with your co facilitators, to compare notes on how your sessions went and the information which you learnt from them. Your co-facilitators could have found useful information that could help you to structure your next session more effectively. Remember, however, not to share individual confidentialities between groups. This is the easiest way to ruin the trust that you have begun to build and to wreck the whole workshop! The next session is about HIV. Try not to start Session E with any peer group until all the groups have finished Session D.

YOUR NOTES ...

THEME 2 – HIV AND SAFER SEX

SESSION E HIV

PURPOSE

To explore our knowledge of HIV and safer sex.

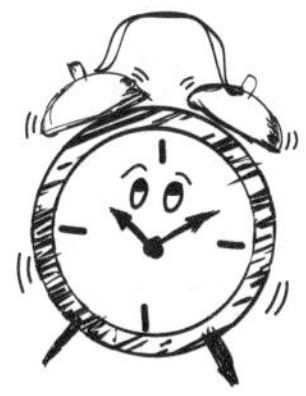

CONTENTS	**TIME NEEDED**
Introduction	
E.1	Muddling Messages
E.2	The Language of Sex
E.3	The TASO Game
E.4	Facts and Feelings about HIV (a long exercise)
E.5	Testing Issues
E.6	Prrr and Pukutu
E.7	Closing Circle

MATERIALS NEEDED: Small pieces of paper, flip-chart paper, strongly coloured crayons, chalk.

PARTICIPANTS: Four separate peer groups.

SPECIAL INFORMATION

- Don't forget to read 'Before You Begin ...!' before using this section of the manual.
- Try to find out the figures for HIV prevalence, as well as the percentage of orphaned children, in your area or country.
- You need to be fully familiar with the issues covered by the HIV quiz before the workshop begins.
- If there is a good local place where people can go for counselling, or for counselling and HIV testing, you should know its location, opening times, and any other relevant information.
- You may find Exercise E.4 needs more than one discussion. If so, agree with the other facilitators to arrange another meeting with your group before any group begins Session F.

INTRODUCTION

1. Sit in a circle with the group, preferably on the ground. Everyone should be at the same level, including yourself.

2. Welcome everyone to the new session. Thank everyone for coming. Enquire about late-comers or non-attenders.

3. Ask each participant to recount quickly something good which has happened to them since the last session.

4. Review the last session. Ask participants to remind us what we learnt then – about risk-taking and our prejudices ... Remind them if they have forgotten.

5. Explain that we are going on to discuss other things in this session, but will start with a game.

EXERCISE E.1: MUDDLING MESSAGES

AIMS: **Energiser. To make people laugh. To help us appreciate in a funny way how easy it is to misunderstand what someone has said.**

DESCRIPTION: **Participants whisper the same message around the circle, one to the next. Then the finished version is compared with the original.**

DIRECTIONS

1. Think of a phrase to whisper beforehand, such as 'many people round here like eating bananas' or 'the sun at this time of year is very hot'.

2. Whisper this quietly to your neighbour and ask her/him to whisper it quietly to the next person.

3. This should be repeated until the phrase has been whispered around the whole circle. Each person should only whisper on what they heard and s/he is not allowed to ask for the phrase to be repeated.

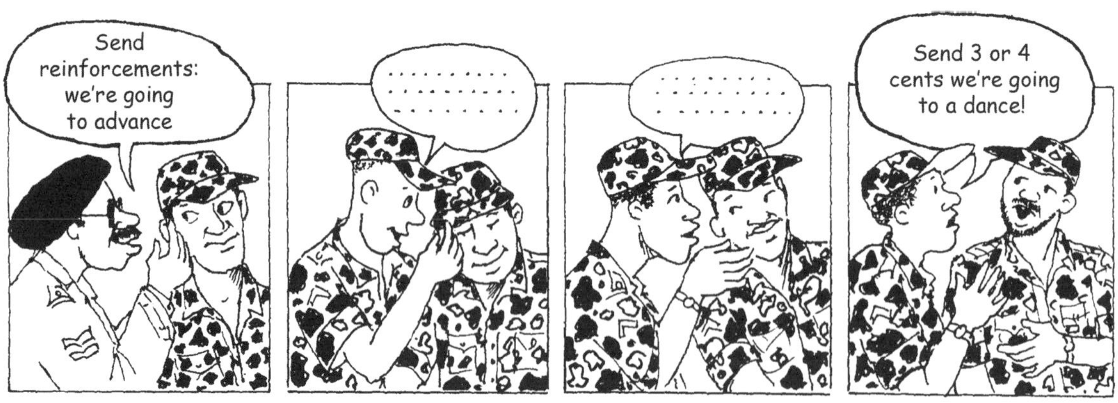

Send reinforcements: we're going to advance
Send 3 or 4 cents we're going to a dance!

4. Finally, when the phrase has been whispered all round the circle, your neighbour on your other side should have received it. Ask her/him to say out loud what s/he heard.

5. Then announce to the group what you originally said. The message normally changes quite a lot as it goes round the circle!

6. If there is time, you could ask someone else to start off another phrase. Point out how easy it is for messages to be misunderstood!

EXERCISE E.2: THE LANGUAGE OF SEX

AIM: **To clarify locally acceptable terminology.**

DESCRIPTION: **A discussion about terms for different sexual organs and sexual acts.**

DIRECTIONS

1. Explain that we are now moving on to talk about things which most people find very embarrassing to discuss in public. But a good way of overcoming the embarrassment is to recognise that we all experience it.

2. Explain that since there is no vaccine or cure for HIV, the only way we have of preventing it spreading is through changes in behaviour and medical practice. Since one of the main routes of transmission is sex, we need to be able to talk about sexual attitudes, behaviour, and safer sex techniques.

3. Explain that you are going to need to talk together about various different sexual parts of the body and different sexual acts. Therefore you need to have a common agreement on acceptable words that you can all use and understand together.

4. Ask the participants to divide into three separate groups for five minutes.

- Ask the first group to brainstorm local words for: male genital organs, semen, pubic hair, female genital organs, skin.
- Ask the second group to brainstorm local words for: vaginal intercourse, vaginal fluids, anal intercourse, orgasm.
- Ask the third group to consider local words for: masturbation, withdrawal (i.e. withdrawal of the penis from the vagina before ejaculation), oral sex, breasts, thigh sex (i.e. mutual masturbation without penetration).

5. Call everyone back into the large circle. Ask each group in turn to report back on the words they want to use.

6. Congratulate everyone on the completion of a difficult exercise.

Feedback and discussion

There may be some denial that, for example, anal sex or oral sex take place. If so, it is probably best to go along with this and just to explain that they are practised elsewhere. But do include them in any future discussions, so that participants know about the risk factors involved in practising them.

In some communities, people may find this exercise really difficult. Some people may get angry and refuse to join in, others may laugh a lot. It would be helpful to explain that this exercise can raise a lot of emotion in people and these reactions are our way of dealing with our feelings about sex being talked about publicly. Encourage participants to set aside their fears or anger and to join in to help one another. In other communities, you may find that you are more embarrassed about using these words than your participants are! Alternatively, you may feel that you and the participants already know all the words involved. But this exercise is worth doing anyway, because the mere public acknowledgement and expression of the words help us to overcome our conventional attitudes towards talking about sex. Use the words that have been decided upon in future exercises.[1]

EXERCISE E.3: THE TASO GAME

AIM: To help people understand how quickly HIV can spread.

DESCRIPTION: Participants are issued with marked pieces of paper. Then they spend a few minutes socialising before responding to instructions according to the mark on their paper.

MATERIALS NEEDED: Slips of paper – one for each participant and one for yourself – 25% marked with '+' and 75% marked with '-'; box or hat.

DIRECTIONS

1. Ask each participant to choose a folded slip of pre-marked paper from a box or hat. Keep one for yourself too, making sure it is one with a '+' sign on it. Emphasise that no-one should look at their slips of paper until the end of the exercise. You should join the participants in following the instructions below.

2. Ask everyone to move freely around the training area, stopping to greet friends.

3. After each person has greeted four or five friends, stop the activity and ask everyone to look at their slip of paper. You should join the participants.

4. Ask all those who have a '+' on their paper to come forward. Explain that this game is **pretending** that these people are HIV-positive. Point out that **there is no risk of acquiring HIV through normal social greeting, and also this is only a game**.

5. Then ask those who greeted any of those who came forward first to come forward to join their friends. Explain that this game is **pretending** that these people are highly vulnerable to acquiring the HIV virus.

6. Next, look to see who is left. Explain that this game is **pretending** that the status of these people is unknown. They may have made friends with others who have only acquired HIV since they met; nonetheless they are still vulnerable.

7. Ask how many people, according to this game:

- originally had HIV?
- are highly vulnerable to acquiring it?
- are vulnerable to acquiring it?
- remain HIV-free?

What does this tell us about the spread of HIV in our community?

8. Now is a good time to give participants figures for HIV and AIDS in your area or country. These could include the percentage of orphaned children. Participants could be encouraged to think what this means for them in terms of the game you have just played.

It is important to include yourself in this game to demonstrate to the participants that you are as vulnerable to acquiring HIV or to having HIV already as they are, and to show solidarity with them in facing the issues related to HIV which we all have to face.

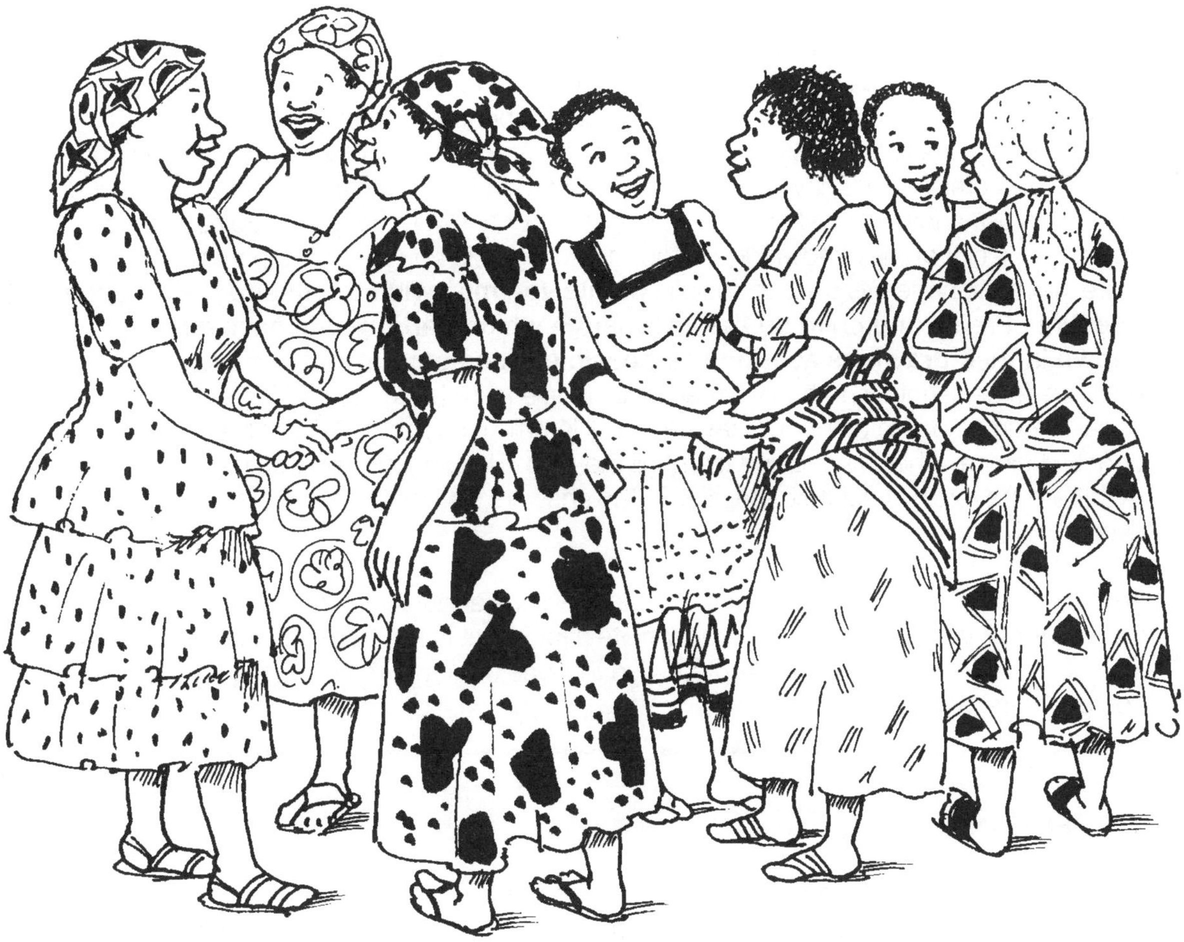

EXERCISE E.4: FACTS AND FEELINGS ABOUT HIV

AIMS: To help participants to assess their own vulnerability and to learn about how they may protect themselves from exposure to HIV. To explore myths, correct misinformation, and accept the limitations of information. To facilitate acceptance of gaps in our knowledge and the need to live and work with uncertainty. To uncover assumptions about, and attitudes towards, particularly emotive issues. To encourage a positive attitude to living, regardless of HIV status and uncertainty.

DESCRIPTION: A discussion session.

MATERIALS NEEDED: Flip-chart paper, strongly coloured crayons, chalk.

DIRECTIONS

Sit in a circle with the participants. Explain to them that you are going to have a discussion exploring facts and feelings about HIV and AIDS. Say that you are going to ask a series of questions and would like them to add their own questions at any stage of the discussion. **Most of the talking in this exercise should be by the participants, rather than you.**

> The guide below suggests questions that you may want to ask to prompt discussion. It is really important that participants are encouraged to **provide and share their own answers** with the group, before you have a go. Encourage them to draw their answers on the ground or on flip-chart paper as often as possible. Drawing helps their explanations and will add interest to the discussion.[2] If their information is good enough, just praise their knowledge and move on to the next question, or encourage one of them to ask another question. Do not impose your answers on the group each time, unless you feel that their knowledge is too limited. To help you if you feel participants need more information there is a list of specific **points you may wish to cover beneath each question. Praise and build on the knowledge which participants have already shown in their drawings as much as possible. Use humour too!** The exercise does not have to be serious and humour can help people learn better by making them feel more at ease. Remember to point out that we are all learning, and that HIV is still a condition about which new things are being learnt all the time. Throughout the exercise, emphasise that there are rarely absolute certainties in the answers and that none of us knows everything!
>
> **NB:** There is another exercise about facts and feelings about HIV in Session O.2, later in this volume. If participants already know quite a lot about HIV, you might use that exercise instead of this one. Alternatively you can use this one here and the one in Session O, when you get there, as a reminder exercise.

THE QUESTIONS

These are some basic questions to prompt the discussion. You can always add extra questions which you feel may be particularly relevant to your context, such as ones about scarification practices, circumcision practices, injecting oneself with drugs, and so on. But try to include everything which is listed here. Note that each question is as open-ended as possible.

a) What is HIV?

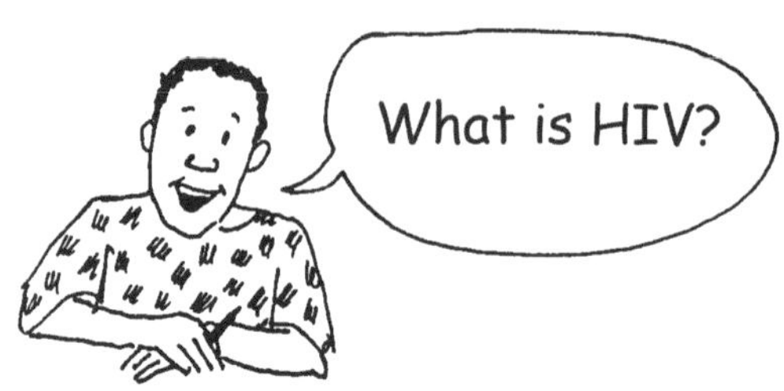

Ask participants to share what they understand about HIV. Encourage them to draw their understanding of how HIV enters someone's body on the ground using chalk, or to use crayons to draw on flip-chart paper. They can draw people's whole bodies or just parts of the reproductive system – whatever they like to help them.

Points you may wish to cover:

- HIV is a small germ called a virus. This is what people catch.
- HIV makes the body weak and less able to fight all kinds of sickness.
- People with HIV in their body often go on to become sick with AIDS, but they do not 'catch' AIDS. AIDS only develops after HIV has stayed in the body for a long time.

- To 'have AIDS' means that someone's immune system is so weak because of having HIV that they can easily get other illnesses too.
- The only way we can tell for certain if we have the virus in our body is through a blood test. If the test shows we have the virus, we are called 'HIV-positive' or said to be 'living with HIV'. If the test shows no evidence of the virus, we are called 'HIV-negative' – but our negative status is not yet certain, because of the window period (see below).
- If someone's HIV develops to AIDS, they can often die of illnesses such as TB, to which they have become more vulnerable because of the HIV virus in their bodies.

The following analogy can help. HIV invades the body like termites invading a mud hut. To begin with, there is no apparent damage. But slowly the termites eat up the poles and thatch which hold the house together. One day a strong wind comes along and knocks the house down. What caused the house to collapse: the wind or the termites?

b) Where do you think HIV came from?

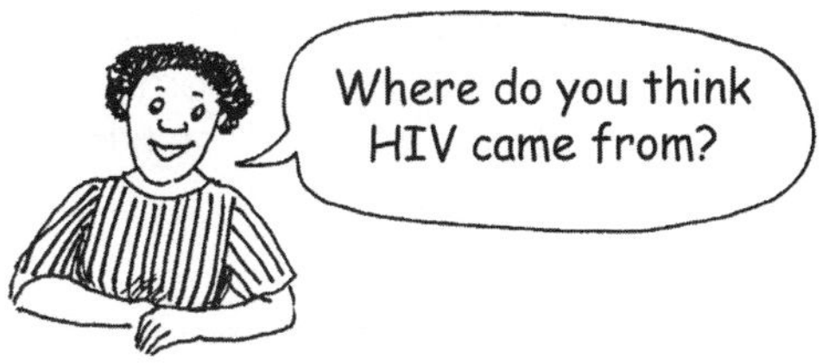

Points you may wish to cover:

- No-one knows. How useful would this information be even if we knew it?
- Just because the HIV epidemic is bad in some places, e.g. Uganda, it does not mean it started there.
- Other things, such as poverty and many years of civil war, have made the situation worse in some countries/places.
- Racism. We always like to blame some other group.
- Blame and prejudice. Remember what we learnt about this already?
- 'Innocent' vs. 'guilty'. Is someone 'guilty' of catching a virus?
- Does it make any difference where other diseases, such as malaria or polio, started?

c) How do you think people can acquire HIV?

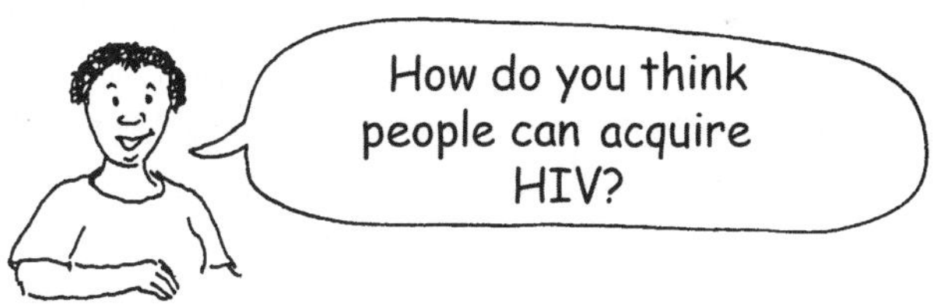

Again encourage participants to make drawings, to share their understanding.

Points you may wish to cover:

For the virus to be transmitted:

- There must be an adequate **quantity** of virus present, and it must be of sufficient **quality**, for a person to acquire HIV. This is most likely to occur with blood, semen, vaginal and cervical fluids, which contain the highest concentrations of virus. It is also true of breast milk, but to a limited extent. Now that ARV medication is available, the chance of HIV being passed on to a baby through breast milk is much reduced if a woman is stable on her ARV medication and has an 'undetectable viral load', which means that the medication is keeping the level of HIV virus in the woman's body very low. The World Health Organization (WHO) therefore still recommends that all mothers in lower income countries should **breastfeed their babies.** This is because the advantages of breast milk (increased immunity against diseases such as measles, polio, and diarrhoea) outweigh the chance of acquiring HIV and exposure to other illness from substitutes given by bottle.[3,4] Studies have also shown that it is safer to breastfeed exclusively for the first six months (without mixing with other foods or fluids), before weaning the baby. For more about breastfeeding, please see Sessions O and Q.
- There must be a suitable **route** for the virus to reach the particular cells for which it has an affinity.

Thus:

- **The blood of someone with HIV** can spread the virus. This can come from a blood transfusion, or from an unsterilized needle or blade. Therefore, care needs to be taken with needles for **injections** and with **razors**, to make sure they are sterilized before **every** new person uses them. This applies whether they are used for medical reasons, for circumcision, for body scarring or any other similar use, where blood is involved. Open wounds should be kept covered by all of us, whoever we are.
- **HIV may be transmitted during sex.** This depends on how people have sex. Safer sex includes:

  - non-penetrative sex, such as masturbation, massage, rubbing, and hugging
  - using a condom for all penetrative sex (vaginal, anal, oral)
  - staying in a mutually faithful relationship, where both partners are HIV-free.

  Some people may like to practise oral sex. This carries little risk of HIV transmission. However unprotected oral sex should certainly be avoided if there are sores present in the mouth or on the genitals, because of other STIs.[5] Oral sex on the penis is safer when a condom is used.

  NB: Certain practices can increase the possibility of HIV transmission. For instance, 'dry' sex, when herbs are placed in the vagina to reduce moisture, may lead to increased friction, causing breaks in the wall of the vagina, and therefore an increased risk of HIV transmission. Open sores on the vagina or penis and STIs also increase the possibility of HIV transmission.

  If people use a cloth to wipe their genital areas after having had sex together using a condom, it is safer for them to use separate cloths. Do wash the cloths afterwards!

- **Women can transmit the virus to their babies, before or during birth.** This has often been the case. Yet with the right care, support and treatment, it is now possible for a woman with HIV to give birth to a child with a 99% chance of the virus not being passed on to the child. The greatest risk factor here is if the woman with HIV has a 'high viral load', which means a high concentration of HIV in her body. This viral load can be kept low ('undetectable') if she takes medication very regularly throughout the pregnancy. This is why it is important to have good supportive testing and care services available, so that women can know their HIV status and adhere to treatment if they have HIV during pregnancy. HIV treatment is the only thing than can reduce viral load and so control the virus. It can take 12–18 months until it is known for sure whether the child is HIV negative or positive. It is possible for a woman with HIV to give birth to some children who are HIV-negative and others who are HIV-positive.

You can read more about all this in Session O.

- **Breast milk:** see above, and below.
- **Vomit, faeces and urine** are all quite harmless, provided that they do not contain any blood. Thus cleaning or bathing a patient is also quite safe, provided all open wounds are covered. Sharing toilets is also quite safe.
- **Kissing** does not spread the virus – unless both partners actually have bleeding gums, when there may be a very small risk.
- **Mosquitoes, fleas and bedbugs** cannot spread the virus either. The body system of the insects does not allow HIV to survive to be transferred.
- **Sweat** does not spread the virus.
- **Sharing food** does not spread the virus.
- **Shaking hands** does not spread the virus.

- **Tears** and **hugging** carry no risk at all. Nor does **sharing sheets, towels, clothes or eating utensils**.

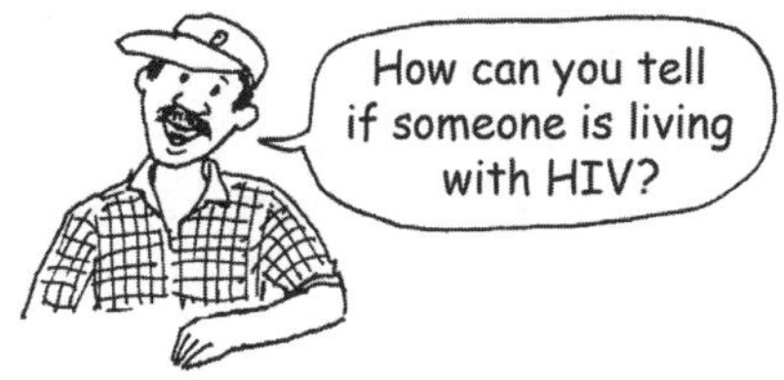

d) How can you tell if someone is living with HIV?

Points you may wish to cover:

- People with HIV can look exactly like you and me.
- On average, about half the people with HIV around the world still have no symptoms of AIDS after ten years. So even though someone may have HIV, provided they are well, they can live a full, healthy and productive life.
- There is a difference between HIV and AIDS. People can carry the HIV virus for many years without knowing they have it. They can look and feel entirely healthy before developing any symptoms of AIDS.
- Many of us do not know whether we have HIV or not. Thus it should be the responsibility of all of us – not just those who know they are HIV-positive – to protect ourselves and others from the virus.

e) If someone has a blood test that says they are HIV-negative, does that mean they are not living with HIV or can't acquire HIV?

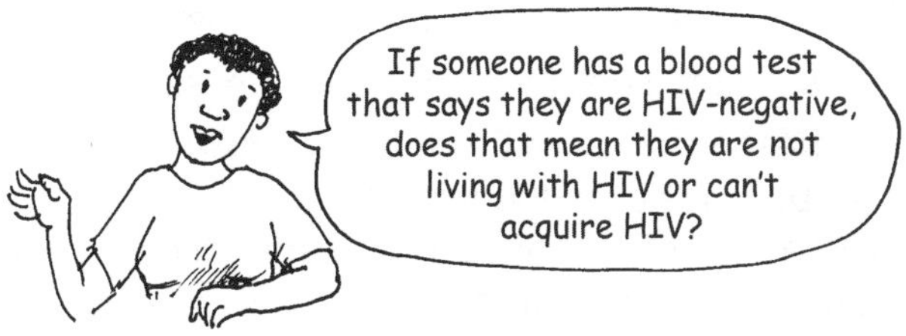

Points you may wish to cover:

- The window period: there are up to three months between the date of acquiring HIV and the date when a test result would normally show positive. So unless we have a negative result twice, in tests spaced three months apart, and we are **certain** that we have not been at risk since before the first test, we cannot safely say that we are HIV-negative.
- Remaining negative: if we are involved in sexual activity, the best way to remain negative is to adopt safer sexual behaviour.

f) What issues do pregnant women who are living with HIV face?

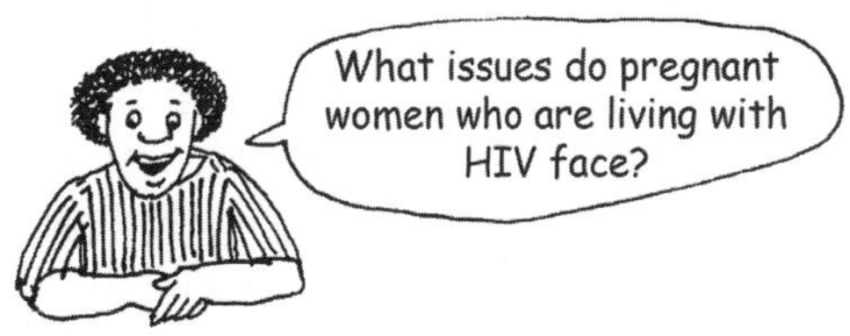

Points you may wish to cover:

- The chance of a woman with HIV having a child born with HIV is about one in three without anti-retroviral therapy. Some children acquire HIV in the womb, some at birth and some through breastfeeding. This means that it is a matter of chance – like a raffle or lottery – whether a child born to an HIV-positive woman acquires it or not. However, if a woman is supported to take anti-retroviral therapy well, there is a likelihood of over 99% that her child will be born HIV-free.[6]
- Remember, it can take 12-18 months for doctors to tell whether a baby of a woman with HIV has HIV or not, depending on availability and quality of tests.
- WHO still recommends that women in low income countries should breastfeed their children, as protection against diarrhoea and other childhood diseases, which can be a greater risk to children than the possible HIV-positive status of their mothers (see question (c) above).
- The health status of a woman living with HIV may deteriorate during pregnancy if she is not supported to take HIV medication. Yet, with the right support and medication, she can keep both herself and her babies happy, healthy and safe. Each woman should decide for herself what choices she wants to make regarding having children or not and she should be given support to follow her choices through.[7]

g) Which activities do you think make HIV transmission most likely?

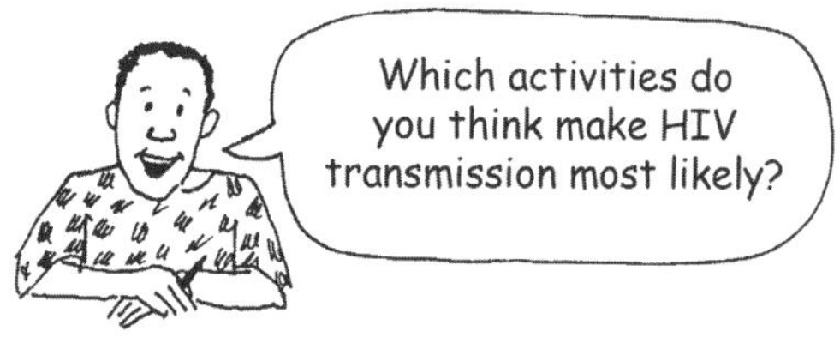

Points you may wish to cover:

- This is a chance for you to review the points discussed after question c) above.
- You may find participants starting to talk about people, rather than activities. If participants say, for instance, having sex with a sex worker, or a young man from the city, is risky ask them whether they think it is the **person** that is the risk or the **activity** involved. Point out that, in many parts of the world, sex workers actively prevent the spread of HIV by always insisting on condom use. But in most places they find this impossible, because their poverty means that they have no power to insist on anything and they have to do whatever their clients want. So is it fair to blame them? Remind participants of the 'Who's Labelling Whom?' exercise. We tend to label people very easily and often forget to recognise our own responsibilities.
- It encourages a false sense of security to assume that only certain people can get HIV.
- We should all work together against the reasons behind the spread of HIV, not people with HIV.
- It is safest to see HIV as **everyone's** issue.
- It is best to talk about **activities** which increase our vulnerability to HIV and not 'high-risk groups'. However, there is one group of people who are very much in danger of HIV. Young women are particularly vulnerable to acquiring HIV through penetrative sex, because their sexual organs are still not fully developed and are more likely to be wounded or torn. This does not mean that young women behave any differently from others. It just means that their young bodies are **physically** most vulnerable to the virus.

h) If a couple are both living with HIV and the woman gets sick first, who must have acquired the virus first?

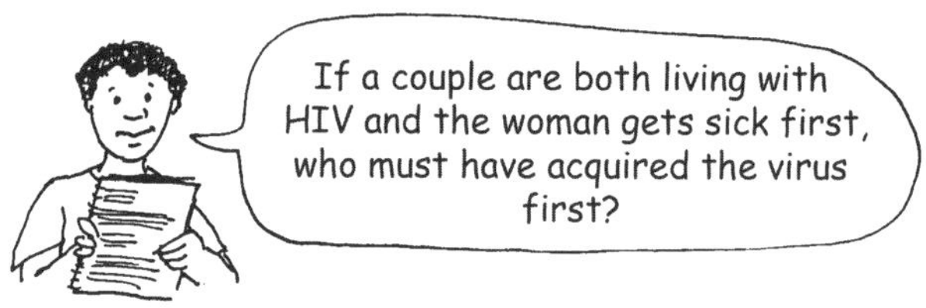

Points you may wish to cover:

- The speed of onset of illness is not always related to who first acquired HIV. Often it can relate to the amount of work which someone has to do, their access to good food and to rest, and their body's natural ability to resist illness. Some people are by nature more prone to illness than others. Since women often have heavy workloads, they can often have poor resistance to illness and can get ill quite quickly. Others can live well and look healthy for 10 years or more.
- Wives are often accused of being to blame if they get sick first. They are then thrown out and sent back to their parents without their children. Is this fair?
- What is the point of blaming? Very few people who have HIV want to give HIV to their partners. Couples who both have HIV could be helped by their relatives and friends to start and stay on HIV treatment when they need it, and be supported with looking after their children and other tasks.

i) How can you prevent sexual transmission of HIV and other STIs?

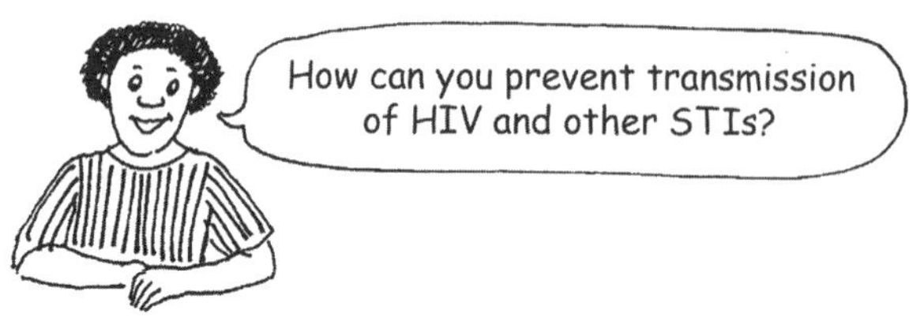

Points you may wish to cover:

- **Never having sex with anyone.** Practising **permanent abstinence**, that is, **never** having sex with anyone, is a safe way of avoiding STIs and sexual transmission of the HIV virus. However, most people, certainly those who want to have children or to get married, find this an inappropriate solution.

- **Temporary abstinence.** This can be a good solution for some people, especially for younger people, those who are not yet ready to have children, and those who are away from their usual partners for some time. However, many people also find this a difficult option, perhaps especially young men because of peer pressure to prove their manhood by having sex with their girlfriends. It is also not a certain way of avoiding HIV or other STIs, unless suitable precautions are taken between the periods of abstinence.
- **Wearing a good-luck charm** is no good at all.
- **Only having sex with one person who only ever has sex with you.** This should work. However, it does not give guaranteed protection, because, in some cases, one partner may have acquired HIV before they started being mutually faithful – or may have been born with HIV – and not be showing any symptoms. The virus can last 10 years or more in the body before making someone ill.
- **Using dry herbs in the vagina.** Drying the vagina by any means makes tearing and bleeding more likely. This makes the risk of HIV transmission greater, not less.
- **Using condoms**. This method is reliable only if the condoms are used correctly (see Session F) and in every act of sexual intercourse. Many people find this option difficult, but others have grown used to it, after practice, and find it helpful. A study[8] of 245 couples in Europe over 22 months, in which one partner had HIV and the other was HIV-negative, found that 123 couples used condoms consistently and correctly. Amongst them, no HIV was transmitted from the partner with HIV to the HIV-negative partner. Among the other 122 couples, where condom use was inconsistent, 12 HIV-negative partners acquired HIV over the same period.
- **Safer sex** should always be practised, even between partners who both have HIV, to avoid repeated exposure to HIV and other STIs, and possible unplanned pregnancy.
- Nowadays, thanks to anti-retroviral medication (ARVs),[9] it is possible for people of different (or unknown) HIV status to have sex with no condom, without HIV being transmitted, if the person who knows s/he has HIV is stable on HIV medication, with an undetectable viral load and/or when the person who knows s/he doesn't have HIV is taking 'pre-exposure prophylaxis' (PrEP). Nonetheless, without a condom, there is still possible exposure to STIs and/or to unplanned pregnancy.
- If we are involved in sexual activities, the safest way for us all to maintain good sexual and reproductive health is for us **all** to adopt safer sexual practices, whether we have HIV or not. Condoms allow us both to **protect and care for others, and to protect and care for ourselves.**
- **Using other contraceptives, such as the pill, IUD or injection** can prevent pregnancy, if taken or used correctly. However they do not protect against HIV or other STIs.
- **Non-penetrative sex.** There is little risk of transmission of HIV during this, provided there is no mixing of body fluids between the couple.
- **Having a vaccine to stop us getting it.** There is no vaccine yet invented to prevent HIV.

j) What worries or fears do you have about condoms?

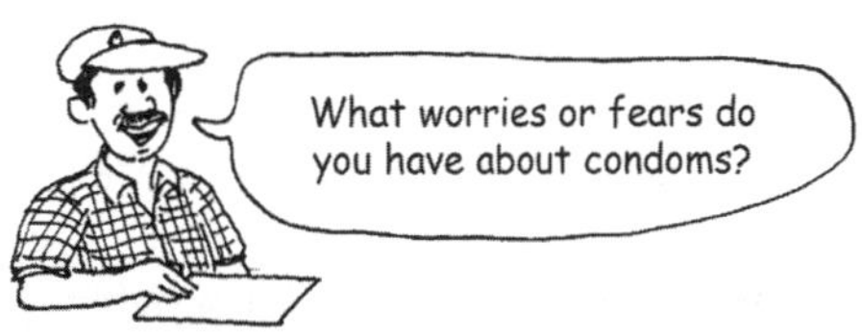

Points you may wish to cover:

- Some participants may say that a condom can get lost inside a woman and hurt or kill her. This is impossible because of the tiny opening between the vagina and the womb. (You could point to participants' own drawings of this, or draw this yourself, to show everyone.) During the birth of a child this opening widens, but at all other times it is far too small to let a condom in.

NB: It is always important to withdraw the penis with the condom still on it before the penis has become soft (see Exercise F.3, when you can explore the importance of this further).

k) Do you think it's any good starting to use condoms if someone thinks they're already living with HIV?

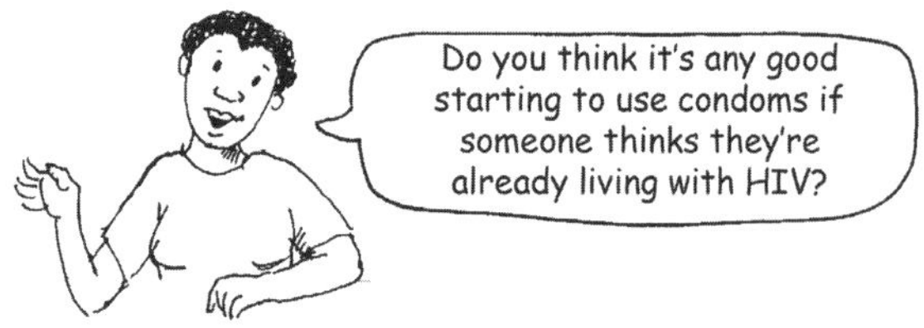

Points you may wish to cover:

- If two people of different HIV status have been having unprotected sex, it is not certain that HIV will have been transmitted. So it is worth starting to use a condom. Also, even if both partners have HIV, they should use condoms if they have sex together to prevent further exposing themselves to the virus. This can hasten the onset of illness. It's also worth using a condom to protect your partner(s), in case they do not have HIV.

l) How do you think people with HIV should be treated?

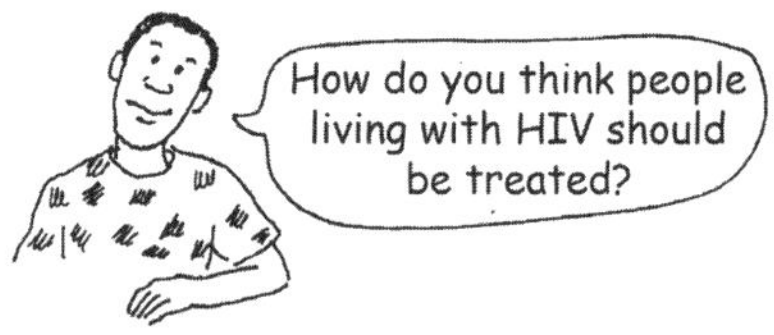

Points you may wish to cover:

- Any of us or any of our family or friends could have HIV. We may even have HIV already without knowing it.
- If we are shunned and avoided, we could quickly fall sick through depression and neglect.
- Just like the house with termites, we can still be fit, active and productive for many years before falling sick. With the support of ARVs when we need them, we can live a full life and have children born HIV-free.
- If we believe ourselves to have HIV, but fear rejection and discrimination from family and friends, we may be less likely to seek counselling and medical care. We are also less likely to use condoms with regular sexual partners, or use ARVs when we need them, because we don't want to arouse suspicion.

This next exercise is on testing so that all workshop participants can learn for themselves what is involved in a good HIV voluntary counselling and testing (VCT) process. While some HIV support services are great, unfortunately, many HIV testing facilities are still not well run. So this exercise can also help participants to learn what they should be expecting from local services and what they could ask for to improve them. **It would be best if you, as facilitator, have gone for an HIV test yourself, so that you know what this experience feels like**. You will need to make sure that local services of some kind are available, and be prepared to support your participants to lobby for the services to be good and for anti-retroviral medication (ARVs) to be available if necessary. Otherwise, people are – understandably – likely not to see the point of being tested.

Members of your peer group who have HIV, or who have friends or relatives who have HIV, may find this exercise particularly difficult, since they may hear people voicing criticism of people with HIV. You need to be aware of this possibility and remind everyone of the ground rules and the exercises in Session D. It may be a good thing to say to your group at the end of this exercise, and again at the end of the session, that anyone who wants to go for individual confidential counselling can do so at a specific local place, its name, location, opening times and so on. People who fear a lack of confidentiality may prefer to go further away from the community for counselling. You could therefore also add the details of other centres in larger towns, or perhaps phone numbers of counselling helplines, if these are available.

EXERCISE E.5: TESTING ISSUES

AIM: To help people think through some of the issues regarding voluntary counselling and testing.

DESCRIPTION: Explanation, then pairs work, followed by group discussion.

MATERIALS NEEDED: Flip-chart, marker pens.

DIRECTIONS

1. Explain that many people wonder whether or not they should go for an HIV test. In this exercise, you are going to discuss how the test works, and then you will help participants to think through some of the issues involved in testing.

2. Ask anyone in the group if they know and could describe to others what the HIV test is and how it works. Encourage them to do so, but don't push people who feel reluctant to discuss it.

Make sure everyone in the group understands the following points:

- The test for HIV is a blood test.
- When someone acquires the HIV virus, it lives in our blood. It can take three to six months before there is enough of the virus to be detected by a test, although we can still pass the virus to others (this is called the window period).
- Therefore, if the test is negative, it shows only the HIV status of somebody three months ago: it cannot say whether that person is definitely HIV-negative at the time he or she takes the test. The person might have contracted the virus one or two months before the test – or the previous night.
- If someone thinks that s/he might have HIV and would like to take a test to find out, it is a good idea to do so. If the test result is negative, the person is encouraged to have another test three months later. If this test is also negative, provided that s/he has not exposed himself or herself to the virus in the meantime, it is most unlikely that s/he has HIV.
- Anyone who has a test should only do so voluntarily and confidentially. This is their right. It is strongly recommended that s/he is counselled both before the test and afterwards. This helps the person to think through what s/he will do in response to the test result. For instance, if the result were positive (which means s/he has HIV), how would s/he cope with the news? Who would s/he want to tell (and, who not)? How could s/he protect his or her partner(s) from acquiring HIV, look after his or her own health, and so on? If the test result were negative, the person would be counselled about how s/he could try to remain negative.

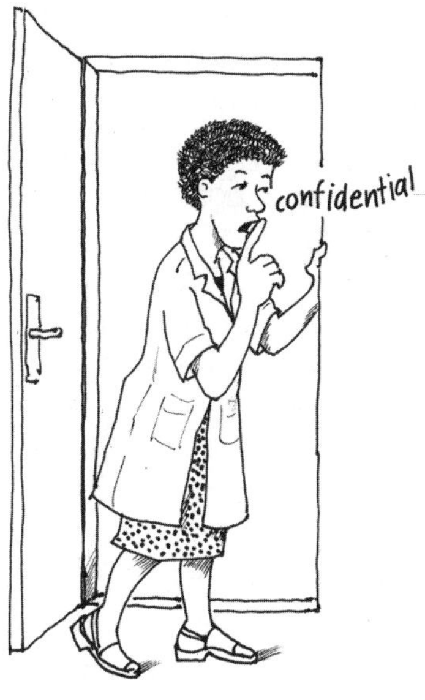

3. Say to the group: 'Some people say that they'll wait to have the test, just to check, before changing their behaviour and, if it's negative, that they're OK and they don't need to take any precautions. What do you think of this?'

Make sure that participants understand the following:

- Having an HIV test cannot be a substitute for behaviour change. As we discussed earlier, no-one who is sexually active can safely call him/herself immune from HIV.
- If someone tests negative, that person needs to make sure that s/he is protecting him- or herself from exposure to the virus.
- If someone tests positive, s/he also needs to protect him- or herself from further exposure to the virus, as well as protecting others from the virus.

4. Say to the group: 'Some people say that, if someone tests positive, everyone should be told of their status, so that we can protect ourselves from him/her. What do you think?'

Make sure that participants understand the following:

- Someone's health status is their own business and not everybody else's. They have a right to confidentiality.
- Remember the exercises we played earlier on taking risks and on labelling. How would we feel if we were told that we have HIV?
- Normal social interaction with someone who has HIV causes no risk to anybody. If we all took responsibility for showing that we care for others, as well as looking after ourselves by, for instance, adopting the safer sexual practices that we have already discussed, this person would pose no greater risk to us than we pose to him or her.

5. Say to the group: 'Some people say that everyone should be tested for HIV. Then we would all know who's safe and who isn't. What do you think of this?'

Make sure that participants understand the following:

- The window period makes this impractical, because it is impossible to say that somebody is definitely HIV-negative at the time of the test, so everyone would have to be tested every three months.
- The effort of mass repeat testing would be totally unaffordable and unmanageable, and open to corruption.
- It goes against human rights to force HIV testing on people. When there is still so much prejudice against people with HIV, people who test HIV-positive may be blamed for having the virus and turned out of their families. Yet experience in many countries has shown that the best educators about the dangers of HIV are people who are themselves living with HIV and who feel confident that, if they talk openly about it, they will still be loved and cared for by their families and friends. Compulsory testing would serve only to isolate people living with HIV from society – and to cut society off from all that people with HIV have to offer.
- Therefore anyone who has a test should do so only voluntarily.

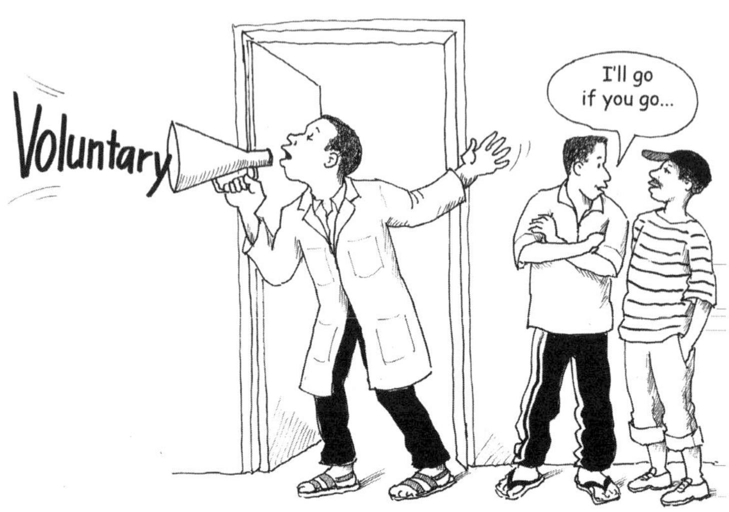

6. Next, ask the group to divide into pairs, working with someone whom they haven't worked with before, if possible. Before they move around, explain that you would like them to consider the following story:

'CATHERINE (or change the name to a common name in this area) visited a health centre when she was expecting a baby. She and her husband already had a 2-year-old daughter and were looking forward to their second child. She had a bit of vaginal discharge, but otherwise felt well and very excited. She was given treatment for the discharge and was also tested for HIV. She was told that she had HIV. She was advised to use condoms, to start taking anti-retroviral medication to protect her own and the baby's health, to bring her daughter and husband for an HIV test, and to return regularly herself for check-ups. When she told her husband all this, he threw her out of the house. Her own parents wouldn't allow her back to live with them, saying she had brought shame on their family. She was prevented from seeing her daughter and turned to sex work in the nearby town to feed herself. Meanwhile her husband, who felt pressure from his parents and his peers to have a son, married another woman.'

Ask participants to think about the following questions:

- What were the consequences of the HIV test for:
  Catherine
  Her husband
  His new wife
  Catherine's new sexual partners
  Her older child
  Her unborn child?
  Her husband's parents?
  Her own parents?
- Did Catherine's test help to prevent HIV?
- What could have happened instead to make the test helpful to everyone concerned and to help HIV prevention generally?

Give everybody about 10 minutes to discuss this story and the questions you have asked in pairs.

7. Call everyone back to the full circle and ask for feedback on the questions. This should take another 30 minutes or so.

During the discussion, encourage participants to consider the following:

- Was Catherine asked whether she would like an HIV test or not?
- Did Catherine receive any counselling before or after the test, or advice about how to talk to her husband or others?
- Was Catherine's husband offered any counselling?
- Why did Catherine's husband marry a new wife?
- Did Catherine's husband wear condoms with his new wife?
- Could Catherine manage to protect her clients from HIV? If not, whose responsibility was that?

8. Say to the group: 'What prejudices do people here have against people who test HIV-positive? In the light of everything which we have been talking about, do these make sense? Are they just?'

Make sure that participants understand that people whose HIV-positive status is known to others can face job loss, home loss, loss of partner or children, social isolation, imprisonment – even murder. This is unjust and hurts individuals and their families. It does not fight the virus.

9. Ask the group: 'What can we do together to change attitudes to people with HIV in our own community and support people like Catherine, her husband and their children?' Encourage participants to come up with specific points,[10] if possible, and to write or draw them on a flip chart.

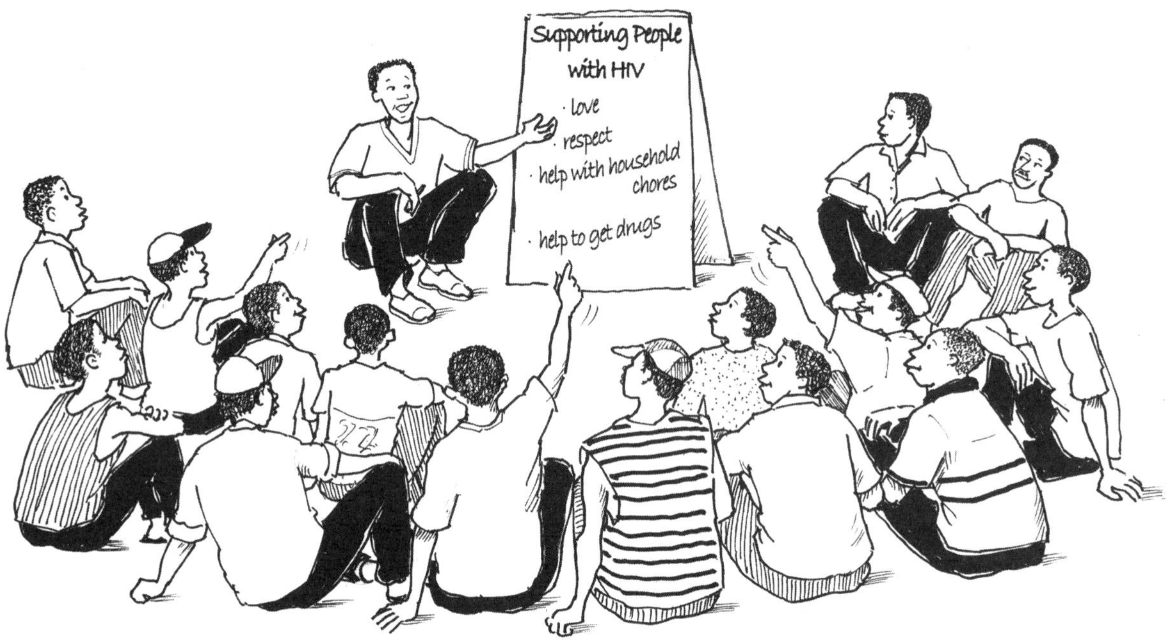
Supporting People with HIV
· love
· respect
· help with household chores
· help to get drugs

EXERCISE E.6: PRRR AND PUKUTU

AIM: A quick exercise to make everyone laugh and move. It is important to have this kind of activity after an exercise that is as thought-provoking as the previous one.

DESCRIPTION: As everyone stands in a circle, they have to react to what you call out.

DIRECTIONS

1. Ask everyone to stand in a circle. Explain that you would like them to think of two birds. One calls 'prrr' and the other calls 'pukutu'.

2. If you call out 'prrr', all the participants need to rise up on their toes and move their elbows out sideways, as if they were a bird ruffling its wings. If you call out 'pukutu', everyone should stay still and not move a feather!

3. Proceed by calling out 'prrr' or 'pukutu'. Anyone who moves when they shouldn't, or who stays still when they should move, has to fall out of the game. They can then help you to watch the other participants. Go on until you have just a few people left in the circle. Everyone should have had a good laugh.

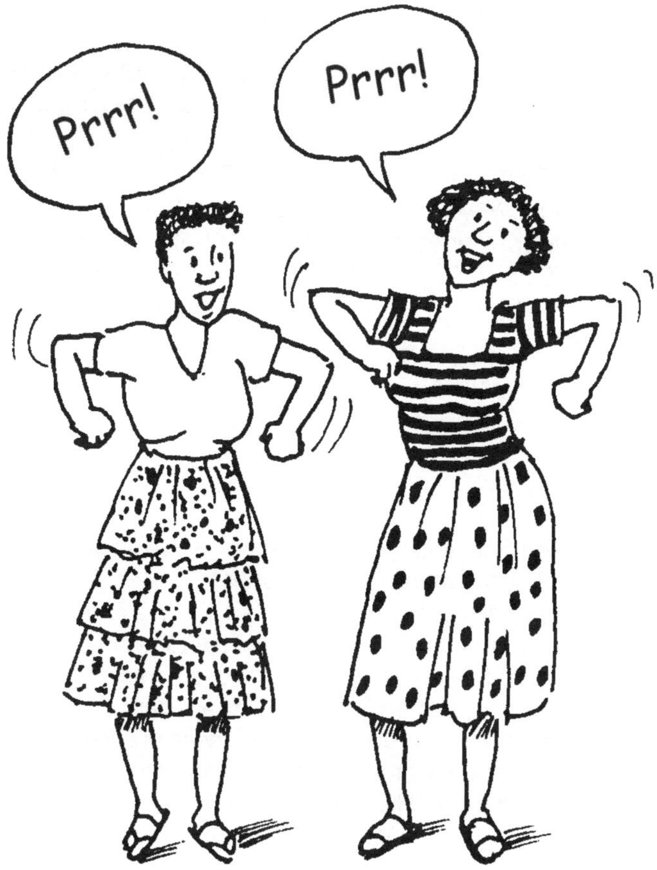

EXERCISE E.7: CLOSING CIRCLE

1. Ask everyone to sit down again in a circle for closing time.

2. Ask each participant to mention one thing which they liked about this session and one thing which they didn't like or found hard.

3. Remind everyone of their role as guardian angel.

4. Encourage participants to talk in general about the kinds of issues they have been discussing in these sessions with their friends and neighbours, if they like, but not to share any confidential information from the peer group with others.

5. Remember to ask for three volunteers to stay behind for a quick session review. (See Annex 4 for details.)

6. Finish off by thanking everyone once more for coming to this session. **Remind participants of a local place where people can go for individual counselling, or counselling and testing (if this service is available in your area).** Arrange a mutually convenient time and place for the next session before saying goodbye.

FACILITATORS' TEAM FEEDBACK

After the end of Session E, meet again with your co-facilitators to compare notes on how your sessions went and the information which you learnt from them. Your co-facilitators could have found useful information that could help you to structure your next session more effectively. Remember, however, not to share individual confidentialities between groups. This is the easiest way to ruin the trust that you have begun to build and to wreck the whole workshop! Remember to check whether there is a good local condom supply before you move on to Session F. The session is likely to create or increase demand, so there should be a good supply available, at a cost which can be afforded by women as well as men.

ENDNOTES

1. Optional additional exercises on STIs and the female reproductive system, including information about the woman's reproductive cycle and when she can best get pregnant, if she wants to, are available in *Stepping Stones – Gambia* – please contact us for these if you would like to use them. There is also more discussion of this in relation to support from health staff to avoid transmission in Session O.4.
2. See Annex 7 for a list of suggested resources to help you use participants' drawings to explore issues. RRA Notes 16 and PLA Notes 23 (IIED1992, 1995) are particularly relevant.
3. In July 2015, WHO stated: 'Antiretroviral drugs now allow these children [of women with HIV] to exclusively breastfeed until they are 6 months old and continue breastfeeding until at least 12 months of age with a significantly reduced risk of HIV transmission.'
4. For more information on breastfeeding studies and recommendations, see Doherty et al. (2010).
5. See i-Base (2013a) for a fuller explanation.
6. See Sessions O and Q for much more information about this. Also see i-Base (2013b) for more information.
7. There is more on this in Sessions O and Q.
8. Clearinghouse (1994).
9. For more information about ARVs and PrEP, see, for example, the i-Base website or information from your Ministry of Health.
10. See Dr Bruno Spire's plenary speech at the Mexico International AIDS Conference, 2008 which discussed the connections between increased love, care and support for people with HIV, consistent condom use, and greater treatment adherence levels, when people need medical treatment.

REFERENCES

Clearinghouse, C.N.A. (1994) 'Facts about Condoms and Their Use in Preventing HIV Infection and Other STDs', *Journal of School Health*, 64: 215–216. doi: 10.1111/j.1746-1561.1994.tb03304.x

Doherty, T. Sanders, D. Goga, A. and Jackson, D. (2010) 'Implications of the new WHO guidelines on HIV and infant feeding for child survival in South Africa', *Bulletin of the World Health Organization*, 89: 62–67. doi: 10.2471/BLT.10.079798

IIED (1992) *RRA Notes* 16, IIED, London, <http://pubs.iied.org/6085IIED.html?k=RRA%20Notes%20 16&r=p> [accessed 7 November 2015].

i-Base, *HIV i-Base HIV treatment advocacy and information* [website], i-Base, London, <http://i-base.info> [accessed 7 November 2015].

i-Base (2013a) *Oral Sex* [website], i-Base, London, <http://i-base.info/guides/testing/oral-sex>[accessed 7 November 2015].

i-Base (2013b) *How and when will I know that my baby is HIV negative?* [website], i-Base, London, <http://i-base.info/guides/pregnancy/hiv-negative> [accessed 7 November 2015]

IIED (1995) *PLA Notes 23,* IIED, London, <http://pubs.iied.org/6092IIED.html?k=PLA%20Notes%20 23&r=p> [accessed 7 November 2015].

Shaw, M. (adapted from Welbourn, A.) (2002) *Stepping Stones – Gambia*, Action Aid, London.
Spire, S. De Zoysa, I. and Himmich, H. (2008) 'HIV prevention: What have we learned from community experiences in concentrated epidemics?', *Journal of the International AIDS Society,* 11 :5. doi: 10.1186/1758-2652-11-5
WHO (2015b) 'Infant and young child feeding' Fact sheet No. 342, WHO, Geneva, <http://www.who.int/mediacentre/factsheets/fs342/en/> [accessed 7 November 2015].

YOUR NOTES ...

SESSION F CONDOMS AND MALE CIRCUMCISION

PURPOSE

To continue our discussions about safer sex and to familiarise participants with use of the condom and the issue of male circumcision.

CONTENTS	**TIME NEEDED**
Introduction	
F.1	Folding Paper Game
F.2	Where do we go from here?
F.3	**DVD Clip 3:** 'The Condom'
F.4	Male Condoms Discussion
F.5	Female Condoms Discussion
F.6	Male Circumcision
F.7	Catch Up Time (optional)
F.8	One New Thing

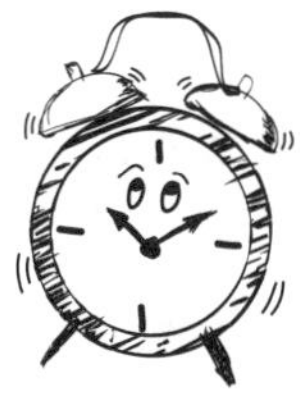

Maximum 4 hours

MATERIALS NEEDED: Four large (A4) sheets of writing paper, flip-chart paper, different coloured marker pens, post-it stickers, chalk, DVD, laptop with DVD player, projector, at least three male and three female condoms in their wrappers for each participant, one banana or dildo for each participant (to use as a model penis), one tube of water-based lubricant.

PARTICIPANTS: Four separate peer groups.

SPECIAL INFORMATION

- Don't forget to read 'Before You Begin ...!' before using this section of the manual.
- You need to have practised the male and female condom demonstrations well.
- If there is a good local place where people can go for counselling, or for counselling and HIV testing, you should know its location, opening times, and any other relevant information.
- In this manual we have not discussed microbicides. But if and when these become available in your area, you should add a discussion of these to this session.
- Some people may be shocked by DVD Clip 3, which is used in this session. If you think this clip is unacceptable for your community, then you may prefer not to show it. On the other hand, facilitators do need to have the courage to challenge people a bit at times! Do remember that the clip will be shown to each peer group separately, which should reduce embarrassment. Facilitators are often amazed by what their groups are prepared to discuss when this degree of privacy is available. But, in the end, you are the best judge of your situation.

INTRODUCTION

1. Sit in a circle with the group, preferably on the ground. Everyone should be at the same level, including yourself.

2. Welcome everyone to the new session. Thank everyone for coming. Enquire about late-comers or non-attenders.

3. Ask each participant to recount quickly something good which has happened to them since the last session.

4. Review the last session. Ask participants to remind us what we learnt then — about HIV and our feelings about it … Check some of the main points and remind participants of any they have forgotten.

5. Explain that we are going on to discuss other things in this session, but will start with a game.

EXERCISE F.1: FOLDING PAPER GAME

AIMS: **To show in a funny way how easy it is for different people to interpret the same instructions in different ways.**

DESCRIPTION: **Four volunteers are asked to close their eyes and fold a piece of paper, according to spoken instructions. Onlookers see how differently they interpret the same instructions.**

MATERIALS: **Four large (A4) sheets of writing paper.**

DIRECTIONS

1. Ask for four volunteers and position them where they can all be clearly seen by the other participants. Ask each volunteer to put on a blindfold or to promise to keep their eyes shut. No participant is allowed to ask any questions during the exercise.

2. Hand each volunteer a piece of writing paper. Each piece should be the same size.

3. Then ask participants to fold their paper in half. Then they should tear off the bottom right hand corner of the paper. Then they should fold the paper in half again. Next they should tear off the lower left hand corner. Remind them not to peep!

4. Then ask all four volunteers to open their eyes, unfold their pieces of paper and display them to the other participants. It is highly unlikely that all four pieces of paper will have been torn in the same way.

Feedback and discussion

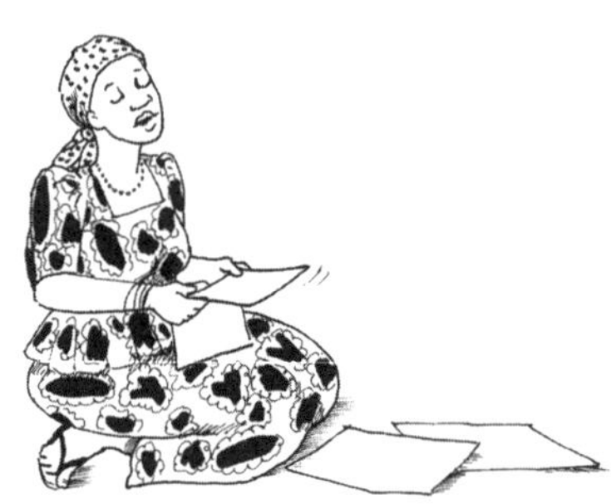

Ask participants what this exercise can show us. One point is to show everyone how even simple instructions can mean very different things to different people. (It makes no difference in this game how literate someone is.) We often think we are saying something clearly to someone, only to discover later that what we have meant and what they have understood have been quite different. Everyone followed the instructions correctly, but the results were very different. This is a useful way of introducing the rest of this session, which is going to give participants a chance to learn about the condom. Encourage them to ask as many questions about it as they like. They will also all have a chance to learn how to use it for themselves.

EXERCISE F.2: WHERE DO WE GO FROM HERE?

AIM: To enable participants to explore questions which may stop us from using VCT services.

DESCRIPTION: Discussion, role play.

MATERIALS NEEDED: Flip chart, marker pens, post-it stickers.

DIRECTIONS

1. Explain that this exercise is about what barriers may stop us from wanting to use facilities and services which may be available in our community, and how we might support one another to overcome these barriers.

2. Remind participants that it is entirely their own right to choose whether or not they go for HIV testing and that no one should tell them otherwise. Then explain that a lot of people would like to be tested, but don't know where to go or what to expect when they go to a testing centre. So here is the opportunity to discuss this a bit.

3. Ask:

- What are the names of the health facilities available in our community?
- What kind of services do they provide?
- How many of us visit these facilities and for what purpose?
- How many of us know about Voluntary Counselling and Testing (VCT) services? Are they available in our community? Are they located in suitable places? Are they open at suitable times?
- Where would we go if we want to find out our HIV status?
- If people around here are tested and found to have HIV, are the medication and care they might need available?

Explain that we sometimes don't go to health facilities and services because we are afraid of what will happen to us if the result is positive.

We are going to discuss and share our views about these fears.

Ask the participants to divide into three or four groups (depending on total numbers in your peer group) to discuss the following:

a) What fears do people here have about visiting a VCT centre?

b) Do local health staff respect the confidentiality of their clients and act supportively? Or do they treat them harshly, talk about them to others, and even tell others who has come in for a test?

4. Ask each small group to role-play one or other of the following two scenes – one or two groups to role-play the positive scene, one or two groups to role-play the negative scene. Imagine a person like them – their gender and age – who recently attended a VCT facility to be tested. In the negative scene, the person tested positive for HIV, and was not supported by the health staff, who had not received the right training or support from their employers. The person with HIV also received no medication to support him or her, even though he or she was sick,

and the health staff were telling others about the test result. In the positive scene, the person tested positive for HIV and was supported by the health staff, who had received good training. They offered the person with HIV more information and support, including information about what medication needed to be taken and when, and also information about a local HIV self-help group that he or she could contact.

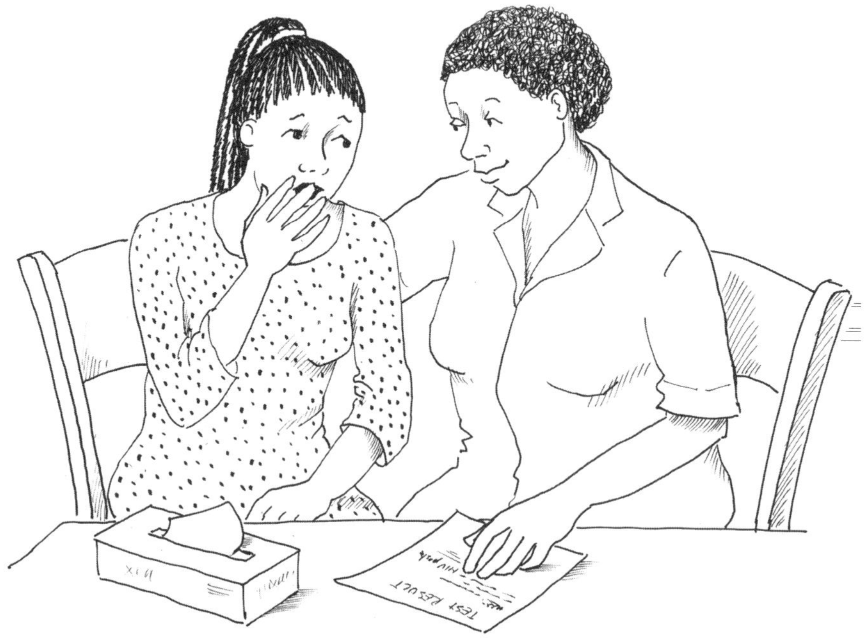

5. The groups present their role plays: the negative scene first, followed by the positive scene. Afterwards, the facilitator leads a discussion by asking the following questions:

- What actions did we see taking place in the role play?
- What was each person doing?
- What are the possible causes of this kind of behaviour?
- Is the behaviour of the health staff good?
- Does this happen in our community?
- What effect does the behaviour have on the person who had the HIV test?
- How does this kind of behaviour affect the use of VCT services?
- How does this kind of behaviour affect the spread of HIV in communities?
- What could we do as a community to improve the use of VCT services nearest us?

> ☞ It may be that some of the members of your peer groups are themselves health staff. Please emphasise that often health staff have not themselves had enough training in these issues, that they are over-stretched and underpaid, and that they too need support to understand these issues because HIV is something which has come along since many health staff were trained and it also affects health staff and their families. **Most health staff acquire HIV through their everyday lives and not through exposure to HIV at work**.

6. Having discussed fears of going to the VCT facility, ask participants to name first the pros and then the cons of knowing one's HIV status, and to suggest possible solutions to each of the cons they mention.

Participants may be encouraged to consider the thoughts in the table below, if they have not already been mentioned. If you like, the group could write or draw their own table.

BENEFITS OF VCT	DISADVANTAGES OF VCT	POSSIBLE SOLUTIONS TO DISADVANTAGES
If you have HIV, you can learn how to take better care of yourself, remain healthy and lead a productive & fulfilling life regardless of your status. If you are HIV-negative, you can learn how to protect yourself so you can remain negative for life.	If you have HIV, you may fear being treated badly by health staff, rejected by your community, thrown out by your husband, partner, in-laws, or parents, and lose all your friends.	Health staff to receive proper training. Health staff with HIV to be kept in post by health centres. All the community to learn about HIV, what it is and what it isn't, and to learn to support everyone with HIV since it can be acquired by anyone – including health staff.
BENEFITS OF WELL TRAINED HEALTH STAFF	**DISADVANTAGES OF POORLY TRAINED HEALTH STAFF**	**POSSIBLE SOLUTIONS TO SUPPORT HEALTH STAFF**
More people feel confident to go to be tested and find out their HIV status. Health staff feel equipped to support clients well. More health staff feel confident to disclose that they too have HIV to employers and colleagues – and clients. More people find out their status and are able to take appropriate action.	People fear going to be tested and avoid it if at all possible. Health staff fear what is happening in their own lives and have no-one to talk with. Health staff feel over-stretched and blame the clients who most need their support.	Request local health officials to provide training for local health staff. Request that both male and female health staff are locally available, to ensure same-gender counselling and testing is available if preferred.

FINALLY ...

Explain to participants that in many countries now, people are learning of their HIV status at times when they are not in a position to prepare for this information or deal with it easily, such as when they are sick in hospital, when they have TB, or when they are expecting a baby. At times like those, their minds are already preoccupied with other concerns and it then becomes extremely tough to deal with an HIV diagnosis as well. Ask them what they think now about the advantages and disadvantages of going for a test at a VCT centre, compared with being offered an HIV test when they are sick or pregnant. You could draw up the table below on another piece of flip-chart paper or on the ground and encourage them to use post-it stickers to write or draw key points on the table.

WHEN TO TEST			
Time of test	**Good points**	**Bad points**	**Conclusions**
No test at all			
Offer of test when attending e.g. TB clinic			
Offer of test when ill in hospital with any problem			
Offer of test when pregnant			
Going for VCT at a time of your own choice			

Next to this table, you also need **another chart**, where participants can place post-it stickers that voice their questions or concerns about the whole testing process, grouped according to similar themes.

Concerns which participants might express include: violence, fear of violence, isolation from friends and family, job loss, rejection by parents, rejection by children, no more children. It would be good to ask participants to remember these, so that they can be brought up again in later discussions. **Please also keep your own note of these concerns, for further reference.**

The hope is that participants' concerns will have already lessened during this session and will continue to reduce through the rest of the workshop. But it is important that the whole community addresses these concerns. It is likely that other peer groups will have similar concerns – and this may make it easier for all community members to support one another to overcome them.

EXERCISE F.3: DVD Clip 3: 'THE CONDOM'

AIM: To overcome embarrassment about condoms, through learning about them in a peer group.

DESCRIPTION: Watching DVD.

ITEMS NEEDED: DVD, laptop with DVD player, projector.

DIRECTIONS

1. Explain to participants that we are now going to watch a DVD clip about how different peer groups can learn about condoms and their use. Ask participants to stand up, have a good stretch, and move round to a new position so that they can all see the screen.

2. Explain that, after they have watched the DVD together, there will be a time for questions.

Make sure that everyone can see and hear the DVD clearly.

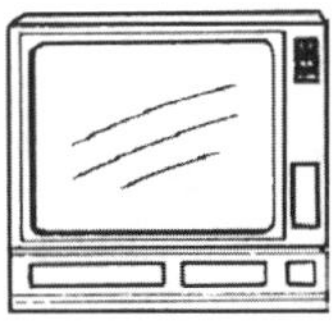

3. Turn on the DVD at the point where it says '3. The Condom'.

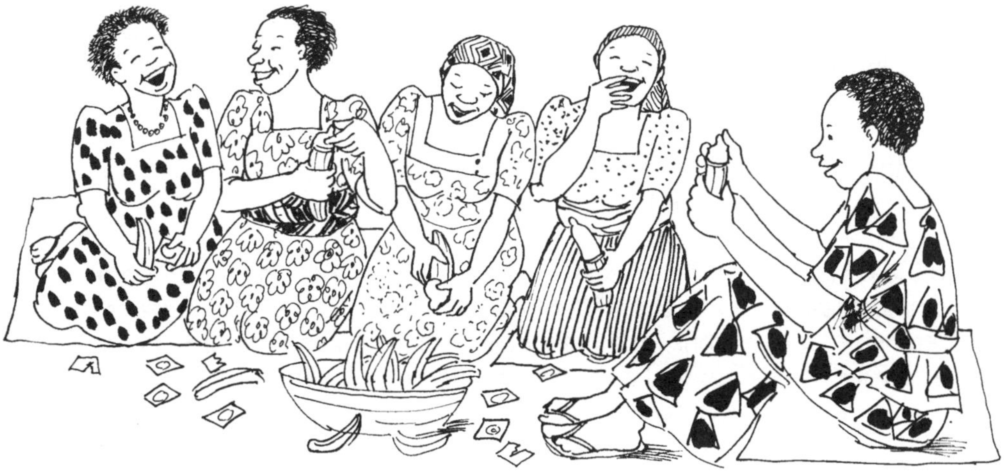

4. Turn off the DVD at the point where the screen goes black.[1]

5. Ask if anyone has any questions they would like to ask before you start the same exercise yourselves. If questions refer specifically to how to use a condom, explain that you are about to go through that with everyone.

> ☞ The main point of the DVD is to encourage people to overcome their embarrassment by showing how the people of Buwenda managed to learn about condoms. The DVD is not a comprehensive guide to how to use a condom: that is what you are going to look at together in the next exercise.

EXERCISE F.4: MALE CONDOMS DISCUSSION

AIMS: To show participants how to use a condom properly and to let them try for themselves on a model.

DESCRIPTION: This exercise enables participants who are interested in learning about condom usage to practise and discuss it openly together. You study some condoms together and discuss how to see if they're recently made, how to put one on, and how to dispose of it safely. Each participant has a go for him/herself.

MATERIALS NEEDED: Enough dildos, bananas, cassava or similar items for each participant to have one. Condoms, enough for a minimum of two each. A tube of K-Y jelly, or other locally available water-based lubricant or spermicide. If it is culturally unacceptable or not possible to use a banana for this exercise, think of something else of a similar shape which is easily available locally.

In many parts of the world, condoms are still not popular for various reasons. This was a problem faced in the Gambia. There, however, a very experienced Stepping Stones trainer, Mamadou Conteh, adopted a new approach. He filmed conversations that he had with local imams (Muslim religious leaders who are highly respected by their communities) about the benefits and challenges of using condoms as a part of a holistic response to HIV, and focused on the use of condoms as a means of protecting men against infertility. Most of the imams began by stating that they were against condoms, largely on religious grounds. But, after some time discussing the religious and health issues, the imams grew to accept that there is nothing in the Qur'an to ban condoms. The imams then agreed that they would not block condom distribution in their communities – and, in some cases, they agreed to become more active supporters of their use.

Then, with the permission of these same imams, Conteh took the video footage back to their communities and, with one of the imams present, played the footage to the village elders, so that they could see the whole discussion and the arguments laid out before them. Then the elders had a chance to talk further with the imam himself, and were able to see the imam's new position. Conteh and his staff team then launched the Stepping Stones workshop in the community, with successful acceptance and uptake of condom use.

DIRECTIONS

Sit in a circle with the participants and explain that you are now going to show one another how to use a condom. Throughout this whole exercise, encourage participants as much as possible to **tell one another the answers to your questions and their own**. Ask those who know something about condoms already to join in and share their knowledge with the others. Only provide the answer to a question yourself if no one knows it, or if you think the answer which has been given isn't accurate enough. This means that **most of the talking in this exercise should be by the participants, rather than you.**

This whole exercise needs to be conducted in such a way that every question leads to a good discussion. Encourage your participants to do as much of the asking and answering as possible – remember you are there just to prompt and guide, not to lead! There is a long list of possible questions below. You may not want to ask them all at one sitting, and you may find that many of them are asked by participants. The list of questions, and the appropriate information which follows each of them, is for your information. Note that some people may have had little knowledge of condoms before this exercise, and it may well need to be repeated two or three times, during or after this workshop, with a bit of new information added each time. As you encourage discussion of each question, produce some condoms in their sealed wrappings and hand them round, one for each participant, so that everyone has a chance to grow used to them. Also, encourage people to draw diagrams to share with one another, if they think this will help them to describe or understand things better. This may be quite a difficult session for some people. Humour helps! Try to keep it light, but make sure that everyone understands each stage.

THE QUESTIONS

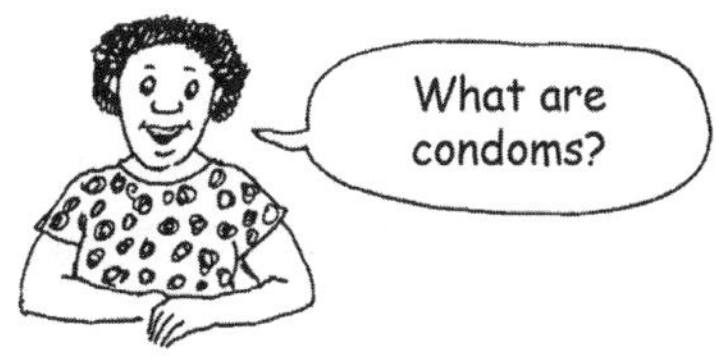

a) What are condoms?

They are made of rubber and are very strong. They are tested in the factory by being stretched and filled with water, to check that they are completely watertight. A condom is worn on a man's penis. A condom will stop his sperm or other fluids coming into contact with a woman's vaginal fluids. So she will not be able to get pregnant and, if either the man or the woman has a sexually transmitted infection, it cannot be passed between them. (*You could fill a condom carefully with water, to show its watertight qualities to everyone.*)

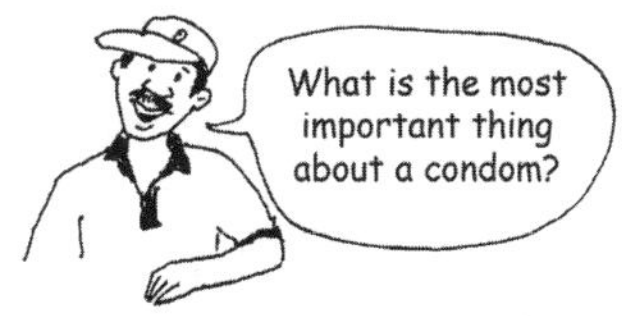

b) What is the most important thing about a condom?

To be sure you have one before you need it! (*Hold the condoms up.*)

c) What can you check about a condom from its packet?

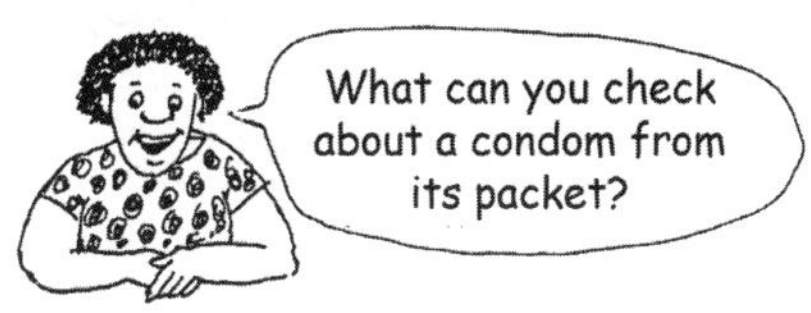

If you have a choice, choose pre-lubricated condoms that come in sealed wrappers and are packaged so that light does not reach them. (*Help everyone to feel how the condom feels lubricated inside the still-sealed wrapper.*) Also check that it is in date!

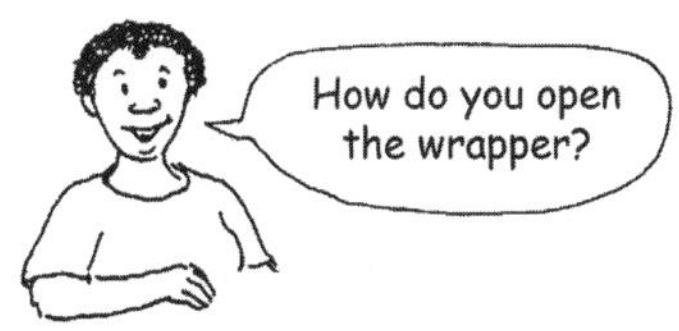

d) How do you open the wrapper?

Carefully, so that the condom does not tear. (*Encourage everyone to do this.*)

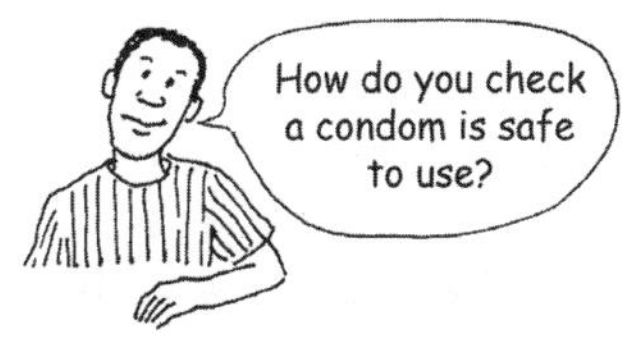

e) How do you check a condom is safe to use?

Look at the condom carefully and feel it to check that it is not discoloured, sticky, brittle, or damaged.' (*Encourage them to inspect it gently.*)

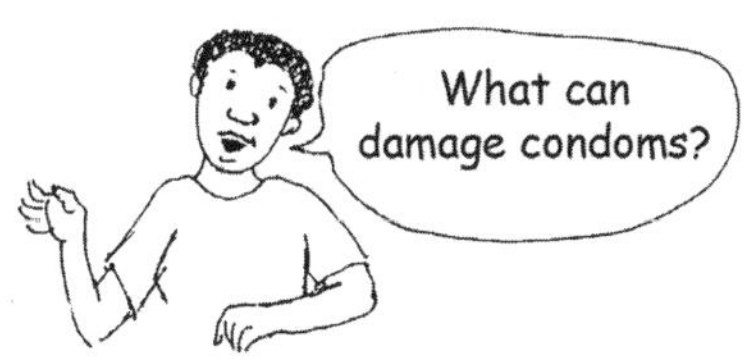

f) What can damage condoms?

Oil-based lubricants, such as Vaseline, damage condoms. Use **only water-based** ones such as KY jelly, glycerine, or spermicides. Lubricants may need to be used if the condoms have no lubricant themselves. However, if both partners make sure that the woman is properly aroused at the start, then her vagina may be moist enough and no extra lubrication will be needed. (*You may need to add an explanation about the importance of foreplay in enabling a woman to feel properly aroused here. For instance, participants may be unclear about the role of the clitoris in sexual arousal and sexual satisfaction for most women. However, it is important to stress that, during foreplay, the penis should not come into contact with the vagina. Also, show a tube of KY jelly, or other water-based lubricant if it is locally used or available.*)

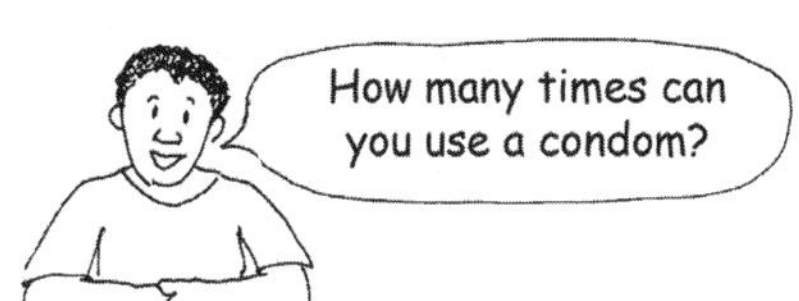

g) How many times can you use a condom?

Once only. Each time you have sex, you must use a new, unused condom on the penis before it enters the vagina or rectum.

h) When do you put the condom on?

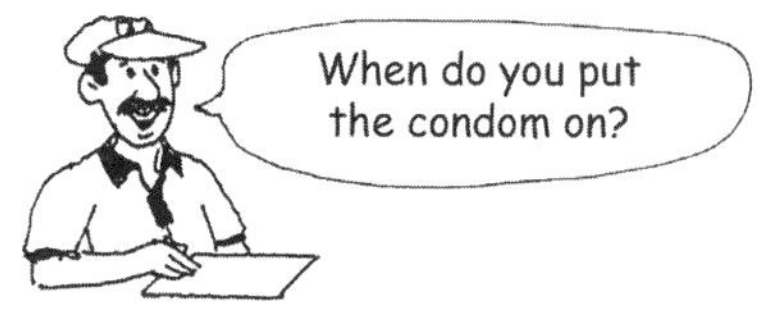

Only when the penis is erect. (*Produce a banana, suitable length of wood, dildo, cassava, or other similar item for each participant. Distribute them to the group, but ask them to wait before putting the condom on.*)

i) What do you do if the penis is uncircumcised?

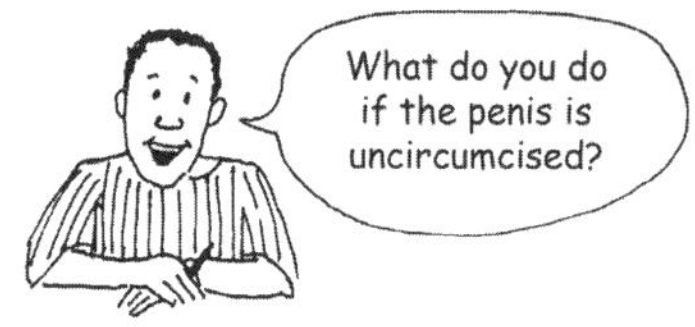

Pull the foreskin of the penis back before putting on the condom. (*If you have a dildo with loose skin, show how this can be done.*)

j) How do you put the condom on?

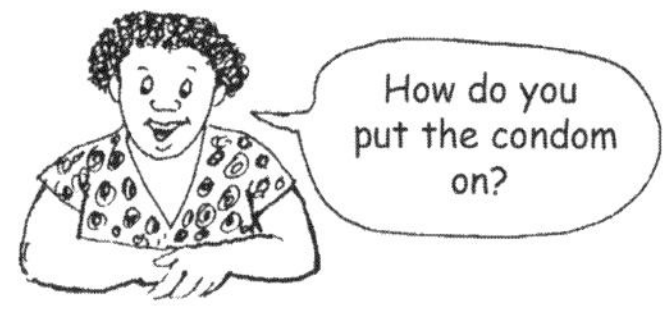

First pinch the top, closed, end of the condom. This leaves a small empty space, to hold the semen. Then unroll the condom down the length of the penis all the way to the base. (*Demonstrate this with your condom. Encourage everyone else to have a go.*) **NB** can participants identify what the facilitator did not do properly in the condom demonstration in the DVD?

k) Then you can enjoy yourselves! Many men find that they reach an orgasm before their partners have been satisfied. Condoms can help men to delay ejaculation Who can explain more what this means?

l) What happens if the condom tears during sex?

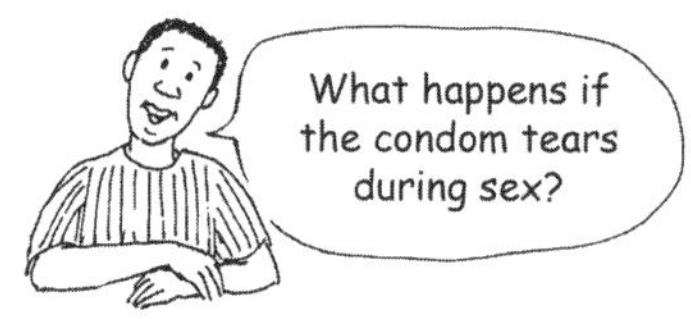

This is less likely to happen if the condom is good quality and if you have put it on properly. However, it does occasionally happen. The best thing to do is to withdraw the penis immediately and put on a new condom. Be careful with very vigorous prolonged sex — if the woman becomes dry, you can use more water-based lubricant or spermicide.

m) What do you do after ejaculation?

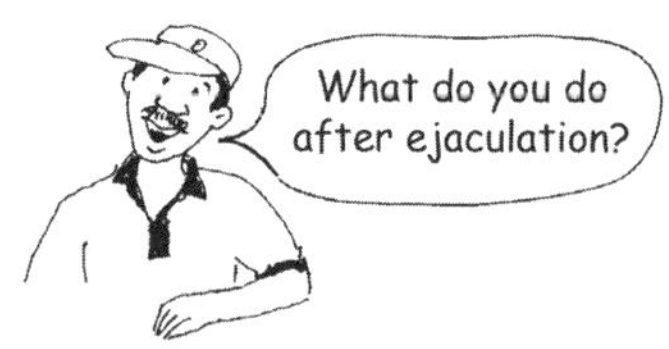

After ejaculation, before the penis goes soft, hold on to the bottom of the condom as you pull the penis out, so that the condom does not slip off, then take off the condom carefully without spilling semen. (*Demonstrate this and encourage participants to copy you.*)

n) How do you dispose of the condom?

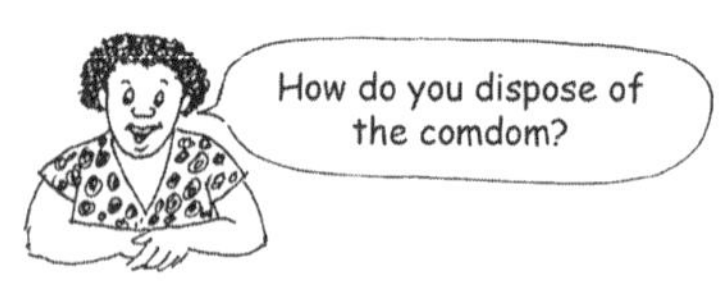

Wrap the condom in paper (such as newspaper) or in a piece of cloth or leaf until you can dispose of it in a toilet or pit latrine, or by burying or burning it. Condoms can damage some sewage treatment methods. Please check with your local services to make sure condoms can safely be put in toilets in this community. Then, if you wipe yourselves after sex, remember to use separate cloths. Condoms should be disposed of away from where children or animals can find them and play with them. Where is a suitable place here for you to dispose of them? (*Wrap up the condom in something easily available locally.*)

o) Where is the best place to store your other condoms?

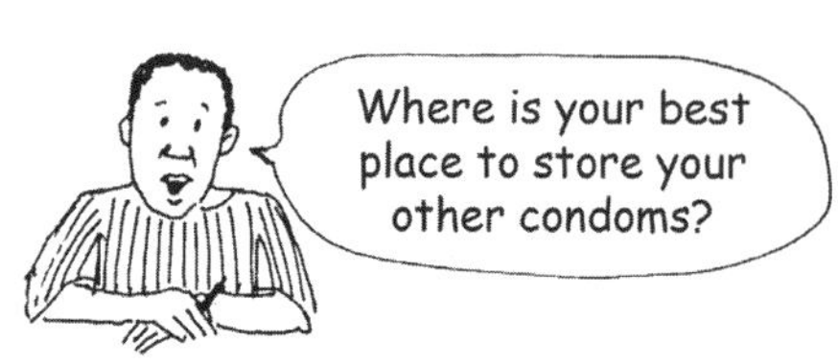

If possible, in a cool, dark, dry place. Heat, light and humidity can damage condoms. Where would be the best place for you to store condoms?

p) What else can a condom protect against?

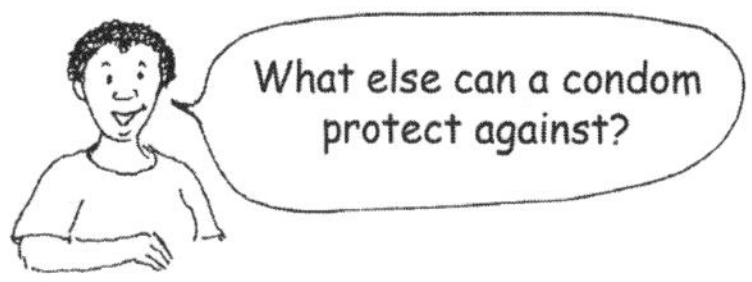

Condoms protect against all kinds of STIs, including gonorrhoea and syphilis. They also protect against unplanned pregnancy.

q) Did you ever imagine you would sit in a circle with your friends and learn how to use a condom?! (*Distribute more condoms for everyone to take away with them, if they like.*)

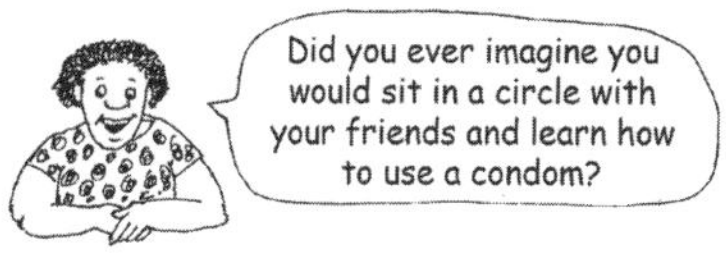

r) Any other questions? (*If you don't know the answers to some of the questions from the group, say you don't know and promise to find out for them, if they would like you to. It's much better to be honest than to give false information!*)

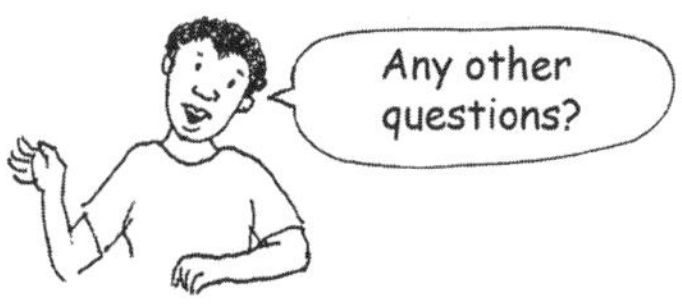

EXERCISE F.5: FEMALE CONDOMS DISCUSSION

Ideally, do this exercise too with all four peer groups.

AIMS: To show participants how to use a female condom properly and to let them try for themselves.

DESCRIPTION: This exercise enables participants who are interested in learning about female condom usage to practise and discuss it openly together. You study some female condoms together and discuss how to see if they're recently made, how to put one on and how to dispose of it safely. Each participant has a go for him/herself.

MATERIALS NEEDED: Female condoms in their wrappers, enough for a minimum of three each.

You will need to practise this exercise with your other facilitators before you do it with participants.

DIRECTIONS

Follow the instructions for the male condom exercise above, but this time help participants to understand everything about the female condom instead.

As with the male condom, pass the female condom around your peer group, so that everyone has the chance to see and feel both of them.

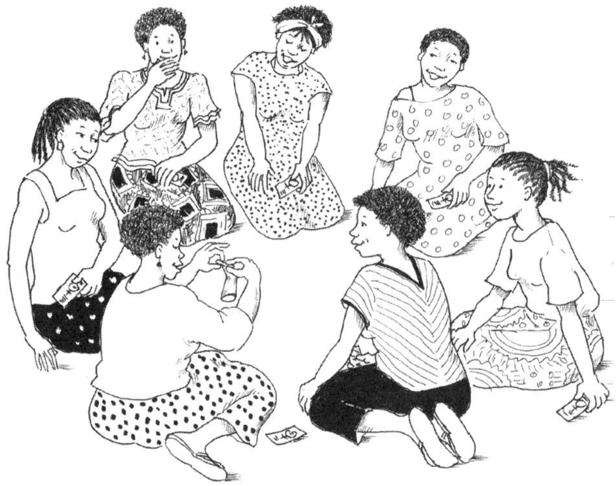

Points to consider with the female condom: Do the male condom exercise first, before the female condom exercise. Make sure that you remind participants to check the sell-by date and the packaging of a female condom, just as with the male condom. Here are some additional comments to add:

a) The female condom can be inserted before people start any sexual activity (even two or three hours in advance of any sexual contact), and must be inserted before penetrative sex starts. Many men find it easier to use than the male condom because they don't have to have an erection before putting it on since it goes inside the vagina (or anus[2]) and not on the penis.

b) The female condom covers a larger area of the body than the male condom, and therefore provides more protection for both partners. Since the larger ring of the female condom fits outside the woman's body, it can't get 'lost' inside. Show how this works by making a circle with your left thumb and middle finger and squeezing the inner, smaller ring of the female condom through the circle, to place it inside the 'vagina'. Then place the outer ring around the 'outer' side of the circle of your finger and thumb. Explain that the muscles in the walls of the vagina keep this outer ring in place outside the body.[3]

c) Once the female condom is placed inside the vagina, many people say that having penetrative sex feels closer to 'natural' sex than when using the male condom, for both partners.

d) Although it makes a crinkly noise to start with, which some people don't like, others find this sexy. This crinkly noise stops once the female condom has warmed up to body temperature.

e) The female condom is not made of latex, so people with allergies to the male condom can use it without problems. This also means that it is safe to use oil-based lubricants or massage oils with the female condom. This is not safe with the male condom, which can be damaged by oil.

f) Encourage participants to experiment for themselves, by giving each participant a female condom of their own, encouraging them to open it and practise inserting it through a hole made by their thumb and finger, as you have done.

Ask participants about local availability of both male and female condoms. If they want to get hold of them and don't know where to find them, see if you can help them to find suppliers, such as the local health clinic, pharmacy, shop, or market stallholder. In other communities where *Stepping Stones* has been used, each peer group has chosen someone in their group to become their condom supplier. Ask participants if they would like the same thing to happen here. Tell participants that they need to create a demand for condoms if they want them, and to bring this demand to the attention of the authorities. If condoms are not available, or are too expensive, the authorities need to hear that the demand is there in order for anything to change. Finish by giving each participant three female condoms if you can. (Research has shown that it's a good idea for people to try them on at least three occasions in order to get used to them.)

EXERCISE F.6: MALE CIRCUMCISION

AIM: To consider male circumcision as a strategy for protection of men and boys against acquiring HIV.

DESCRIPTION: Group discussion.

Male circumcision is an issue which raises strong emotions. If the participants are from a community where all males are circumcised, either at birth or around puberty, then this exercise should be compulsory in order to help everyone understand that male circumcision, while it has some benefits, is not a cure for HIV, nor does it offer total protection against HIV.

If the participants are from a community where male circumcision is not traditionally practised, participants should also be encouraged to do this exercise in order to help them understand more about what it can and can't do in relation to HIV. However, if participants are very resistant to the idea of male circumcision, don't force them to do this exercise.

Before you facilitate this exercise, you need, as usual, to discuss it thoroughly with your co-facilitators and to explore fully what male circumcision means to you in your own lives. You may come from a community where all males are circumcised and so, if you are a male, it is a part of your identity and, if you are a female, it is normal to have a sexual relationship only with a man who is circumcised. Or you may come from a community where no males are circumcised and so, if you are a male, it is a part of your identity not to be circumcised; and if you are a female, it is normal never to have a sexual relationship with a male who is circumcised. All of these attitudes are considered normal and natural in their respective communities so, as a facilitator, you need to respect the fact that your views may be very different from those of the participants in your group. There are no 'rights and wrongs' of male circumcision.

You also need to be clear that this exercise is about male circumcision only. No authority is suggesting that there are any health benefits associated with *female* 'circumcision'. (Indeed, female circumcision can cause serious, life-long genito-urinary and other health problems for many girls and women — including problems during and after childbirth.)

DIRECTIONS

1. First of all it will be useful to you to find out the participants' views about male circumcision in relation to their own community. Are they members of a community where male circumcision is the norm and you are not considered a proper member of this community, as a male, unless you are circumcised? If so, when are males circumcised? Is it at birth, age 6–8, puberty, or some other time? What ceremonies are associated with male circumcision in this community? What do participants see as the benefits of circumcision for the individual male and for the rest of the community? Why?

Alternatively, are they a community where the opposite is true and where male circumcision is definitely not practised? If so, would anyone there ever even consider male circumcision? If so, at what age? If not, why not?

Or is this community made up of some who have been circumcised and others who haven't? What factors decided who was circumcised and who wasn't? What benefits can people see in male circumcision? What benefits can people see in not being circumcised?

2. Next, it will be useful for you to explore with the participants what they already know about male circumcision in relation to HIV. Ask them: 'Who can tell me something about male circumcision and HIV?' Encourage everyone who wants to to say something about it. This will help you to understand more clearly what correct information people already have, and what information needs to be further discussed and explained, so that everyone understands accurately what male circumcision can and can't do for their whole community.

3. When you have spent some time exploring the two questions above with your participants, you will have a much clearer idea of what their views are and will be able to shape the rest of the exercise more effectively. Now encourage people to listen to the following as you read it out to them. **Try to read this quite a few times to yourself beforehand**, so that you are familiar with what it says and feel more comfortable about reading it out.

After each paragraph, check if the participants have understood what you have read, and ask if they have any questions for clarification. If you think the answer is coming up further ahead, then just ask them to remember their question and ask it again later if they still feel they haven't had a full answer.

Read this out:

MALE CIRCUMCISION: *Research has shown that men who have been medically circumcised are up to 60% less likely to acquire HIV after sex with a woman living with HIV than men who are not circumcised. Voluntary male medical circumcision programmes are now widespread, especially in resource-poor countries where HIV prevalence is high and circumcision prevalence is low, mainly in sub-Saharan Africa.*

This exercise is to help everyone understand more about this procedure and to explore its many dimensions for ourselves. Here are some common concerns which people have raised.

a) **Medical risk to males:** *Circumcision carries the risk of bleeding and infections. Although the formal research studies were conducted under very high quality supervision, there were still some men who bled from the wound after the operation or developed wound infections with delayed healing.*

- *What local healthcare provision is there here? How well are staff trained to carry out male circumcision and look after the man or boy if things go wrong?*

- *What would be the consequences for a man's family if he were to get sick after the operation?*

It is really important for a man or boy to be circumcised by an experienced practitioner who uses sterile techniques. Otherwise there is a risk of bleeding from the wound and infection. Circumcision of boys when they are babies also needs to be conducted under sterile conditions. There do seem to be fewer complications when boys are circumcised as infants,

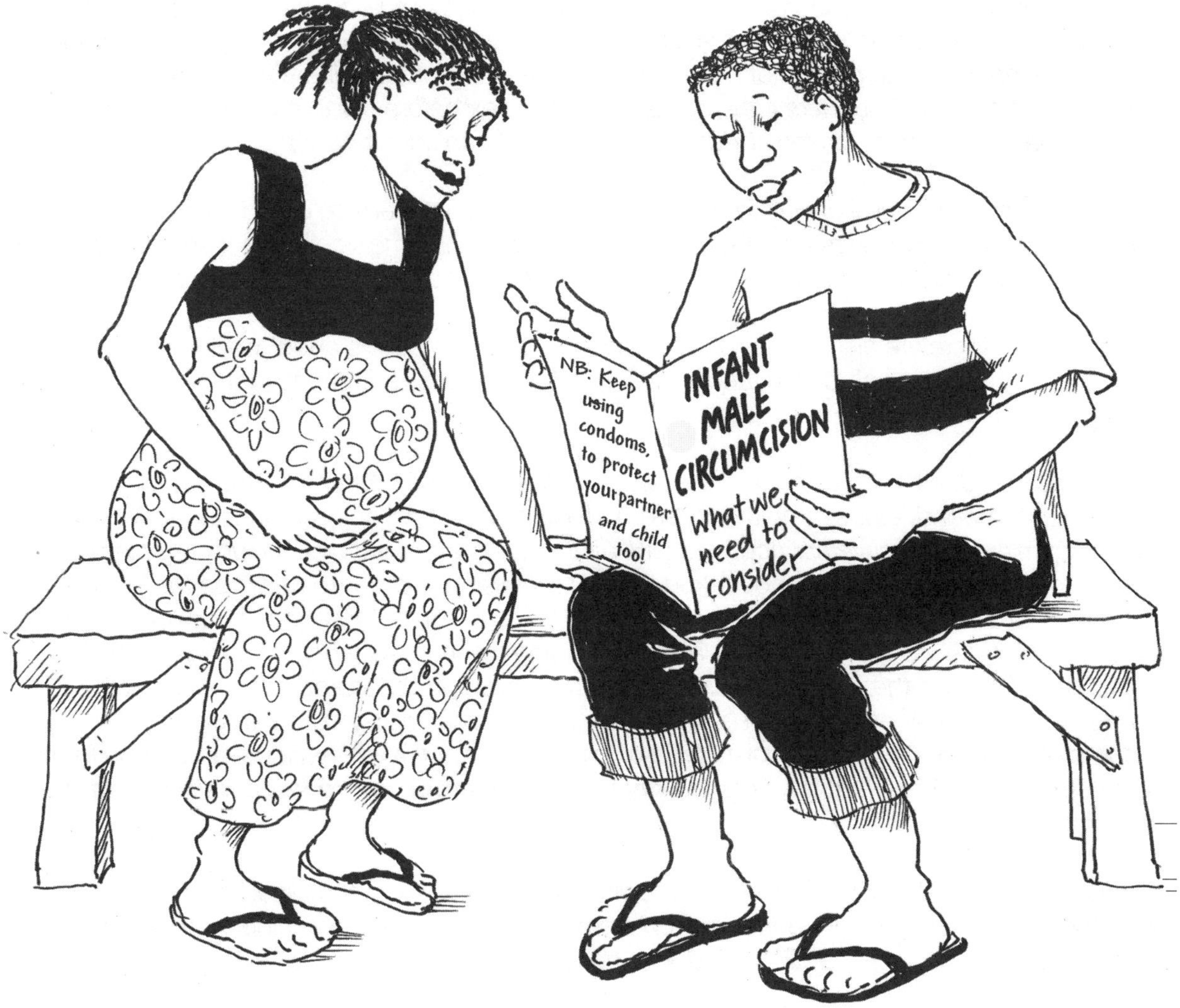
NB: Keep using condoms, to protect your partner and child too!
INFANT MALE CIRCUMCISION
what we need to consider

rather than when they are older. But if a baby boy has acquired HIV at birth, being circumcised will not cure the HIV. So all women with HIV need to be given proper care and support during their pregnancies and after the birth, in order to minimise the risk of HIV transmission at birth. (Many exercises later in this volume address how they can do this.)

Many traditional male circumcision ceremonies are conducted by a respected older man in the community who uses one knife, which has been used for many generations, to cut all the boys' or men's foreskins. But in this time of HIV, what was traditionally seen as a strong and powerful symbol of brotherhood and connection between peers and across generations can actually itself contribute to the spread of HIV. So it is really important, even in these traditional male circumcision ceremonies, to ensure that each boy or man is circumcised by the elder with a clean, sharp blade which is used only on him to avoid contracting HIV or other blood-borne conditions from others' blood, and to avoid passing anything to others through his blood.

Fit teenage boys, when circumcised traditionally, are kept in seclusion from their family for a good month to six weeks after the procedure, are fed on nourishing food and given a lot of rest until the wound heals. This is all for good reasons – it gives the wound time to heal properly and those circumcised can fully recover their health and energy.

b) ***Medical risk to females:*** *Reducing the number of men acquiring HIV would mean that, in the longer term, fewer women also would be exposed to HIV and this would also be something to celebrate. However, it is not yet clear how women fit into the story. This is unfortunate, since men mostly have sex with women, so women have to be part of the story. Although the WHO/*

UNAIDS guidelines on male circumcision agree that male circumcision is a complex issue, no-one yet knows for sure what the real challenges are going to be. But one study in Uganda has suggested that circumcision of males who already have HIV can increase the risk of passing the virus to their sexual partners if the couples resume sex before the circumcision wound is totally healed. (This usually takes about six weeks, but it can take longer.)[4]

It seems clear that the level of HIV prevalence in the population needs to go down quite a lot before women will experience any direct benefits from male circumcision. Even then, a woman will not benefit from male circumcision if the man already has HIV and if they don't use a condom.

4. Explain that there are also key issues in relation to people's beliefs about what male circumcision can and can't do for them which need to be explored, because there is a lot of wrong information around. For example:

a) Circumcision does not give a man total protection against HIV. There are many men throughout the world – for example, in Muslim, Jewish and Christian communities – who have been circumcised and have still acquired HIV. All the normal precautions, including male or female condom use, still need to be taken after circumcision in order to minimise the risk of acquiring HIV or of passing it on to others. In fact, if a man could only choose between using a male – or female – condom properly and having unprotected sex when circumcised, he would be safer using the condom, which provides on average 90% protection – for both partners – against HIV and other STIs and unplanned pregnancy. By contrast, being circumcised but not using a condom can provide only up to 60% protection – and this is for him alone, not for his female partner. ***This is why it is really important to keep using condoms after circumcision.***

It is perhaps helpful to think of male circumcision and condom use combined as similar to travelling in a car. People can reduce the chances of getting hurt in an accident by wearing a seat belt and by keeping at a low speed. But even with both these precautions, people still get badly injured or killed in accidents. Neither the seat belt nor the low speed, even if combined, cuts out all risk. And when travelling by car, it is always much better if the driver and all the passengers involved talk with one another along the way, to make sure the driver stays awake, to make sure everyone's seat belt is fitted properly, to agree on the best route, and to avoid potholes in the road, low overhanging trees, stray goats and chickens ... A journey shared is not only safer for all, but also more enjoyable for all – just like life. So the question of male circumcision is also one better discussed and agreed amongst all those concerned, so that everyone can enjoy the journey together and reach their destination safely.

b) Male circumcision is also not a cure for HIV. If a man or boy already has HIV, he is not going to stop having HIV once he has been circumcised. Therefore he and his partners need to go on making sure that condoms are being used during sex, to minimise the risk of his passing HIV to others. In fact, WHO guidelines recommend that it is better for any man who is considering circumcision to be tested for HIV before going ahead with the operation. But many do not agree with these guidelines because they feel that any man should have the right to be circumcised, if he would like to be, irrespective of his HIV status. (It is worth knowing that circumcision can also offer men some protection against other sexually transmitted infections, so that is a reason why males with HIV should be circumcised if they want to be.)

c) As mentioned above, studies have shown that, if a man has sex with a woman before the wound is fully healed, and if he already has HIV, the woman is more likely to acquire HIV through blood from the unhealed wound. These are all issues which a man needs to consider and discuss with those around him before he opts to be circumcised.

d) A study in Kenya in 2007 showed that, of 90,000 men tested in 15,000 households, 13.9% of uncircumcised males had HIV, whereas only 4.3% of circumcised males had HIV. However, 'cross-sectional prevalence' data, as this is called, is not proof that being circumcised is what protected these males from HIV: many other behaviours, such as having fewer sexual partners before a certain age, might be associated with the practice of circumcision amongst those tested. The difficulty is that, while they are often well funded, scientific medical studies do not necessarily include the social science dimension – especially the gender-specific social science dimension – of the issue. When gender-specific social science studies are also conducted, the findings normally reveal a much more complex picture than do the purely medical results.

*e) In several parts of the world, male circumcision is now becoming freely available through the health services. However, do remember that you still need all the other health services that you had previously – and which are your right. If you find other services might be suffering, it would be good to call a meeting with your local political or community representatives, to see what can be done to make sure that **existing** service levels for **other** health issues are maintained alongside the new male circumcision services.*

5. This is a lot of information to take in! A useful way of getting participants to summarise the points is to consider the case of an adult man who is thinking of being circumcised. The questions below cover some of the things he needs to think about. Ask participants to talk about their views on each one, then see if they can add others of their own for the group to discuss.

- Who is going to pay for the operation? Has the man planned ahead financially to cover all the expenses involved?
- Do the participants think being circumcised should be a confidential issue for an individual or not? If not, why not?
- Has the man discussed his plan to be circumcised with his wife or partner, or with other family members (such as his sisters or mother), and worked out who will look after him and nurse him until he is better?
- How will he raise the subject with women in his family if it is taboo to talk about such things with them?
- Does he have the capacity to take time off work?
- Can he and his wife or partner take time off work together to go for couple counselling beforehand?
- Does his partner/sister/mother have time to look after him? What will her workplace say if she needs time off work?

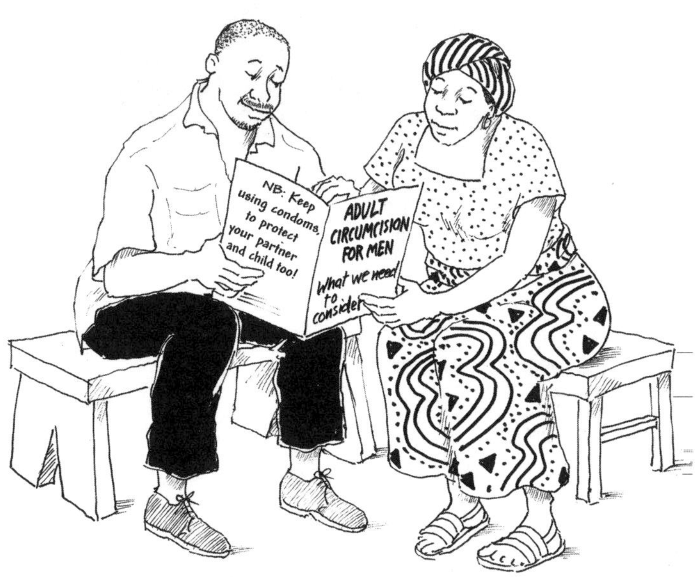

NB: Keep using condoms to protect your partner and child too!
ADULT CIRCUMCISION FOR MEN
What we need to consider

- Does he have access to painkillers?
- After the operation, he must then ensure that he waits until the wound is fully healed – and then, ideally, another two weeks – until he has sex again with anyone. He should then use – and continue to use – a male or female condom with all his partners.

6. After all this, ask participants what they think they would like to do in their own community. Would they like to continue with male circumcision as they already do it traditionally? What changes will need to be made to the traditional ceremony to make it medically safe? If they don't already do it, would they now want to consider introducing it for baby boys, or for young men, or older men? Or all three? Explore options with the participants. The important thing is for them to be aware of the facts about the issue as they are known so far – and for them then to make up their own minds about whether or not to change anything in their community.

7. Lastly, encourage participants to talk about what they have learnt and discussed with their partners or other family members, neighbours or work-place colleagues but for them not to reveal anyone's personal details. This issue needs to be discussed carefully across the community, so that everyone understands the full picture about what male circumcision can – and can't – offer in an effective response to the HIV pandemic.

EXERCISE F.7: CATCH UP TIME (optional)

AIM: **To enable participants to ask and discuss more questions regarding HIV, condoms, and other issues to do with sexual health and safer sex.**

DESCRIPTION: **A general discussion.**

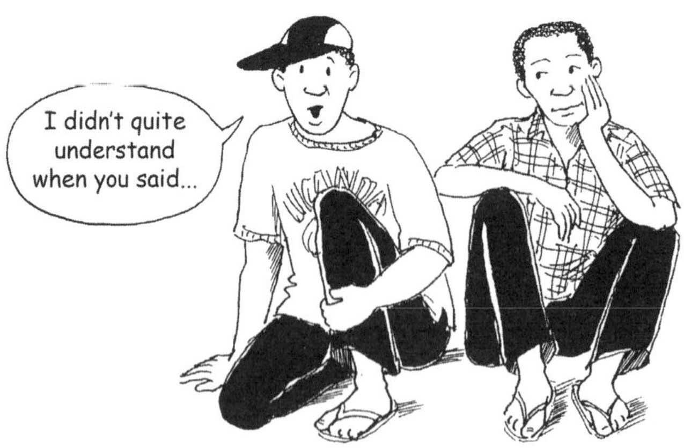

DIRECTIONS

1. Ask participants if they have thought of any questions since the previous session that they would like to ask or to discuss with other participants.

2. Remember to encourage participants themselves to provide answers for one another as much as possible. Only join in if asked to, or if you think there is a need for more accurate information to be provided. Remember to encourage the use of drawings to help people explain ideas to one other.

3. When you feel that participants' interests are flagging, move on to the last exercise of this session.

EXERCISE F.8: ONE NEW THING

AIM: Winding-down exercise.

DESCRIPTION: Everyone sits in a circle and shares one new thing which they have learnt.

DIRECTIONS

1. Explain that this has been a session with a lot of new information. Say that you would now like to bring the session to a close with a reminder of how much knowledge and experience we already have to share among ourselves.

2. Ask the participant to your right to share with the group something they have learnt beginning 'One new thing which I have learnt today is ...' Then ask the next person to speak. Go round the circle, finishing with yourself, so that everyone has made a contribution.

3. Remind everyone of their role as guardian angel.

4. Encourage participants actively to talk about the issues they have been discussing in these sessions with their friends and neighbours, but not to share any confidential information from the peer group with others.

5. Remember to ask for three volunteers to stay behind for a quick session review. (See Annex 4 for details.)

6. Finish off by thanking everyone once more for coming to this session. **Remind participants of a local place where people can go for individual counselling, or counselling and testing, if they would like it (if this service is available in your area).** Arrange a mutually convenient time and place for the next session before saying goodbye.

FACILITATORS' TEAM FEEDBACK

After the end of Session F, meet again with your co-facilitators, to compare notes on how your sessions went and the information which you learnt from them. Your co-facilitators could have found useful information that could help you to structure your next session more effectively. Remember, however, not to share individual confidentialities between groups. This is the easiest way to ruin the trust that you have begun to build and to wreck the whole workshop!

ENDNOTES

1. Participants may want to view the DVD clip again. If so, it is usually best for them to have some discussion about it first, then to have a further discussion after the second viewing.
2. **NB** the female condom can also be used for anal sex by both men and women and by men who have sex with men.

3. If you want to use further illustrations, you can access them on the Female Condom website (Female Health Company 2013).
4. See also an article entitled 'What do you Mean I've Got to Wait for Six Weeks?!' (Toefy et al 2015) Read WHO's webpages about male circumcision to learn more about it (WHO 2015c).

REFERENCES

Female Health Company (2013) *FC2 Single Use Only*, The Female Health Company, London, <http://www.femalecondom.org/wp-content/uploads/2015/01/FC2-generic-instructie-leaflet-highres-for-download.pdf> [accessed 7 November 2015]

Toefy, Y. Skinner, D. and Thomsen, S. (2015) "What do You Mean I've Got to Wait for Six Weeks?!" Understanding the Sexual Behaviour of Men and Their Female Partners after Voluntary Medical Male Circumcision in the Western Cape', *PLOS ONE*, 2015: 10(7) at, <http://www.ncbi.nlm.nih.gov/pubmed/26176946> [accessed 7 November 2015]

WHO (2015c) *Voluntary medical male circumcision for HIV prevention in 14 priority countries in East and Southern Africa: Progress brief*, WHO, Geneva, <http://www.who.int/hiv/pub/malecircumcision/brief2015/en/> [accessed 7 November 2015]

YOUR NOTES ...

THEME 3 – WHY WE BEHAVE IN THE WAYS WE DO

SESSION G OUR OPTIONS

PURPOSE

To consider different choices which we may have in our lives.

CONTENTS	TIME NEEDED
Introduction	
G.1	Spider's Web
G.2	Possible Futures (this is a long exercise)
G.3	**DVD Clip 4:** 'Hopes and Fears: The Young Women'
G.4	**DVD Clip 5:** 'Hopes and Fears: The Young Men'
G.5	Jungle
G.6	If I Were an Animal

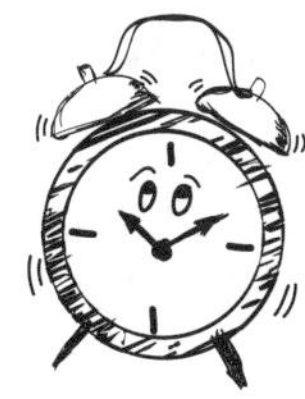

3–4 hours

MATERIALS NEEDED: Ball of string, DVD, laptop with DVD player, projector.

PARTICIPANTS: Four separate peer groups.

SPECIAL INFORMATION

- Don't forget to read 'Before You Begin ...!' before using this section of the manual.
- The meeting after this one will be the first full workshop meeting. This will involve only members of the four peer groups: nobody else. This needs to be explained to everybody.
- You need to make sure that all four peer groups have completed all the sessions up to and including this session, before they hold the first full workshop meeting. See the notes about the workshop duration in 'Before You Begin ...!' for a further explanation of this.
- You also need to liaise between the four peer groups to arrange a convenient time and place for the first full workshop meeting and Session H after it.

INTRODUCTION

1. Sit in a circle with the group, preferably on the ground. Everyone should be at the same level, including yourself.

2. Welcome everyone to the new session. Thank everyone for coming. Enquire about late-comers or non-attenders.

3. Ask each participant to recount quickly something good which has happened to them since the last session.

4. Review the last session. Ask participants to remind us what we learnt then – about HIV, condom use, testing ... Remind them if they have forgotten.

5. Explain that we are going on to discuss other things in this session but will start, as usual, with a game.

EXERCISE G.1: SPIDER'S WEB

AIMS: Energiser. To remind everyone that they are each an important part of the group.

DESCRIPTION: A ball of string is unravelled and held taut by everyone, like a spider's web.

MATERIALS NEEDED: Ball of string.

DIRECTIONS

1. Make sure everyone is sitting in a circle. Produce a big ball of string. Hold on to the end of the string, then roll it across the ground to someone sitting opposite you, saying his/her name as you roll it to him/her. Keep holding on to your end, tightly.

2. Ask the recipient to hold on to the string so that it makes a taut line on the ground between you both. Then ask him/her to roll the ball back across the circle, along the ground, to someone else, saying that new person's name as it rolls to him/her.

3. Everyone keeps on with this, until the circle is full of taut criss-crossing lines. Each person should be holding on tightly to a bit of string. The ball of string should finally be rolled back to you, so that you hold the beginning and the end of the string.

4. Next ask everyone to look at how the string connects you all, like a spider's web. You are all dependent on one another to keep this web firm and supported. If anyone were to take their hand away from the web, that part of it would collapse.

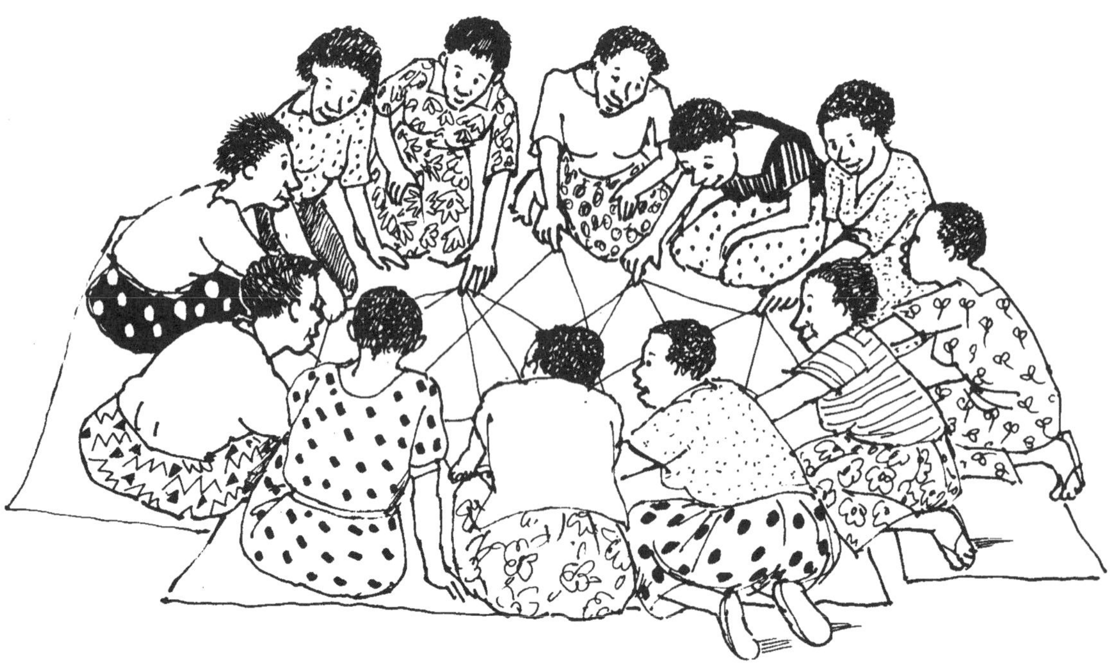

5. Ask people to suggest how this spider's web exercise relates to our real lives.

6. After a few comments, ask everyone to let go of the string. Gather it up in a loose pile so that it can be rewound later. Ask everyone to think about our dependence on one another – and our need to support one another – during the course of today's session.

EXERCISE G.2: POSSIBLE FUTURES

AIM: To help participants think about different possible futures for themselves.

DESCRIPTION: Using tableaux,[1] and role play, participants develop two possible future scenarios for a typical person like themselves in their own community. One is what they consider to be their most likely future, the other a less likely, and perhaps more hopeful, future. The aims of this are to encourage participants to think about the possibilities of a better future, and visualise what that means. The process of doing this can lead participants to an assessment of the choices they have in their own lives, and empower them to see that they can change the direction of their lives.

DIRECTIONS

1. Divide participants in your peer group into three small groups. Ask each group to make up a character based on a mixture of themselves and of the same gender and similar age. Give her/him a name. Point out that this should not be a real person, but rather someone made up by them, who is similar to themselves. (If it were a real person, this could be hurtful to them.)

2. Ask each group to think about this imaginary person, and work out a story, describing him or her, using the following questions:

- How does s/he behave at present?
- What do they think his/her future holds, if s/he continues to behave in exactly the same way as s/he has until now?
- What do they see as the likely progression of his/her life?
- What will his/her relationships with his/her friends, partner(s), and children be like?
- What will s/he achieve in his/her life?
- Who will s/he be living with?
- Will s/he have any income? If so, from what kind of work?

In Buwenda, one of the small groups in the older women's peer group thought up a story about a woman like them, who was preparing to leave her husband and children, take a few belongings, and return to her parents' home. The women said that, if it was not for the fate of their children, many of themselves would have already done this.

3. After discussion, each group creates a tableau which gives a frozen visual representation of their ideas about their imaginary character's likely future. They will need to decide where they are placing the character and so on. Is s/he at home? In a bar? On the streets? With friends?

They do not need the tableau to show every idea they have had. The tableau is merely a summing-up of their general understanding about what their character's future looks like.

For example, if the group consider that s/he is likely to end up penniless, having to beg for money, their tableau could show him/her on the street in a city, begging. The tableau will not necessarily explain why s/he is there – it is up to the audience (i.e. the other groups – see 6 below) to find that out at the end by questioning the participants. Alternatively, the group may want to show what made him/her turn to begging, in which case they could, for instance, present instead a tableau of him/her being thrown out of home for some reason.

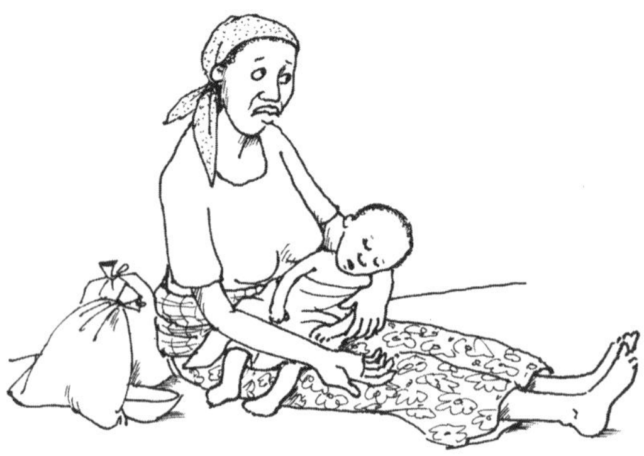

Members of the group take up positions in the tableau, with someone taking the imaginary character's position. Encourage the group to use as many members as possible in the scene. If their perception of the character's future is that s/he is totally alone, and no-one else comes into the picture at all, they could still use people representing the family and friends s/he has lost – by placing them standing apart from him/her and looking away, for example.

In Buwenda, the small group described above created their own tableau of the woman leaving home, by showing her standing in the middle of a crowd of people. She was looking miserable and had one hand held to her head, which was piled high with her few clothes and belongings. The crowd around her represented her children and other relatives and friends. They were tugging at her clothes and were looking very sad, silently begging her not to leave them. The woman's husband was absent from the scene.

4. Participants then move on to prepare a second tableau. They stay in the same small groups. The second tableau of each group will be a representation of the future that their imaginary character could have if s/he changed direction. The group need to think about what could happen if their character stopped behaving in the way s/he is at present.

- What could his/her relationship with his/her partner(s), friends, and children be like?
- How could they be treating each other? What would happen to these relationships if their imaginary character behaved differently?
- What kind of work could s/he have? What kind of home life?

Encourage each group to think about a future for their imaginary character which is hopeful and fulfilling. Discourage them from discussing too much how their partner(s) need to change: this exercise should be focusing on the imaginary character who is like themselves!

In Buwenda, the older women then created a new tableau, where the same woman now looked happy and contented. She was resting and being looked after by her family, while her husband was milking the animals.

5. Each group then creates a tableau which sums up these ideas. For example, they could hope that their imaginary character gets on well with everyone, has a safe source of income, and is respected. A tableau of this could show him/her at home with his/her family and friends. The group would then decide what the imaginary character is doing in the scene and how to show the rest of the family relating to her/him in a way which shows that they are getting on well with each other.

6. When all the groups have practised their two tableaux and are ready (after about half an hour), get the first of your three small groups to show their two tableaux to the rest of the peer group.

To start off with, the small group shows the two tableaux it has prepared straight after each other, without making any comments. Once the audience has seen both tableaux, they have an opportunity to ask questions.

The **aim** of this questioning is to explore the ideas which the tableaux express, and for the participants to clarify anything they are not sure about. The participants in the tableau being considered can either stay in position while the questioning is going on, and answer from the perspective of the person whose role they have taken on or, if they would rather, they can come out of the tableaux and answer as themselves.

Encourage everyone to think about the differences between the likely future and the possible future for the imaginary person at the centre of the tableau.

Here are some useful lead questions:

- What kind of things would their imaginary character have to do to make sure that his/her life didn't follow the less fruitful path?
- What difficulties would s/he be likely to encounter?
- What do the participants think would make the character want to change the direction of his/her life?

In Buwenda, one of the older women actors in the second tableau was asked by the audience what she was doing. She said: 'I am a child of this family, taking a cup of tea to my father. We are now happy and contented as a family because my parents are now cooperating so well in the household work …'

7. Each of the other two small groups then takes it in turns to have 30 minutes or so to present their two tableaux to the others and to have a discussion along the lines described above.

8. For the last stage of this exercise, all participants together take a few minutes to consider each imaginary character in turn.

What one first step could s/he take which would take her/him off the path s/he is on and lead her/him in a new direction?

The only rule for the first step for any of the imaginary characters is that it must be something specific and practical which can actually be tried out.

For example, the first step for a male character may be that he offers his wife some money for herself from his earnings.

The first step for a female character may be that she and other women form a group to generate income which they themselves keep.

If the participants make general suggestions like 'S/he's just got to change her/his attitude', help to turn it into something specific and practical by asking questions. For instance, how would we know that she had changed her attitude? What would we see her doing?

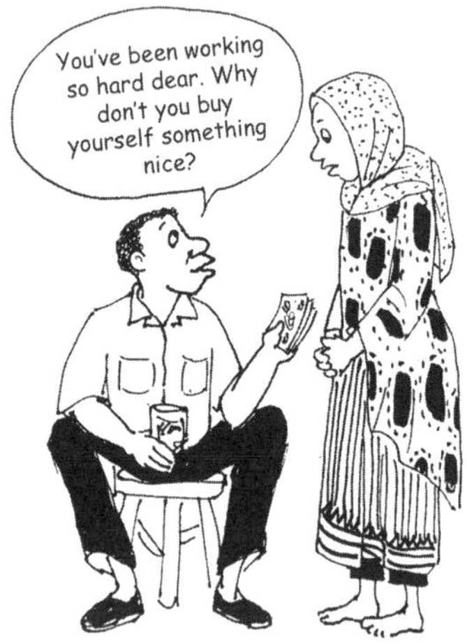
You've been working so hard dear. Why don't you buy yourself something nice?

9. Finally, explain that the next time you will meet will be at the first full workshop meeting, where members of other peer groups will also be present. At this meeting, each peer group is going to have an opportunity to present one set of two tableaux to the other peer groups.

Explain that there will not, unfortunately, be time for every small group to present their two tableaux. Therefore each peer group is being asked to select one set of tableaux to present to the other peer groups.

Ask participants to decide for themselves now which small group's work they would like to show to the other peer groups. Suggest that they choose the one which feels most representative to them of the kind of concerns which most of the peer group members face.

Participants may feel nervous about presenting their tableaux in front of members of other peer groups. However, encourage them by reminding them that every peer group has been working on the same exercises as their own. Also, every group will be feeling equally nervous!

EXERCISE G.3: DVD Clip 4: 'HOPES AND FEARS: The Young Women'

AIM: To explore possible futures for the young women in our communities.

DESCRIPTION: Watching the DVD clip, followed by a group discussion.

MATERIALS NEEDED: DVD, laptop with DVD player, projector.

DIRECTIONS

1. Explain to participants that we are now going to watch a DVD clip about two young women in Buwenda. Ask participants to stand up, have a good stretch, and move around to a new position so that they can all see the screen.

2. Say that while they are watching the clip, you would like them to think about how the situations of these two young women in Buwenda compare with those of young women in their own community.

- If they are older men or women, they could think of their own daughters or younger sisters.
- If they are younger men, they could think of their girlfriends, or wives, or sisters.
- If they are younger women, they can think of themselves!

3. Explain that there will be a chance to talk about what they have seen after they have watched the DVD.

Make sure that everyone can see and hear the DVD clearly.

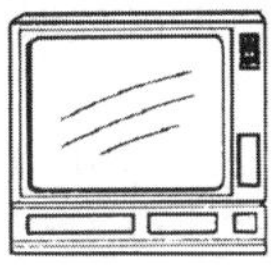

4. Turn on the DVD at the point where it says '4. Hopes and Fears: The Young Women'.

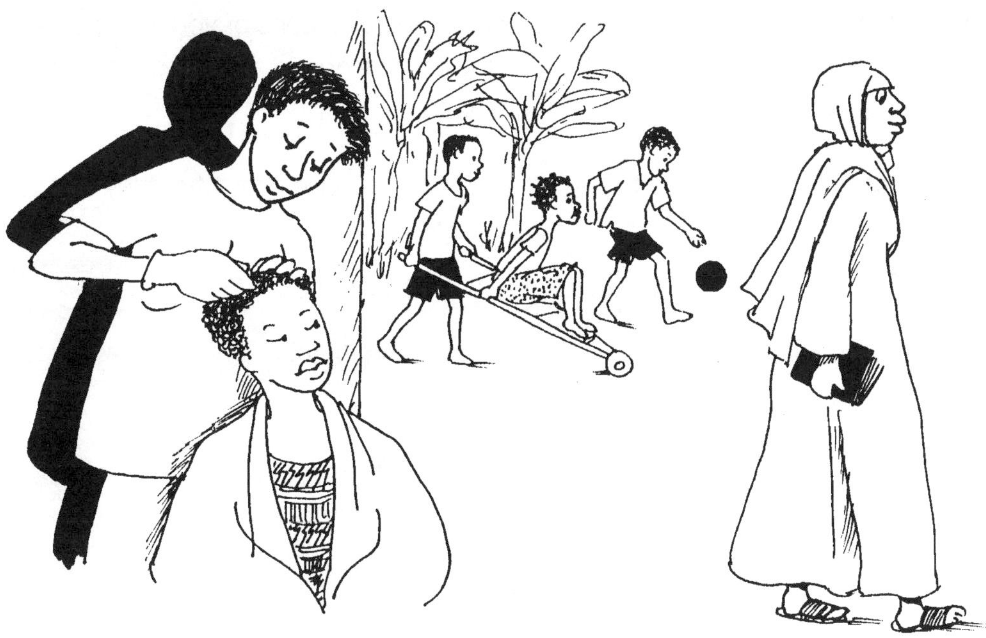

5. Turn off the DVD at the point where the screen goes black.

6. Next, ask participants the following four questions:

- Can they summarise the hopes and difficulties or fears of each of the two young women from Buwenda?[2]
- In what ways are the situations of these young women relevant to their sexual health?
- What are the hopes and fears of young women in your **own** community? In what ways do you think they are similar to or different from those of the young women in Buwenda?
- Can you suggest what could be done in your own community to improve the future for young women?[3]

EXERCISE G.4: DVD Clip 5: 'HOPES AND FEARS: The Young Men'

AIM: To explore possible futures for the young men in our communities.

DESCRIPTION: Watching the DVD clip, followed by a group discussion.

MATERIALS NEEDED: DVD, laptop with DVD player, projector.

DIRECTIONS

1. Explain to participants that we are now going to watch a DVD clip about two young men in Buwenda. Ask participants to stand up, have a good stretch, and move around to a new position so that they can all see the screen.

2. Say that while they are watching the clip, you would like them to think about how the situations of these two young men in Buwenda compare with those of young men in their own community.

- If they are older men or women, they could think of their own sons or younger brothers.
- If they are younger women, they could think of their boyfriends, or husbands, or brothers.
- If they are younger men, they can think of themselves!

3. Explain that there will be a chance to talk about what they have seen after they have watched the DVD.

Make sure that everyone can see and hear the DVD clearly.

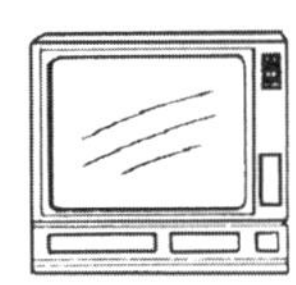

4. Turn on the DVD at the point where it says '5. Hopes and Fears: The Young Men'.

5. Turn off the DVD at the point where the screen goes black.

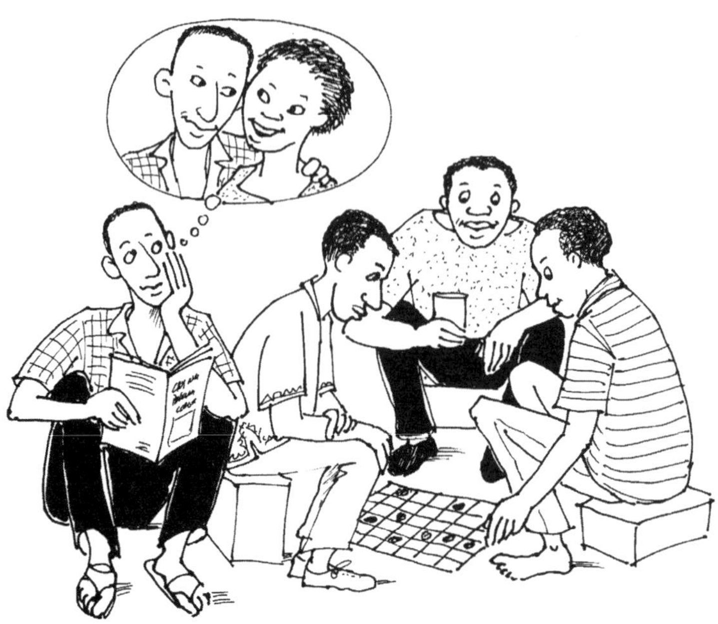

6. Next, ask participants the following four questions:

- Can they summarise the hopes and difficulties or fears of each of the two young men from Buwenda?
- In what ways are the situations of these young men relevant to their sexual health?
- What are the hopes and fears of young men in your own community? In what way do you think they are similar to or different from those of the young men in Buwenda?
- Can you suggest what could be done in your own community to improve the future for young men?

EXERCISE G.5: JUNGLE

AIM: **To lighten the mood. To energise everyone with laughter and movement.**

DESCRIPTION: **Variation on 'Fruit Salad', but with three animal names instead of fruit names!**

DIRECTIONS

See exercise C.1 for details.

EXERCISE G.6: IF I WERE AN ANIMAL

1. Ask each person in turn in the circle to say 'One thing I have learnt from today's session is ...'; and 'If I were an animal, I would like to be a ... because it is ... Start with yourself.

2. This should be quite a quick game. Encourage participants not to spend too long on their choice.

3. As a going-home exercise, you could ask participants to reflect on their choice of animal, on the basis of what they have learnt at these sessions. Ask them to think at home about whether they would like to be another animal instead of or as well as, the one each of them has just chosen.

4. Finish off by thanking everyone once more for coming to this session. Remind them that the next time you meet will be at the first full workshop meeting, where each peer group will show the others a set of two tableaux. Remind the group chosen from your peer group to be ready to present their tableaux again at this next meeting.

5. Remind everyone of their role as guardian angel.

6. Encourage participants to talk in general about the kinds of issues they have been discussing in these sessions with their friends and neighbours, if they like, but not to share any confidential information from the peer group with others.

7. Remember to ask for three volunteers to stay behind for ten minutes for a quick review of this session. (See Annex 4 for details.) Make sure that everyone has agreed a mutually convenient time and place for the first full workshop meeting, before saying goodbye.

FACILITATORS' TEAM FEEDBACK

After the end of Session G, meet again with your co-facilitators, to compare notes on how your sessions went and the information which you learnt from them. Your co-facilitators could have found useful information that could help you to structure your next session more effectively. Remember however not to share individual confidentialities between groups. This is the easiest way to ruin the trust that you have begun to build and to wreck the whole workshop! The next meeting is the first full workshop meeting. Remember that this is only for the members of the four peer groups, not the general public.

ENDNOTES

1. A tableau is a frozen scene representing people in a situation. No-one speaks, but their positions and expressions tell the story of what is happening to them. See Annex 1 for more detail.
2. See Annex 3 for a synopsis of each film clip.
3. Participants may want to view the film clip again. If so, it is usually best to have some discussion about it first, then to have a further discussion after the second viewing.

YOUR NOTES ...

FIRST FULL WORKSHOP MEETING

PURPOSE

To share peer group ideas so far.

TIME NEEDED: Maximum 2 hours.

MATERIALS NEEDED: None.

PARTICIPANTS: Members of the four peer groups, all meeting together. (No general public.)

SPECIAL INFORMATION

Don't forget to read 'Before You Begin ...!' before using this section of the manual.

AIMS: To enable all members of the four peer groups to meet together and share some ideas. To help participants realise that they do share some similar concerns with other peer groups.

DESCRIPTION: Members of all four peer groups meet together. Each peer group shows the others a set of two tableaux from the 'Possible Futures' exercise. Each tableau is followed by discussion.

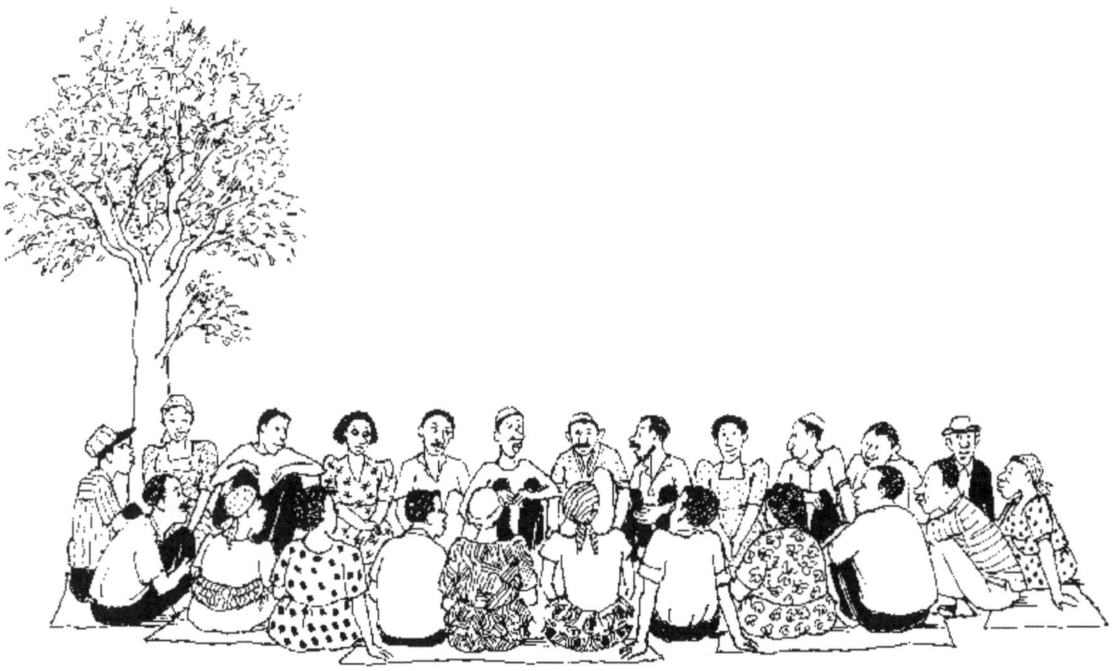

DIRECTIONS

The lead facilitator and/or one other facilitator should:

1. Thank everyone for sparing the time to come to the meeting. Explain that all peer groups have been working on their tableaux and that they have produced some fine ideas and acting. Now they have a chance to see each other's work and to present their own ideas to the full assembly. Explain that this is not a competition, but an opportunity to share ideas. Explain

that you know some groups are feeling nervous about presenting their ideas in public, but encourage them to be brave and encourage the whole audience to support each presentation.

2. Peer groups should be asked to decide amongst themselves which peer group should go first and so on.

In Buwenda, the young men were very nervous of acting in front of their mothers, and the older women were feeling similarly nervous about acting in front of their sons. But their facilitators reassured them that everyone was feeling nervous. Afterwards, the young men were thrilled to have performed so well. Both the young men's group and the young women's group were pleased to have had attention paid to them by the other groups.

3. Each peer group should present their 'bad future' tableau first. Once they are in their frozen position, the audience should be encouraged by the facilitators to ask questions of the actors in the tableau.

For instance:

- Who is each main character?
- What are they doing?
- How have they come to this situation?
- Why has this situation developed?
- What could they have done to avoid this situation?

The actors should be encouraged to answer the questions themselves whilst holding their position in the tableau.

4. Once the discussion of the 'bad future' tableau is completed, the actors should then present their 'good future' tableau. Facilitators should then encourage the audience to ask similar questions of the actors: who is who, what is happening, how, why, etc., as above.

5. After the discussion of the second tableau is complete, the next peer group should take up their positions and repeat instructions 3 and 4, above. Continue until all peer groups have presented their tableaux and had them discussed.

6. Next, ask participants whether they noticed any **similar** of themes across all the peer group presentations. What differences emerged among the peer groups?

7. Finally, thank all participants for their fine acting and explain that next time you will go on to Session H. Each facilitator should arrange a mutually agreeable time and place for Session H with his/her own peer group.

8. Each facilitator should remind everyone in his/her peer group of their role as guardian angel.

9. Encourage participants to talk in general about the kinds of issues they have been discussing in these sessions with their friends and neighbours, if they would like, but not to share any confidential information from the peer group with others.

10. Each facilitator should then remember to ask for three new people from their own peer group to stay behind for an instant review of this meeting. (See Annex 4.)

This meeting is important because it allows participants to voice their own concerns to other community members for the first time. It also enables them to realise that, with regard to shared hopes and fears, they have more in common with other members of their own community than they realise. This is valuable groundwork for developing greater trust and cooperation between different sections of the community. But it is also important for participants to go back to working in their peer groups. Don't be tempted to abandon this principle now! There is still a lot of sensitive material to be covered in later sessions, and participants will need the privacy and safety of a peer group.

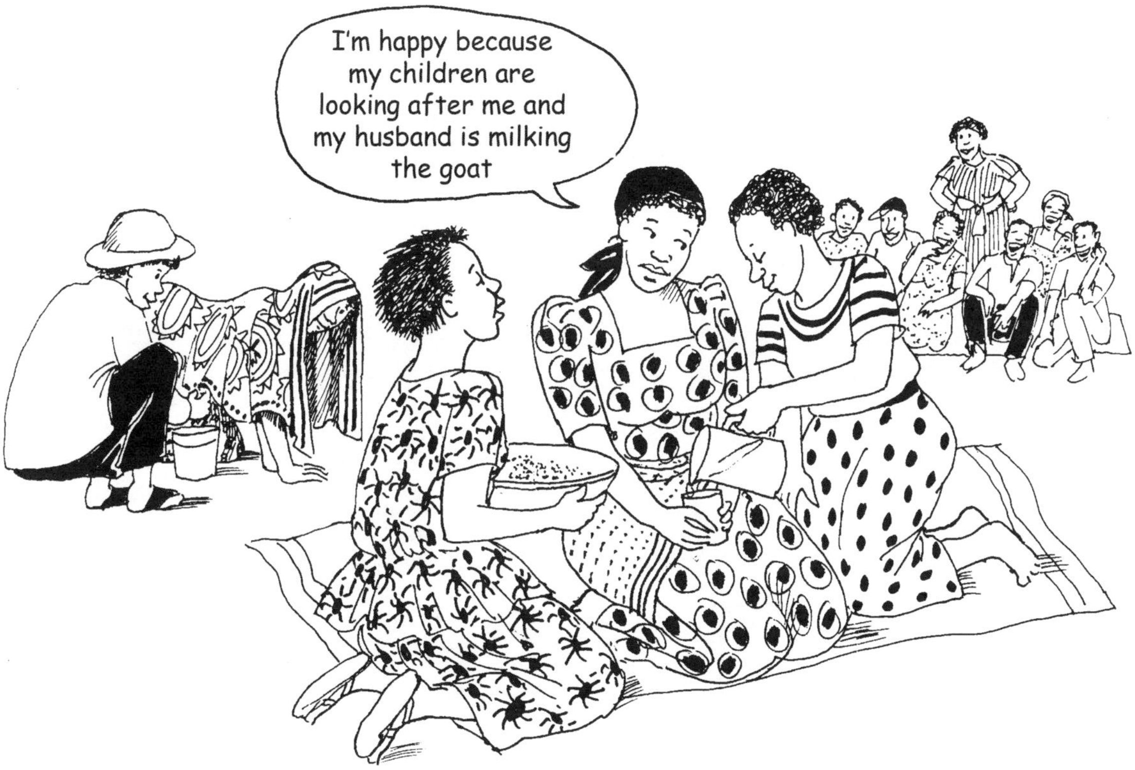
I'm happy because my children are looking after me and my husband is milking the goat

FACILITATORS' TEAM FEEDBACK

Don't forget to have another feedback session now! Some interesting similarities or differences will emerge in the tableau presentations. You may well be able to build on these in further workshop sessions. Over the next few sessions, we will be helping participants to analyse their own patterns of behaviour in relation to alcohol, traditional expectations, money, social pressure to behave in certain ways, and personal styles. There are several DVD clips for use in these sessions. Remember to encourage participants to compare what they see with their own experiences, so that the clips are used most effectively – that is, as springboards for discussion of participants' **own** concerns.

YOUR NOTES ...

SESSION H LET'S LOOK DEEPER: PART 1

PURPOSE

To study why we behave in the ways we do.

CONTENTS	TIME NEEDED
Introduction	
H.1	Oh Henry!
H.2	Exploring Why (this is a long exercise)
H.3	**DVD Clip 6:** 'Alcohol'
H.4	Community Likes
H.5	Happy Song and Closing Circle

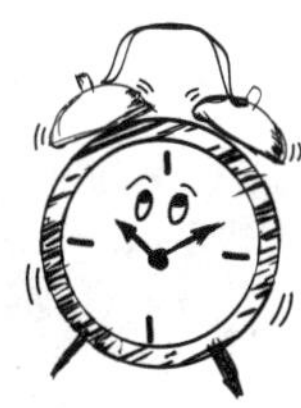

3–4 hours

MATERIALS NEEDED: DVD, laptop with DVD player, projector.

PARTICIPANTS: Four separate peer groups.

SPECIAL INFORMATION

Don't forget to read 'Before You Begin ...!' before using this section of the manual.

INTRODUCTION

1. Sit in a circle with the group, preferably on the ground. Everyone should be at the same level, including yourself.

2. Welcome everyone to the new session. Thank everyone for coming. Enquire about late-comers or non-attenders.

3. Ask each participant to recount quickly something good which has happened to them since the last session.

4. Review the last session. Ask participants to remind us what we discussed at the meeting – the tableaux of the other peer groups, ways in which they were similar to or different from this group's tableaux ... Remind them if they have forgotten.

5. Explain that we are going on to discuss other things in this session, but will start once more with a game.

EXERCISE H.1: OH HENRY!

AIMS: Energiser. To make people laugh. To help people realise the power of the way in which we express language to communicate our feelings to others.

DESCRIPTION: Participants each have to say 'Oh Henry!' (or appropriate name) round the circle, one after the next.

DIRECTIONS

1. Stand in a circle. Explain that, as we learnt together in our first session, there are many different ways of communicating with our bodies.

2. Explain how this game will illustrate how different uses of our voices combined with our bodies can also communicate a lot to others.

3. Take a common name in the community – perhaps you could use the name chosen by one of the peer group for their character in Exercise G.2. Using this in place of the stars, show how you can say 'Oh ********!' with anger, with fear, with sexiness, with laughter. You give an example of these first!

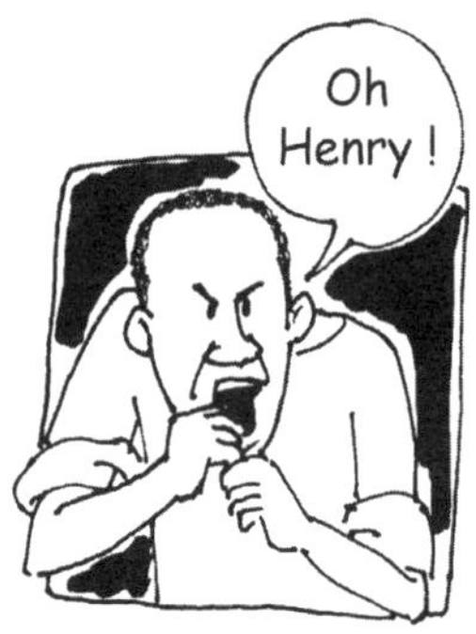

4. Ask each participant in turn in the circle to say 'Oh ********!', using the same name each time. Ask each one to try to say it in a different way, expressing a different feeling. **NB:** If in your community, a husband and wife are not allowed to use each other's names to each other, perhaps you could also do this exercise using the locally acceptable word for 'Oh wife' or 'Oh husband'.

5. When everyone has had a go, ask participants to analyse what they have learnt from this. Things they have noticed may include loud or soft voices, confident or unconfident voices, emphasis, facial expressions, eye contact, body language, and so on.

6. Encourage everyone to repeat the phrase in turn again. This time they should convey a different message through the phrase than the one they previously conveyed.

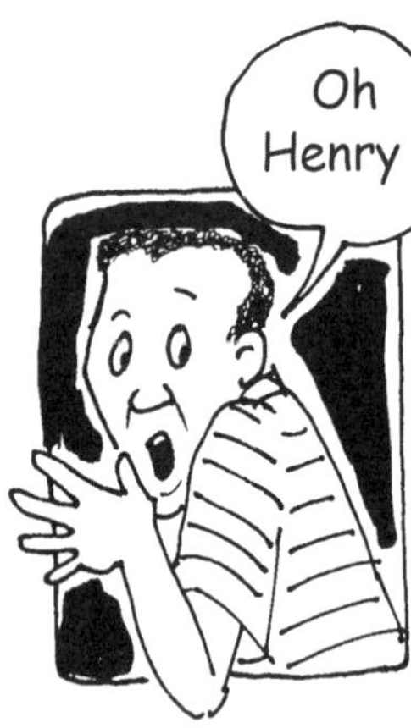

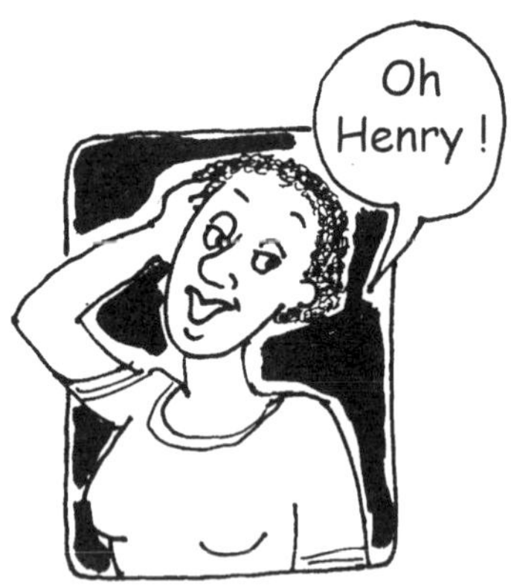

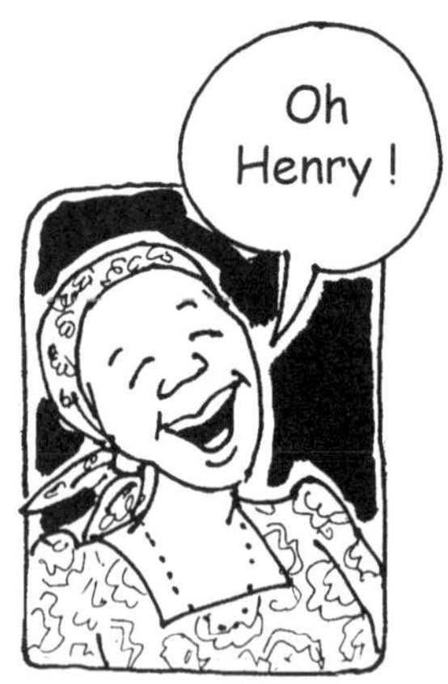

EXERCISE H.2: EXPLORING WHY

AIMS: To help participants consider situations which involve sex and risk-taking in their own experiences. To help them think of other ways of handling such situations through analysis of the circumstances.

DESCRIPTION: Role plays, followed by plenary discussion and analysis.

DIRECTIONS

1. Begin by recalling previous exercises: remind participants that we have discussed concerns which they have about sex; situations where they have been in arguments; times when they have felt themselves to be taking risks; and likely or less likely possible futures for a typical person in their community.

2. Explain that in this session we are going to explore some of these issues in more detail by thinking specifically about typical sexual encounters experienced by **characters like themselves** in their community. Emphasise that you don't want anyone actually to describe themselves and that you would much rather they just made up something on the basis of their general knowledge of people like them without labelling individuals. Refer to some of the examples of issues around sex and personal dilemmas which were discussed during Session B. **NB:** Only refer to examples which were brought up by the peer group which you are working with. Don't refer to fears of the other peer groups, even though you may know them!

It would be good to come up with, say, four different situations. There are some examples below of things which each peer group may mention.

OLDER WOMEN:

- widow having to sleep with her dead husband's brother
- wife having to sleep with her husband who has come home after a long journey

YOUNGER WOMEN:

- young wife wanting a child when her husband has other sexual partners as well as her
- sugar daddies tempting teenage girls

OLDER MEN:

- old man fearing that he may be impotent
- man approached by a woman in a bar

YOUNGER MEN:

- young man wanting to use a condom but fearing that his girlfriend/wife may be angry

3. Explain that you would now like to ask everyone to work in four different groups. Ask each group to choose one of the situations they have just described and plan a quick role play – using words, song, dance, or just body language – which describes a typical scene that could lead to sex for someone like them in their community. It could be set anywhere: in the house, in a field, in a bar, outside school … wherever they think sex – or the actions or words leading up to it – takes place in their community. In this way, each of the examples will be acted out by a different group.

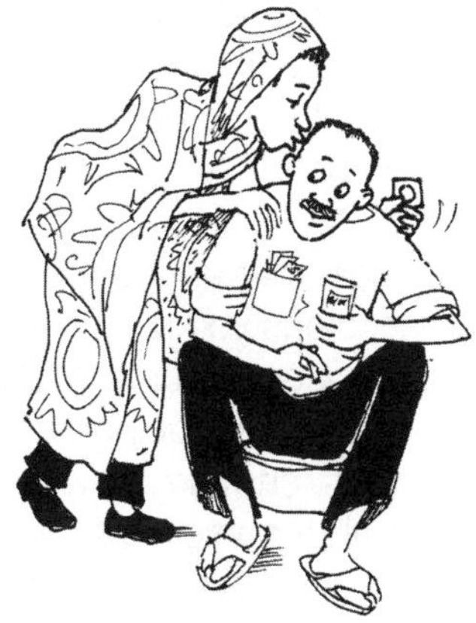

One person needs to play the character most like themselves, another needs to play his or her potential sexual partner. Other members of the group can act as friends of each of these or as other people, such as a father.

Ask them to plan a scene which will clearly show everyone else who is who, what the situation is, and how they react to one another. They don't have to act out the sex scene itself – just the circumstances which lead up to it! Give the groups 10 minutes to work on their scenes. Say that you want each group to produce a scene which is a maximum of 3 minutes long.

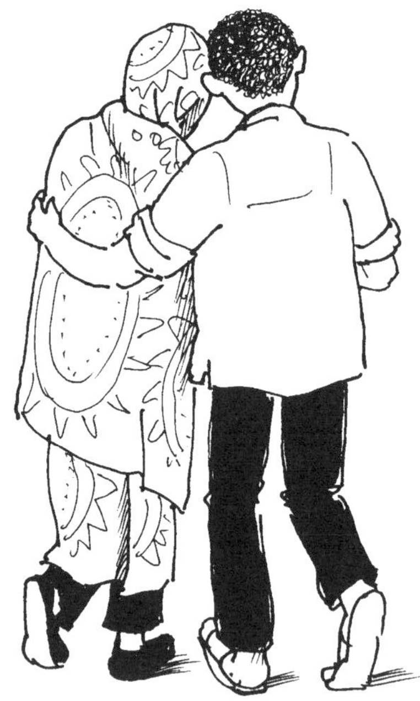

Reassure people also: explain that they may feel all this pretty embarrassing stuff to role-play, but remind them that we all feel fear and embarrassment at times. If we accept that we all feel this and try to find the courage to overcome it, we may help one another to face the issues more effectively.

4. After 10 minutes, call everyone back together. Explain that we are now going to watch all the four different role plays. Say that this is not a competition, so we are not going to judge who are the best actors. Instead, we are just going to have a chance to see a variety of different situations in our own community. Ask who would like to begin.

5. Encourage each group in turn to act out their scene. After each has been shown, encourage participants to discuss the following:

- **Why** did these characters have sex?
- **What** were the good things (if any) about them having sex?
- **What** were the bad things (if any) about them having sex?
- Did the character who was most like them **want** to have sex?
- Could they imagine what might make the character like them feel differently about having sex in this situation?
- Could the character who was most like them have been able to **say no** to sex if s/he had wanted to?
- What were the **factors** which influenced her/his control (or lack of control) of the situation? Was s/he drunk? Did s/he fear being beaten or ridiculed? Did s/he need the money? Did s/he find the other person too attractive to resist ...?
- What about the person with whom someone like them was about to have sex? Repeat the last four questions for her/him.

6. After each of the four role plays has been analysed, ask participants to discuss which of them illustrated safer sex. It is possible that none of them did. You may need to spend 10–15 minutes in discussion after each role play. Encourage actors and audience together to discuss what they have seen. There will clearly be overlaps in the discussion. This is good as it helps people to recognise patterns in expected behaviour.

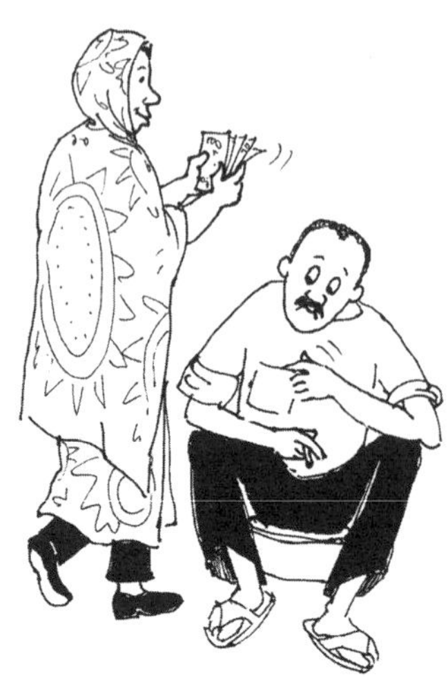

7. Explain that during the rest of this session and in the next few sessions you are going to consider together several factors which influence our sexual behaviour. Explain also that, in a later session, participants will have a chance to re-enact their role plays, showing how they could ensure safer sex – or no sex at all, if participants have decided that their character/the person most like them would prefer that.

8. Say that the first factor which you are going to consider is alcohol. Ask participants whether they would like to ask any further questions about today's session, before you move on to the next discussion.

This exercise acts as an introduction to discussions, later in this session and in the next session, about several factors that influence who people have sex with. The issues which may be relevant to participants' experiences are likely to include:

- **Drinking alcohol.** How it makes us feel. Whether its combination with sex is helpful or otherwise.
- **The community's beliefs and expectations** regarding sex. Local circumstances, such as: brides sleeping with their husband's father at marriage; arranged marriages; widows sleeping with a stranger on the death of their husband; widows marrying their dead husband's brother; men being expected to have a lot of wives and children to gain respect etc.
- **Ideals of men and women** and their behaviour. What is expected of women in their community, what is expected of men in their community.
- **Sexual obligations** of men to women, and women to men. How often and when must a man sleep with his wife, and how often and when must she sleep with him?
- **Enjoying sex**. Do women enjoy sex? Are women allowed to show it if they enjoy sex? Do men enjoy sex?.
- **Having children**.

EXERCISE H.3: DVD Clip 6: 'ALCOHOL'

AIM: To help participants consider the advantages and drawbacks of drinking alcohol. (In your community, alcohol may not be drunk, or there may be another drug which influences sexual behaviour in use as well or instead. You can adapt this exercise accordingly.)

DESCRIPTION: Watching DVD, followed by discussion.

MATERIALS NEEDED: DVD, laptop with DVD player, projector.

DIRECTIONS

1. Explain to participants that we are now going to watch a DVD clip about some members of Buwenda village. It starts with some women singing a song about alcohol. We will then see a scene acted by the older men about one of the consequences of excessive drinking. Finally, we will see a group who are sitting in the banana plantation tasting some newly brewed banana beer and talking about drinking.

Ask your participants to stand up, have a good stretch, and move around to a new position so that they can all see the screen.

2. Say that while they are watching the clip, you would like them to think about the use of alcohol in their own community.[1]

Make sure that everyone can see and hear the DVD clearly.

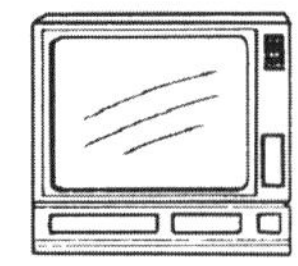

3. Turn on the DVD at the point where it says '6. Alcohol'.

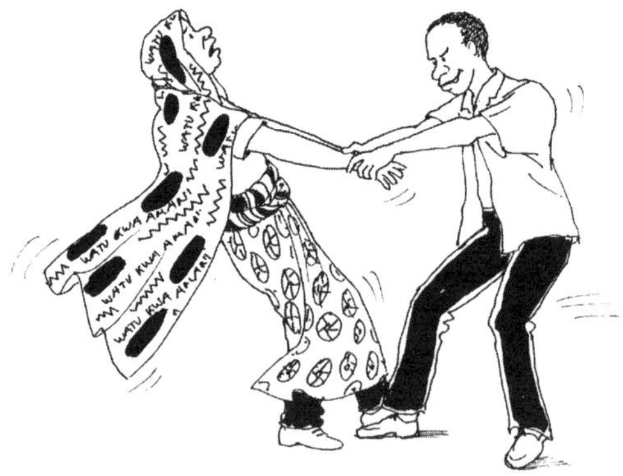

4. Turn off the DVD at the point where the screen goes black.

5. Ask participants to summarise what they saw and heard in the clip.[2]

Here are some points to help you guide the discussion about alcohol.

- *Many makers of alcohol are women who sell it to earn an income for themselves, for school fees, to pay taxes, and so on. In Buwenda this brewing is legal, but in many places it is done illegally. If people drink too much alcohol, who is it fair to blame: the maker or the drinker? If alcohol is banned, what alternative income is there for the makers?*
- *Some people viewing the older men's rape scene would blame the woman for being there, rather than the man for being drunk and behaving so badly. Is it fair to blame the woman for being there?*
- *Some people may say that the woman should have struggled even more and shouted out. But, in many places, women being attacked are afraid of screaming for fear of being cross-questioned and blamed, which would bring shame on their family. Is this fair?*

6. Then ask participants to divide into pairs and to consider the following questions in relation to their own community and their own use of alcohol – or its use by their partner, or father, or mother, if they don't drink alcohol themselves.[3]

- **Why** does the alcohol-maker in your community (if there is one) make alcohol?
- For what **reason(s)** do you (or your partner or parents) drink alcohol?
- What are the **good** things about drinking alcohol?
- What are the **bad** things about drinking alcohol?

7. Ask everyone to return to the large circle and go over each of these four questions again, asking the participants to share what they discussed.

8. Next, say to the participants: 'At the end of the DVD clip, one of the men said, '*There are good things about alcohol. Our ancestors used it to make friends. They used it when they proposed. They made use of it in everything.*' Another man responded, '*Yes, if you can control it and don't let it control you.*' What do you all think of these remarks?'

9. Finally, ask participants, 'What role do you think alcohol has to play in terms of influencing sexual behaviour?'

- In many societies, alcohol has traditionally played an important role in weddings, funerals, and other ceremonies, being used as a form of blessing. It has also been an important way of thanking people who lend their labour to one another. But it would normally have been drunk in small quantities and not over-used, as it often is today. What was the case in your participants' community in the past?

- Why do some people drink so much alcohol? In many parts of the world, people often start drinking alcohol because of **peer pressure**: it is a way of being accepted and liked by their friends. Alcohol **over-use** has increased alongside unemployment and poverty. People often turn to drinking more alcohol because of stress, depression, or lack of alternative means of enjoyment. They see drunkenness as a way of escape from their worries. Yet they often then discover that **over-use** leads to many additional problems. But the addictive qualities of alcohol mean it is then very hard for people to stop over-drinking. Is this relevant to your community at all?

- In many places where alcohol sales have been banned (such as in the USA several decades ago), people continue to make and sell it illegally, often producing dangerous mixtures. And others go on drinking it. So this is not a realistic solution.

- In some parts of Africa, the drinking of alcohol has been reduced by limiting the length of weddings, for instance, or limiting bar opening times to daylight or early evening hours. But some say that drinking is then just concentrated in to a shorter time. There are no simple solutions. But one thing is clear: when any of us has drunk too much alcohol, it is very difficult for us to act responsibly or keep control over our actions.

EXERCISE H.4: COMMUNITY LIKES

AIMS: **To bring people back to the present. To remind them of good things about their community after the difficult previous exercise.**

DESCRIPTION: **Each person describes one thing s/he likes about her/his community.**

DIRECTIONS

Sit in a circle with the participants. Ask each in turn to say 'I like my community because ...' Start with yourself and encourage participants to say anything they like about it. They may like other people, or the trees, the river, or whatever. They just need to mention one thing each.

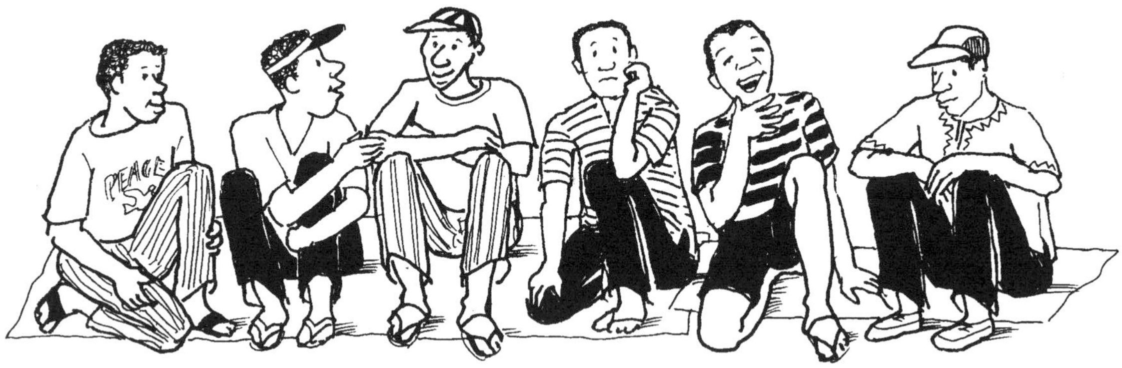

EXERCISE H.5: HAPPY SONG AND CLOSING CIRCLE

AIM: To finish the session on a happy note.

DESCRIPTION: The participants sing a happy or funny song of their choice.

DIRECTIONS

1. Ask participants to sing a song, preferably one to which they can dance, that they find happy, or funny, or both.

2. Join in as best you can, dancing too if possible.

3. Thank everyone again for coming. Ask each member of the group in turn to mention one thing that they have learnt today and one thing that they are looking forward to doing before the next meeting.

4. Ask if there are any more questions about today's session.

5. Remind everyone of the time and place for the next meeting and say you look forward to seeing them all again there.

6. Remind everyone of their role as guardian angel.

7. Encourage participants to talk in general about the kinds of issues they have been discussing in these sessions with their friends and neighbours, if they like, but not to share any confidential information from the peer group with others.

8. Remember to ask for three new volunteers to stay behind for an instant review of the session. (See Annex 4 for details.)

FACILITATORS' TEAM FEEDBACK

After the end of Session H, meet again with your co-facilitators, to compare notes on how your sessions went and the information which you learnt from them. Your co-facilitators could have found useful information that could help you to structure your next session more effectively. Remember however not to share individual confidentialities between groups. This is the easiest way to ruin the trust that you have built and to wreck the whole workshop!

ENDNOTES

1. Other common drugs can also be discussed here, after alcohol, if participants like.
2. For a synopsis of the clips, see Annex 3.
3. Participants may want to view the clip again. If so, it is usually best for them to have some discussion about it first, then to have a further discussion after the second viewing.

YOUR NOTES ...

SESSION I LET'S LOOK DEEPER: PART 2

PURPOSE

A development of the previous session.

CONTENTS	**TIME NEEDED**
Introduction	
I.1	Shout, Whisper, Sing
I.2	**DVD Clip 7:** 'Traditions'
I.3	Touch Something Blue
I.4	**DVD Clip 8:** 'Money'
I.5	Hand Push
I.6	Testing the Water
I.7	Closing Circle

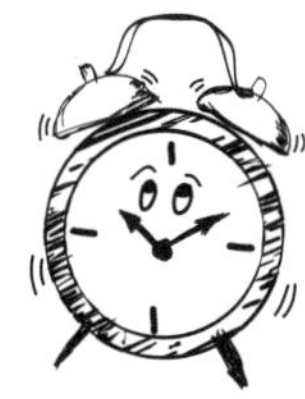

3–4 hours

MATERIALS NEEDED: DVD, laptop with DVD player, projector.

PARTICIPANTS: Four separate peer groups.

SPECIAL INFORMATION

Don't forget to read 'Before You Begin ...!' before using this section of the manual.

INTRODUCTION

1. Sit in a circle with the group, preferably on the ground. Everyone should be at the same level, including yourself.

2. Welcome everyone to the new session. Thank everyone for coming. Enquire about late-comers or non-attenders.

3. Ask each participant to recount quickly something good which has happened to them since the last session.

4. Review the last session. Ask participants to remind us what we learnt then – about potential situations leading to sex and the role of alcohol in our lives. Remind them if they have forgotten.

5. Explain that we are going on to discuss other things in this session but will start, as usual, with a game.

EXERCISE I.1: SHOUT, WHISPER, SING

AIMS: To energise the group. To have fun.

DESCRIPTION: Participants move around the group and call another's name, or adjectival names.

DIRECTIONS

1. Ask participants to stand in a circle. Explain that you are going to call out someone's name as you cross the circle towards them. S/he should then move from her/his position in the circle to the place where you were standing. As s/he does so, s/he should call out someone else's name. That person should then move, calling out another name ... and so on. You could use the adjectival names from Session A, if you would rather.

2. When your name gets called again, continue with the game, but this time whisper the name of the person you choose next and ask everyone else to whisper too when it's their turn.

3. Finally, when your name is called again, say that this time the name of the next person must be sung out. Continue until everyone has had a go.

EXERCISE I.2: DVD Clip 7: 'TRADITIONS'

AIMS: To help participants think about local traditions which may influence HIV transmission and how those traditions might be changed.

DESCRIPTION: Watching DVD, followed by discussion.

MATERIALS NEEDED: DVD, laptop with DVD player, projector.

DIRECTIONS

1. Explain to participants that we are now going to watch a DVD clip of the older women's group from Buwenda village. They are doing a role play about a tradition in their community whereby a widow is remarried to her dead husband's brother. Ask participants to stand up, have a good stretch, and move around to a new position so that they can all see the screen.

2. Say that while they are watching the clip, you would like them to think about whether or not there are similar traditions in their own community.

Make sure that everyone can see and hear the DVD clearly.

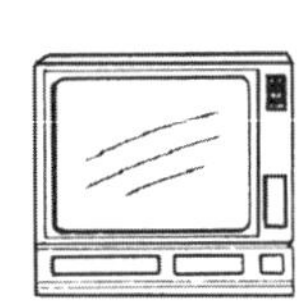

3. Turn on the DVD at the point where it says '7. Traditions'.

4. Turn off the DVD at the point where the screen goes black.[1]

5. Ask participants:

- To summarise what they saw and heard in the clip. Emphasise that the practice of a widow marrying her dead husband's brother (known in English as 'the levirate') is normal in this community.
- What do they imagine the widow feared about marrying her dead husband's brother?
- What fears might the brother have?

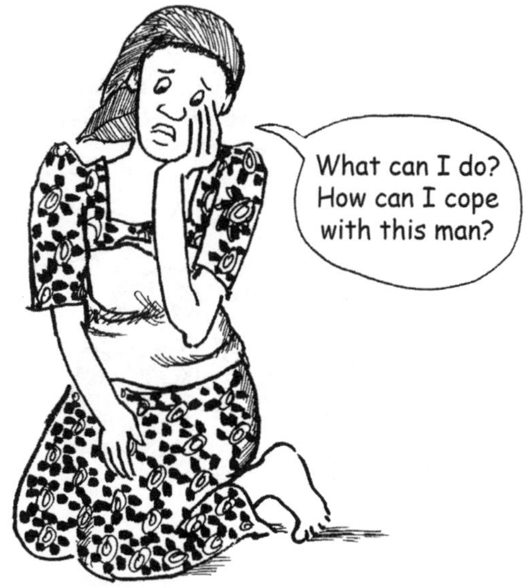
What can I do? How can I cope with this man?

☞ If participants do not include fear of HIV or other STIs in the discussion, you should suggest adding it.

6. Then ask participants to divide into pairs and to consider the following questions in relation to their own community and their own traditions:

- Are there traditions in our community, which involve sex and could help the spread of HIV or other STIs?
- What are these traditions and why are they risky?
- Is there a way in which these traditions could be changed to reduce the spread of HIV? Is there a way of getting everyone to agree to these changes?

7. After pair work, call everyone back to the centre.

- First ask people to name all the different traditions of their community that involve sex and which may influence the spread of HIV or other STIs.[2]
- Next, for each tradition, ask participants why they think it could influence the spread of HIV. Make sure everyone understands one another.
- Third, ask for participants' ideas on how these traditions could be changed to reduce the threat of the spread of HIV. Encourage participants to be as specific as possible in their suggestions.

8. If participants come up with some suggestions which they feel hopeful about, you could suggest that they may like to air them at the next meeting of all the peer groups. There they could be discussed more widely.

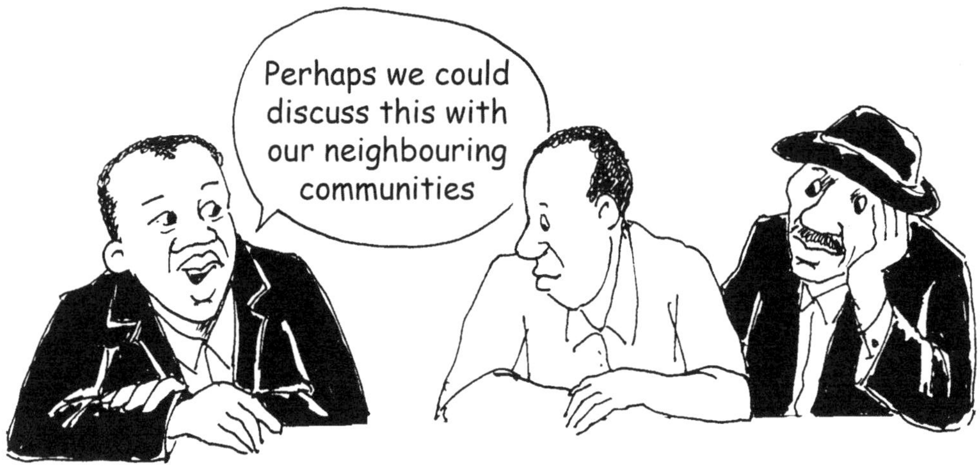

In different parts of Africa there are very different traditions about sexual practice. Even in one country there can be a lot of variation in what different groups of people think is the good and right thing to do.

- In some areas, people believe that it is right for a widow to marry her dead husband's brother.
- In some areas, people believe that a man should always marry his cousin.
- In some areas, people believe that it is fine for old men to marry young women.
- In some areas, people believe that a new bride should have sex with her husband's father before she has sex with her husband.
- In some areas, people believe that a widow should have sex with a stranger after her husband has died.
- In some areas, people believe that a widow should have sex with someone from her dead husband's family after he has died.
- In some areas, people believe that a woman should have sex with anyone of her husband's age group, if he comes to stay.
- In some areas, people believe that at initiation ceremonies, or at weddings or funerals, people should have sex with a number of other people.

Each of these traditions is considered to be the totally **normal**, good thing for people who behave correctly and properly in that community to do. Not to have sex according to these traditions would be very hard for an individual since s/he would be breaking society's rules or expectations.

Yet in some places, communities have decided to adapt – or even break with – tradition and permit people to behave differently because of the threat of HIV. The local chiefs have altered the tradition to cope with modern circumstances. For instance, in one area in Zambia, widows can now jump over the legs of their dead husband's relative instead of having sex with him. This has been a big 'jump' for them, but it can be done. This whole exercise therefore is designed to help **your** participants begin to think of possible alternatives too.

Finally, people often feel that their traditions are under threat in this kind of discussion. Therefore, it is also important to point out that **all societies** have some good traditions and some bad traditions. For instance, in some areas, girls and boys are given strict rules about not having sex before initiation rites which take place around puberty. Initiation rites for young women have often included education by older women about sex, childbirth, parenting, and so on. If young women became pregnant before such rites had taken place, they and their child would be thrown out of the community. However, in recent years, such rites, rules, and the teachings connected with them are dying out.

Also, many traditions may have been good ones until HIV arrived. For instance, the tradition shown in the DVD is considered by many to have been a good way of providing for the widow and her children before HIV. It may be useful to help participants also think of some good traditions in their community – ones which anyone would value and which carry no potential threat to anyone.

EXERCISE I.3: TOUCH SOMETHING BLUE

AIM: An energiser to get people moving around and laughing.

DESCRIPTION: A game of tag.

DIRECTIONS

1. Ask everyone to stand up. Then explain that when you call out, everyone is to find something blue around them and touch it. This could be someone's blue shirt or scarf, a shoe or whatever.

2. Do this, then call out, 'Touch something green!' and everyone should run to touch a green object. Next, 'Touch your toes!' or, 'Touch someone's ear!', 'Touch that tree over there!', or whatever.

3. Ask other people to join in with their own suggestions.

EXERCISE I.4: DVD Clip 8: 'MONEY'

AIM: To help participants explore the links between money and the spread of HIV, and how these links might be changed.

DESCRIPTION: Watching DVD, followed by discussion.

MATERIALS NEEDED: DVD, laptop with DVD player, projector.

DIRECTIONS

1. Explain to participants that we are now going to watch another DVD clip of the groups in Buwenda village. They are doing role plays about the use of money in the household. Ask participants to stand up, have a good stretch, and move around to a new position so that they can all see the screen.

2. Say that while they are watching the clip, you would like them to think about whether or not there are similar issues in their own community.

Make sure that everyone can see and hear the DVD clearly.

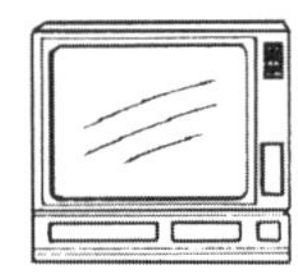

3. Turn on the DVD at the point where it says '8. Money'.

4. Turn off the DVD at the point where the screen goes black.[1]

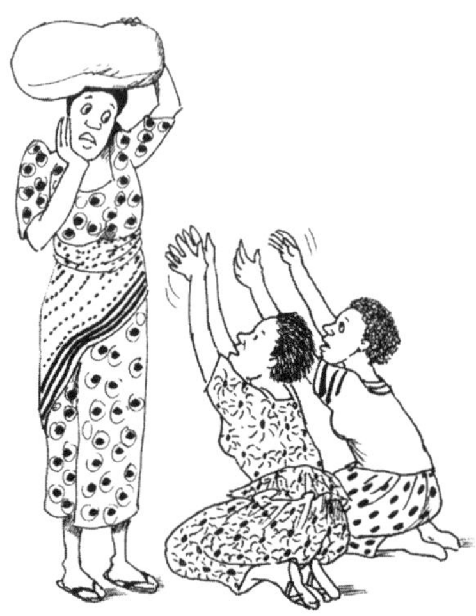

5. Ask participants first to summarise what they have seen.[3]

6. Next ask participants to move into **threes** and discuss the following points:

- What are the main costs facing you and your family?
- Who takes responsibility for these costs amongst you and your partner(s)?
- How is access to money relevant to the spread of HIV?

7. Call everyone back to the full group and go through these three questions again.

8. Then ask the full group for their comments on the following questions:

- What were the good things about the couple's relationship at the end of the DVD?
- What were the bad things about the couple's relationship at the end of the DVD?
- Do you know of partners in this community who have arguments over paying for things?
- What could the community do to help them stop arguing?

EXERCISE I.5: HAND PUSH

AIMS: To energise the group. To introduce the idea of conflict.

DESCRIPTION: Two lines of participants push against each other, followed by analysis.

DIRECTIONS

1. Ask participants to form two lines facing each other. Each participant touches palms with the person facing her/him in the other line. Call one line 'Line 1' and the other 'Line 2'.

2. Ask all the participants in Line 1 to start pushing against the person opposite them in Line 2, only using their palms. People in Line 2 can respond in any way they like.

3. After 30 seconds or so, ask everyone to stop and then to change roles. This time Line 2 members should push against Line 1 members, and Line 1 members can respond as they choose.

4. After another 30 seconds or so, ask everyone to sit down in a big circle. Ask people how they felt doing this exercise. Did they respond by pushing back or by giving in, or what? How did this relate to their real life experience of conflict?

EXERCISE I.6: TESTING THE WATER

AIMS: To encourage participants to reflect on common patterns of their own behaviour. To look at how our behaviour varies according to changes in circumstances.

DESCRIPTION: An individual exercise in personal reflection.

DIRECTIONS

1. Explain to participants that we have been looking a lot at things which happen **around** us in our communities, and which shape our lives. We are now going to start to look at things which happen **inside** us.

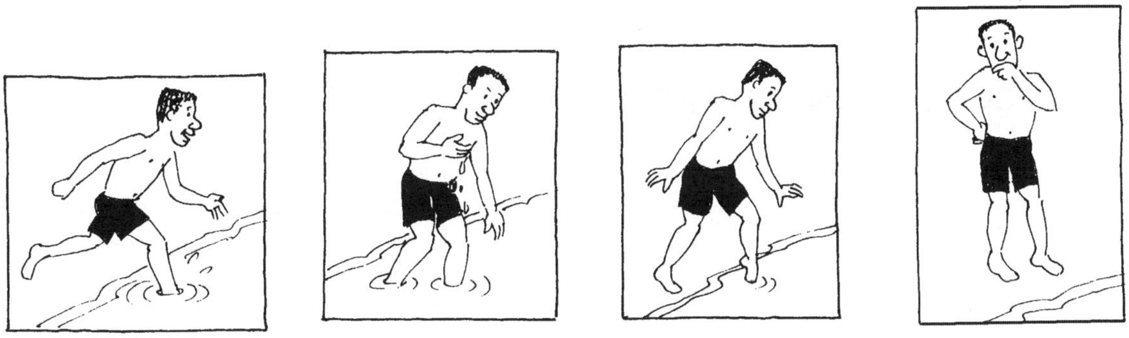

Ask participants this question: 'If you went to the sea,[4] or to a river, or lake, and you really wanted to get cool in the water, which is the most likely way for you to get into the water?' Would you:

- Just run towards the sea and dive in?
- Walk in slowly, wetting your body bit by bit and getting used to the temperature?
- Dip your toe in the water, then decide if you'll go in or not?
- Stand on the beach contemplating the view and surroundings, while considering what you will do next?

(You could act out these actions as you are saying them, to help people laugh a bit!)

Point to four different corners of the training area, one for each action described above. Ask participants to move to the corner matching the action which each of them thinks is most likely for him/herself.

2. Once everyone in the group has moved to a corner, give each type of response a title, such as 'plunger', 'wader', 'tester', 'delayer'. Ask participants the good and bad things about each of these types of behaviour.

3. Now ask each participant to consider whether the type of behaviour they chose is the way they behave most often. If they find that they behave differently in different circumstances, get them to think of a particular situation and a response. Once they have thought about this, they could share their thoughts in groups of three or so.

Feedback and discussion:

In what ways does our behaviour change in different circumstances? What sorts of conflicts could arise when a 'plunger' has to work or live alongside a 'tester'? In what ways could the two actually benefit from each other? What are the positive aspects of each approach? For what reasons do people adopt these different approaches?

> The assumption here is that a greater awareness of how we respond in different situations increases our understanding of the dynamics involved in conflict situations. It also encourages attention to the behaviour of others, and an understanding of the needs underlying their behaviour. Remind participants of the 'Taking Risks' exercise which they did in Session D.

EXERCISE I.7: CLOSING CIRCLE

1. Thank everyone again for coming. Ask each member of the group in turn to mention one thing that they have learnt today and one thing that they are looking forward to doing before the next meeting.

2. Ask if there are any more questions about today's session.

3. Remind everyone of the time and place for the next meeting and say that you look forward to seeing them all again there.

4. Remind everyone of their role as guardian angel.

5. Encourage participants to talk in general about the kinds of issues they have been discussing in these sessions with their friends and neighbours, if they like, but not to share any confidential information from the peer group with others.

6. Remember to ask for three new volunteers to stay behind for the instant review of the session. (See Annex 4 for details.)

FACILITATORS' TEAM FEEDBACK

In this session, you have addressed the roles of local traditions and money in the spread of HIV. You have then begun to look at different ways in which individuals behave. This will be explored further in the next few sessions. After the end of Session I, meet again with your co-facilitators, to compare notes on how your sessions went and the information which you learnt from them. Your co-facilitators could have found useful information that could help you to structure your next session more effectively. Remember however not to share individual confidentialities between groups. This is the easiest way to ruin the trust that you have built and to wreck the whole workshop!

ENDNOTES

1. Participants may want to view the clip again. If so, it is usually best for them to have some discussion about it first, then to have a further discussion after the second viewing.
2. Here we are only asking people to focus on traditions involving sex. If scarification or circumcision are practised in your community as well, it would be good for you to add an exercise on this to the session. However, please try to keep the discussions about them separate.
3. See Annex 3 for a summary.
4. If people in your community fear water, this may not be a very good example. Instead you could ask them to consider how they behaved when they met new people, or went to a new place for the first time, or when strangers came to their area, or when they were asked to do a new task…

YOUR NOTES …

SESSION J LET'S SUPPORT OURSELVES

PURPOSE

To find new skills to change the ways in which we behave.

CONTENTS	**TIME NEEDED**
Introduction	
J.1	Statues of Power
J.2	Attack and Avoid
J.3	**DVD Clip 9:** 'Saying 'Yes'?'
J.4	Taking Control
J.5	The Yes/No Game
J.6	Supporting Ourselves to Regain Control
J.7	Closing Circle

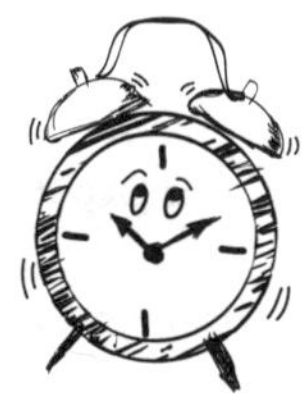

3–4 hours

MATERIALS NEEDED: DVD, laptop with DVD player, projector.

PARTICIPANTS: Four separate peer groups.

SPECIAL INFORMATION

Don't forget to read 'Before You Begin ...!' before using this section of the manual. In Exercise J.2, you will need to speak aloud a list of words describing different types of behaviour. Work through this list beforehand with your co-facilitators to make sure you all understand these words and have common words in your local language for them.

INTRODUCTION

1. Sit in a circle with the group, preferably on the ground. Everyone should be at the same level, including yourself.

2. Welcome everyone to the new session. Thank everyone for coming. Enquire about late-comers or non-attenders.

3. Ask each participant to recount quickly something good which has happened to them since the last session.

4. Review the last session. Ask participants to remind us what we learnt then – about local traditions, about sharing money, and the influence of each of these on the spread of HIV and other STIs. Remind them if they have forgotten. What else did the last session explore?

5. Explain that we are going on to discuss other things in this session, but will start with a game.

EXERCISE J.1: STATUES OF POWER

AIM: To look at the emotions we associate with power and how they affect us.

DESCRIPTION: A physical exercise, in pairs, using tableaux.

DIRECTIONS

1. Divide the group into pairs. Each pair is going to produce a tableau (frozen image) showing one person in a position of power and the other in a powerless position. Allow them a few minutes to prepare their tableau, then ask them to swap around (so that the powerful figure becomes the powerless and vice versa) and prepare a second tableau.

2. When they have prepared both tableaux, give each pair the opportunity to show them to the rest of the group. Ask for quick comments about what people observe. Ask both members of each tableau to express what they are feeling in one word (proud, scared, humble, or whatever).

Feedback and discussion

Which of the two positions felt more familiar to participants? Can they relate any of the emotions they felt to situations in their lives? What did they feel for the powerless person when they were in the powerful position, and vice versa?

> This exercise can quickly activate strong associations and emotions, and you should be conscious of this. Those who have strong emotional reactions might welcome an opportunity to talk about them. If so, it can be a good idea to have feedback in small groups.

EXERCISE J.2: ATTACK AND AVOID

AIMS: To gain an understanding of assertive and unassertive behaviour. To recognise the kinds of behaviour which are familiar to us. To remind ourselves of verbal and body language clues which warn us of an attitude or type of behaviour in others. To notice these signs in ourselves and see it as an opportunity to recognise what kind of response we are likely to use and check that it is appropriate.

DESCRIPTION: A group exercise introducing assertiveness, looking at aggressive and defensive behaviour.

DIRECTIONS

1. Sit in a circle with the participants. Ask participants to listen to the list of actions which you are going to read out.

- If they think they do something often, they should put both hands in the air.
- If they think they do something sometimes, they should put one hand in the air.
- If they think they never do something, they should keep both hands down.

Join in with these actions yourself. (If you feel participants are ready to be more active, you could ask them to move to different corners of the training area in response instead: e.g. frequent doers on the right, never doers on the left, sometimes doers in the middle.) The actions appear in two columns. Read out the first column first, then the second. Ask participants to react after each word.

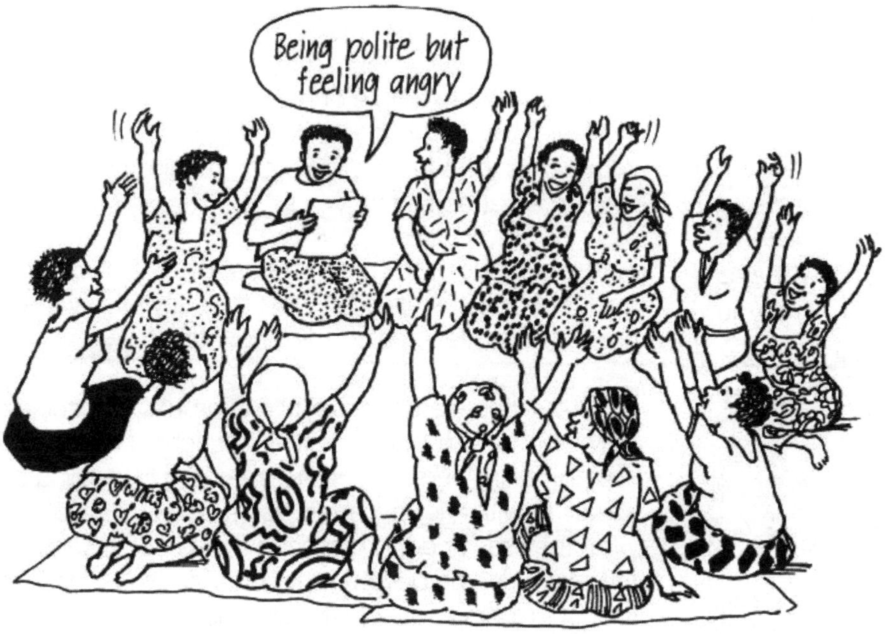

LIST OF ACTIONS

First column:	Second column:
Nagging	Withdrawal
Shouting	Sulking in silence
Interrupting	Taking it out on the wrong person
Exploding	Declaring that you are being unfairly treated
Warning (If you don't do this ...!)	Talking behind someone's back
Correcting (Look at the facts ...!)	Trying to forget about the problem
Persisting (I am right ...!)	Feeling ill
Insulting	Not wanting to hurt the other person
Being sarcastic	Feeling low and depressed
Threatening revenge (I'll get you back for this!)	Being polite but feeling angry

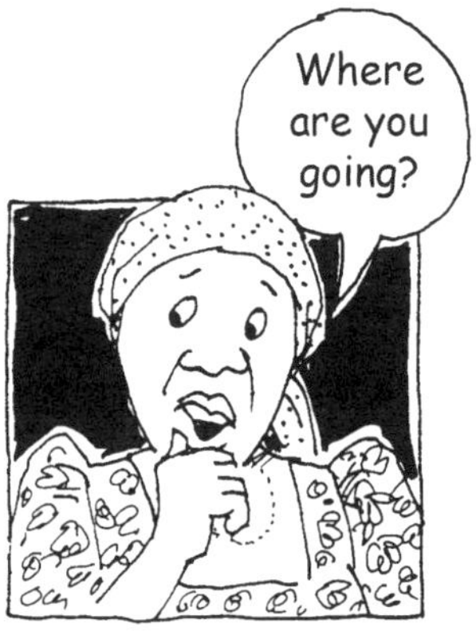

2. Point out to everyone that the words you read out first (from the first column) are attacking behaviour, and the second lot of actions are avoiding behaviour. Ask everyone to note for themselves which they found they do more often.

3. **What?** Brainstorm the word 'attack' and then the word 'avoid', allowing one minute for each word. Ask participants to call out anything which each word means for them. There may well be good and bad feelings expressed about each word.

4. **Why?** Then ask participants to think of one reason they themselves would behave in an attacking or avoiding way. Ask a few participants to describe their examples to everyone.

5. **How?** Ask participants to consider how attacking or avoiding would be expressed – what they would say, how they would say it, and how they would say it with their bodies.

6. **For instance?** Ask everyone to think of one word or phrase that they use when either avoiding or attacking, whichever is their most frequent behaviour. They should consider how it is said and the body language which accompanies it. An example of avoiding behaviour might be, 'Where are you going?' said in a soft, uncertain way which indicates that the questioner is expecting an angry answer, and accompanied by hunching the shoulders and turning away the head. Ask how the same phrase could be said in an attacking way.

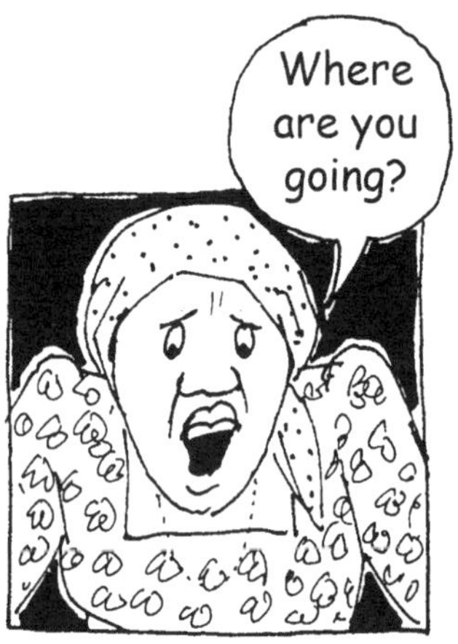

7. Ask somebody to give theirs as a practical example. You might point out how the effect of what they say is very much dependent on what they do – their body language.

With the 'where are you going?' example, you could suggest that they try using the phrase without hunching their shoulders, looking straight at the person they are speaking to, smiling strongly and speaking with a loud, certain voice. This will have a big effect on what they say and the message that is being communicated. In this example, the person may find that, when they stop hunching their shoulders and look straight ahead, what they actually say is interpreted much more positively.

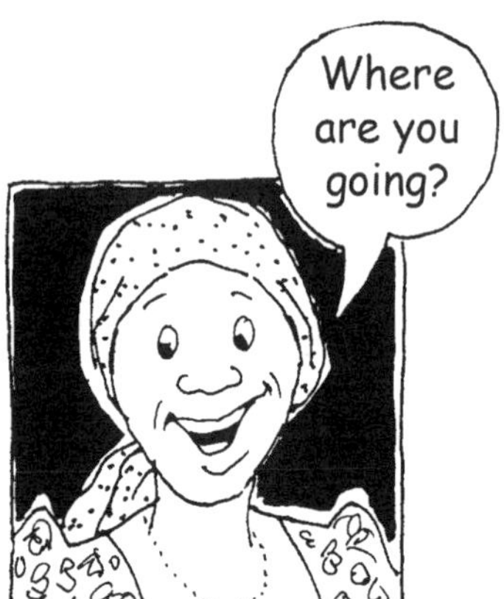

8. In groups of three, get everyone to give their example while the other two in the group offer suggestions about how they might alter their body language to make their response an assertive rather than an attacking or avoiding one. Other examples to try could be: 'What time are you coming back?', 'How much does this cost?', and other ideas of their own.

Feedback and discussion

What signs can help us to recognise and even predict others' behaviour? What signs can we learn to recognise in ourselves which warn us that we are embarking on an unassertive approach? How can we alter our ways of reacting and begin to learn a new response? How does it feel to change our body position?

Assertiveness has as much to do with body language as with what we say. And what we say is often unconsciously influenced by our own body language. If we adopt defensive physical postures, such as looking down or hunching our shoulders, we are unlikely to speak assertively. On the other hand, adopting assertive body language can make it easier for us to speak assertively.

An assertive response is a centred response. We are balanced – not leaning forward in an attack mode, not shrinking back in an avoiding mode. Although most of our confrontations are verbal rather than physical, there are often visual signs, even if they are tiny, of our body going on the attack or becoming defensive. This exercise is a step towards using the signs we get to build a more assertive response rather than reacting immediately.

EXERCISE J.3: DVD Clip 9: 'SAYING 'YES'?'

AIMS: To help participants consider a common situation. To show the difficulties in being clear about people's wishes or intentions.

DESCRIPTION: Watching DVD, followed by discussion.

MATERIALS NEEDED: DVD, laptop with DVD player, projector.

DIRECTIONS

1. Explain to participants that we are now going to watch a DVD clip of the young women's group from Buwenda village. They are doing a role play of a situation which is familiar to them. Ask participants to stand up, have a good stretch and move around to a new position so that they can all see the DVD screen.

2. Say that while they are watching the clip, you would like them to think about the relevance of this clip to their own community.

Make sure that everyone can see and hear the DVD clearly.

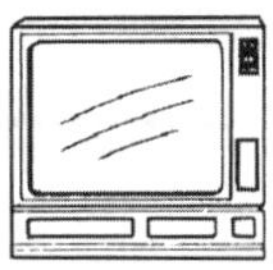

3. Turn on the DVD at the point where it says '9. Saying 'Yes'?'.

4. Turn off the DVD at the point where the screen goes black.

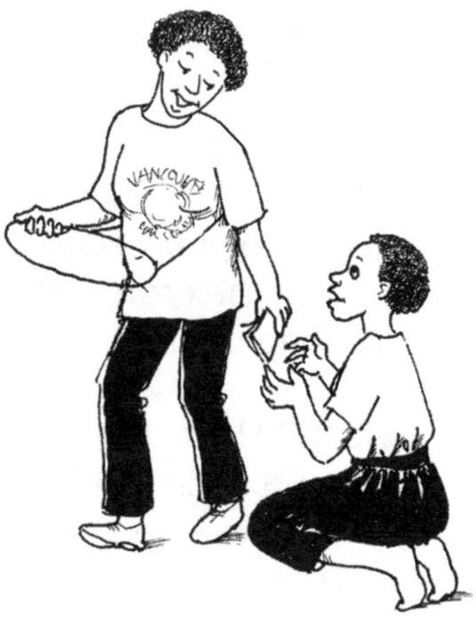

5. Ask participants to summarise what they saw and heard in the clip.[1] Remind participants that, in Buwenda, it is quite normal for a woman to kneel before a man as part of their greeting.

6. Then ask participants to divide into pairs and to consider the following questions in relation to their own community and their own reactions to what they saw:

- Who was in control of the situation?
- Who was acting responsibly?
- Who was responsible for the baby?

- What were your own reactions to what you saw?
- How does this story relate to our community here?

7. Back in the full circle, review participants' answers to these questions.

By this stage, we hope that all participants will agree that:

- The man was in control of the situation.
- The young woman was vulnerable. She might have wanted money for her school fees, but was unaware of the all the likely implications and consequences of her actions.
- Neither the man nor the young woman was acting responsibly.
- The man, the young woman, and the communities from which they came were all responsible for the baby.

If you find that any participants disagree with this analysis, you may find it helpful to:

- Refer back to previous exercises, such as 'What is Love', 'Ideal Images and Personal Destroyers' and so on.
- Ask, 'Was she really asking for it? Did she think he looked great? Or was it too rude for her to say no? Or was she longing for the possibility of some money and status?'
- Did he really have a right to have sex with her and then reject her?
- Finally, consider community responsibility: if she had had some sex education, at her school or from other people, could this have helped? If their communities had discouraged liaisons between men of his age and schoolgirls, would this have helped?

Some of you may find that the incident in this clip is different from local experiences. In some areas it is common for a young woman to be approached by an older man and for her to be glad to have sex with him in return for money and other support. Parents may expect their daughters to pay their way like this. Yet these young women are vulnerable to unplanned pregnancy, HIV, and STIs. If this is the situation in your area, these questions of shared responsibility are still relevant and it is important to discuss them here. Would she have been able to say, 'Yes – with a condom!' for instance?

If you need more time to talk now, do so. If not, you can go on to the next exercise... .

EXERCISE J.4: TAKING CONTROL

AIMS: To explore ways of taking control or feeling in control. To rehearse these ideas in front of the group. To increase confidence. To find more appropriate ways of presenting oneself.

DESCRIPTION: A group exercise looking at ways of using our own power in group and social situations.

DIRECTIONS

1. As a warm-up, ask participants to lie on the ground. Ask them to imagine that they are feeling completely useless, with no resources, no confidence, no control. Then, to slowly rise and start to feel better about themselves. They move up a sliding scale from 1 (feeling completely useless, no control) to 10 (confident and totally in control). Everyone walks around the training area, slowly changing as they move up their scale. When *everyone* has reached their 10 you can stop. You could ask a few participants to demonstrate their movement from 1 to 5, others from 10 to 5, and a third group from 5 to 10. How often do they feel they do this in everyday life? What do they feel as they move up or down the scale?

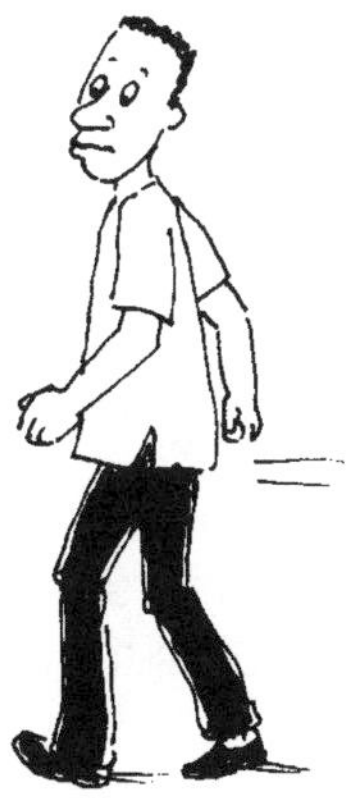

2. With everyone in a circle, ask one person at a time to enter the circle and to take control, to feel confident, to have a presence in the group. It is a good idea to create two gaps in the circle: an entry point and an exit point. Each individual must decide for her/himself what kind of control s/he wants to exercise and how s/he will establish it. S/he might, for example:

- Enter the circle quietly, pause, look round the circle making eye contact with everyone, and depart quietly.
- Rush in and, with great excitement, tell us what s/he has seen.
- Come in with confidence, look at one person and request that they move from one side of the circle to the other side of the circle. (The request will be followed if it is issued with the necessary control and authority.)

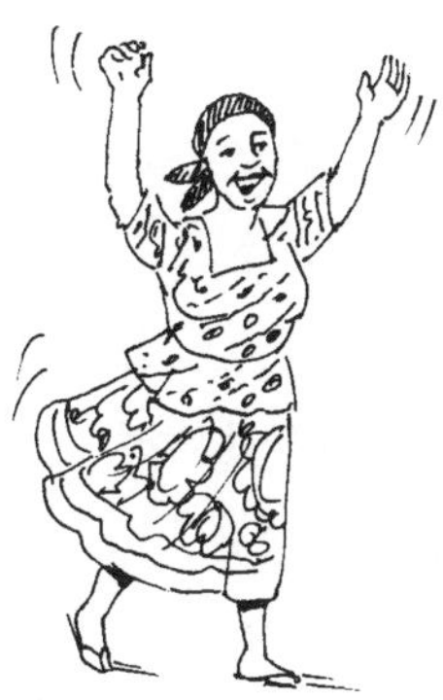

These are three very different ways of taking control, each of which would suit a different personality, but they are all effective. You could demonstrate them to the participants before encouraging them to have a go.

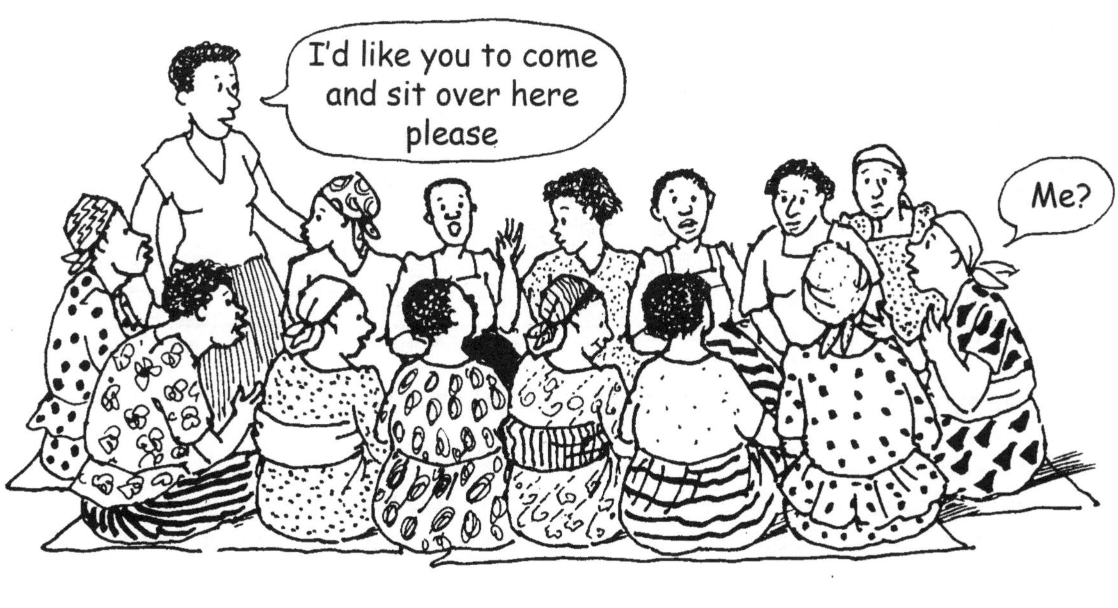
I'd like you to come and sit over here please
Me?

Feedback and discussion

What difficulties did participants encounter when attempting to take control? How did they overcome them? What kind of comment or observation from the group would they find useful? Did people get any new ideas from watching the range of approaches? What would participants like to practise or improve?

Some participants may need to be challenged, or need a lot of help. A good way is to sit in the middle of the circle and challenge them to make you move. Move only when you feel they have achieved the necessary control and authority. Stay seated, giving them tips about how to improve, until you feel you really would shift! For others, being too aggressive may be the problem. You may need to use a similar technique to encourage them to be less aggressive but more assertive.

You could encourage participants to consider how domination and submission relate to the colonial experience in some countries, or the relationship between some fathers and their sons. Or ask them for more relevant examples.

By contrast, you could relate the concept of sharing power – being assertive – to President Mandela in his conciliatory attitude towards former President de Klerk when apartheid rule finished in South Africa. Being assertive does not mean that you lose control – although many aggressive people think that listening to and respecting others threatens their own power. Thinking of highly respected people may help participants to see that this is not the case.

EXERCISE J.5: THE YES/NO GAME

AIMS: Cheerful exercise. To show how many different ways we have of making use of these two common words.

DESCRIPTION: Participants have an argument with each other, using one word each.

DIRECTIONS

1. Ask participants to stand up and split into two groups. One group should stand in a line facing the centre of the training area, and the others should stand in a line facing them.

2. Explain that one group is the 'yes' group and the only word they can use is 'yes'. The other group is the 'no' group and this is the only word they can use.

3. Each group needs to try to convince the other group of the truth of its own statement, but each can only use the one word, yes or no.

4. After a minute or so, get the groups to swap roles, with the 'yes' group saying 'no' and vice versa.

5. After another minute, ask participants to describe how they felt doing this exercise, including comments on body language, use of attacking or avoiding stances, laughter etc. Explain how laughter is an other important means of expression: it can be a good equaliser sometimes, but at others can be very harmful.

Feedback and discussion

There are many different ways of saying yes and no, across the full range of emotions. It is good for us to have a go at saying them in different ways. Each different way can have its own effect on others.

EXERCISE J.6: SUPPORTING OURSELVES TO REGAIN CONTROL

AIM: To analyse how we can take responsibility for our actions.

DESCRIPTION: Plenary discussion followed by pairwork and a summary plenary.

DIRECTIONS

1. Start this exercise with the following explanation:

When we have done something wrong, we often feel uncomfortable about what we have done, but don't really know what we can do about it. It is often much easier to blame someone else, or to say that things were out of our control, than it is for us to take responsibility for our actions. We can probably all think of times when we have regretted doing or saying something and have felt frustrated about it. We often end up blaming someone else to try to make ourselves feel better.

But are we then really in control of the situation, or is the situation in control of us?

2. Ask the group if they have any ideas about how the sugar daddy in the DVD clip, or any man in this situation, such as a teacher, a work manager, or a male relative, could have taken responsibility for his actions after the scene.

> ☞ If you are working with the younger women or older women, you may instead like to think here of how the young woman in the clip could have been supported to take responsibility for her actions, or spend a few minutes discussing each of them. But since this situation can often end up with the young woman blaming herself, and taking on the responsibility and costs of looking after the baby, it would be better here to focus mainly on what the man could have done.

3. Once participants have made a few suggestions, you can propose the following **four-point plan** which could help us all to take responsibility for the things which we do:

a. **ACKNOWLEDGE** what we have done.
b. **ACCEPT** responsibility for it.
c. **ACT** appropriately to limit the damage done (have any necessary conversations, sort out the mess, or, in this case, help the young woman with financial support for their child).
d. **MAKE SURE** we won't do it again.

4. Ask participants what they think of this four-point plan.

5. Next, ask participants to divide into pairs. Each person in the pair should take it in turn to think of a situation in which they have found themselves during the last month. It could have been with a partner, a son or daughter, an employer – anyone. The problem may have been big

or small. The important thing is that the participant feels that s/he handled the situation badly and didn't take enough responsibility for his or her own actions. They should then:

- Describe the situation to the other person in the pair.
- Explain how s/he handled it.
- Say if s/he blamed someone else: if so, who?
- Explain how s/he feels about it now.
- Describe how s/he might have handled it better, using the four-point plan above.

Encourage the **listening** member of the pair to help with suggestions if the one **talking** feels stuck on the last two points of the four-point plan (i.e. how to act to limit the damage and how to prevent a repeat). Ask listening participants to take care that they make constructive suggestions and don't become too critical of the talking participant.

Time the activity so that each member of the pair has five minutes in each role, i.e. as talker and as listener/adviser.

6. Call everyone back to the circle. Ask if anyone would be prepared to share their experience with the whole group. If so, ask them to explain quickly what they discussed in their pair. Ask others what they think of what the participant chose to do and perhaps to make alternative suggestions.

7. Point out that it is often easier for people to discuss things with a friend when they feel they have handled things badly and that this four-point plan enables us to think through a situation more clearly so we can **regain control of the situation for ourselves**. Encourage participants to try it out for themselves over the coming week and to bring an example with them to next week's session.

> ☞ This exercise is an important step in helping people to change how they react when things go wrong for them. It is likely to provoke a lot of discussion.

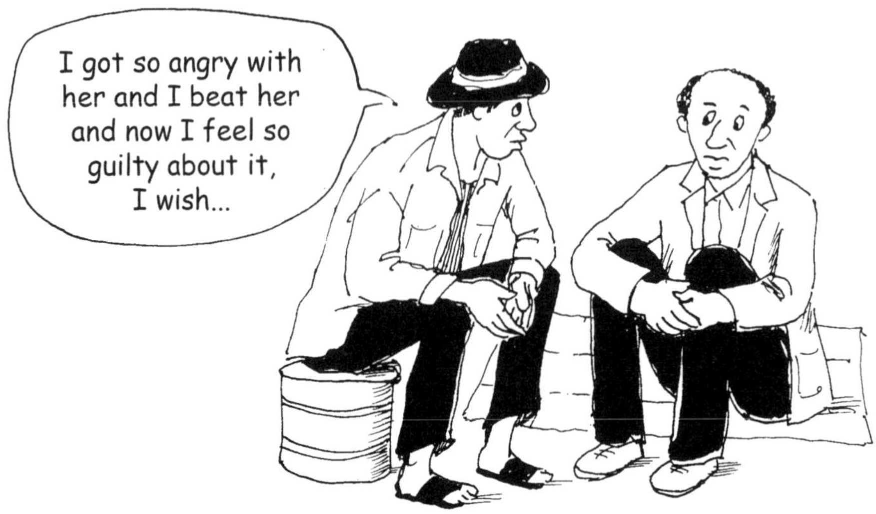
I got so angry with her and I beat her and now I feel so guilty about it, I wish...

EXERCISE J.7: CLOSING CIRCLE

1. Thank everyone again for coming. Ask each member of the group in turn to mention one thing that they have learnt today and one thing that they are looking forward to doing before the next meeting.

2. Ask if there are any more questions about today's session.

3. Remind everyone to think about the four-point plan for taking responsibility for our own actions, and encourage them to make use of it at least once before the next session.

4. Remind everyone of their role as guardian angel.

5. Encourage participants to talk in general about the kinds of issues they have been discussing in these sessions with their friends and neighbours, if they like, but not to share any confidential information from the peer group with others.

6. Remind everyone of the time and place for the next meeting and say you look forward to seeing them all again there. Remember to ask for three new volunteers to stay behind for a quick instant review of this session. (See Annex 4 for details.)

FACILITATORS' TEAM FEEDBACK

After the end of Session J, meet again with your co-facilitators, to compare notes on how your sessions went and the information that you learnt from them. Your co-facilitators could have found useful information that could help you to structure your next session more effectively. Remember however not to share individual confidentialities between groups. This is the easiest way to ruin the trust that you have built and to wreck the whole workshop!

ENDNOTE

1. Participants may want to view the clip again. If so, it is usually best for them to have some discussion about it first, then to have a further discussion after the second viewing.

YOUR NOTES ...

THEME 4 – WAYS IN WHICH WE CAN CHANGE

SESSION K LET'S ASSERT OURSELVES

PURPOSE

To develop more assertiveness skills.

CONTENTS	**TIME NEEDED**
Introduction	
K.1	Tugs of War and Peace
K.2	**DVD Clip 10:** 'Saying 'No'?'
K.3	Opening a Fist
K.4	**DVD Clip 11:** 'Coming Home'
K.5	'I' Statements
K.6	Closing Circle

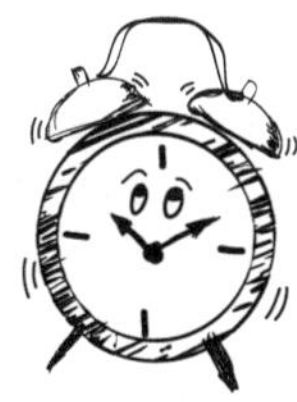

3–4 hours

MATERIALS NEEDED: A **strong** rope, DVD, laptop with DVD player, projector.

PARTICIPANTS: Four separate peer groups.

SPECIAL INFORMATION

Don't forget to read 'Before You Begin ...!' before using this section of the manual.

INTRODUCTION

1. Sit in a circle with the group, preferably on the ground. Everyone should be at the same level, including yourself.

2. Welcome everyone to the new session. Thank everyone for coming. Enquire about late-comers or non-attenders.

3. Ask each participant to recount quickly something good which has happened to them since the last session.

4. Review the last session. Ask participants to remind us what we learnt about accepting responsibility for our actions. Remind them if they have forgotten. Ask a few people to describe briefly how they have used the four-point plan during the week. Thank and praise those who share their experiences with the group.

5. Explain that we are going on to discuss other things in this session, but will start with a fight!

EXERCISE K.1: TUGS OF WAR AND PEACE

AIMS: Warm-up exercise. To illustrate benefits of working together.

DESCRIPTION: Everyone pulls together on a rope.

MATERIALS NEEDED: A length of strong rope.

DIRECTIONS

1. Divide the group into two teams. Ask these two teams to stand up and hold opposite ends of a long strong rope. Mark a line across the middle of your training area over which each team must try to pull the other.

2. When you have said 'One, two, three, go!', the teams should start pulling against each other. Let them go on until one team has ended up falling over the dividing line.

3. Next, ask everyone to sit in a circle. Now tie the same strong rope in a large circle and hand it to the participants, so that they are sitting round the edge of it.

4. Ask all the participants to pull together on the rope so that they can all stand up.

5. Ask participants what this illustrates.

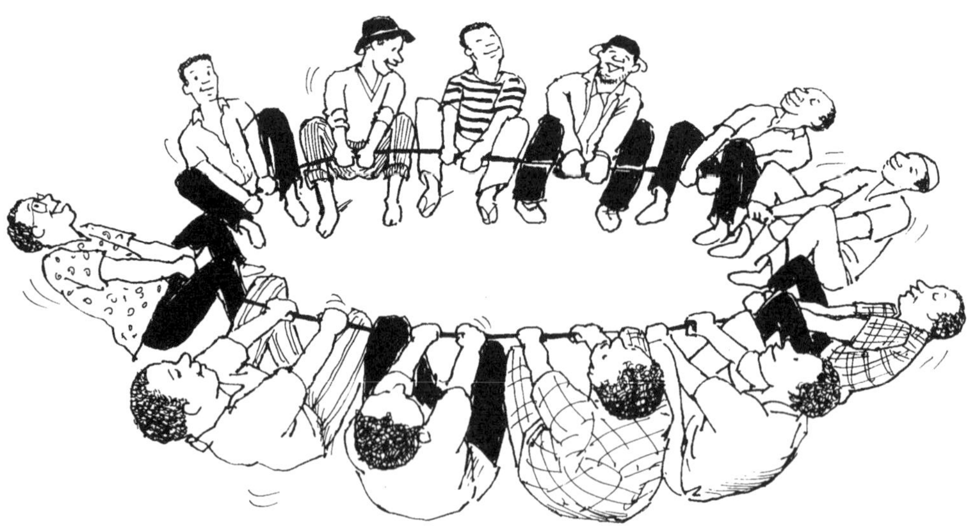

The idea is to show how, instead of pulling on opposite ends – a tug of war, where only one team wins – we can respond to situations in a win-win way, so that everyone benefits and feels good about the result. True, the tug of war might feel more fun for the victors – but how do the losers feel?

EXERCISE K.2: DVD Clip 10: 'SAYING 'NO'?'

AIM: To help participants consider one way in which women can handle sugar daddies, teachers, male relatives, bosses, and so on.

DESCRIPTION: Watching DVD, followed by discussion.

MATERIALS NEEDED: DVD, laptop with DVD player, projector.

DIRECTIONS

1. Explain to participants that we are now going to watch another DVD clip of the young women from Buwenda village. They are repeating the sugar daddy pick-up clip – but this time with a different result. Ask participants to stand up, have a good stretch, and move around to a new position so that they can all see the screen.

2. Say that while they are watching the clip, you would like them to consider what they would think about this kind of outcome in their own community.

Make sure that everyone can see and hear the DVD clearly.

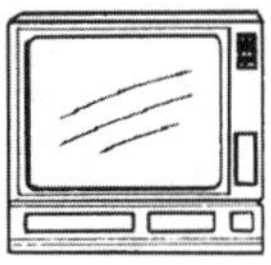

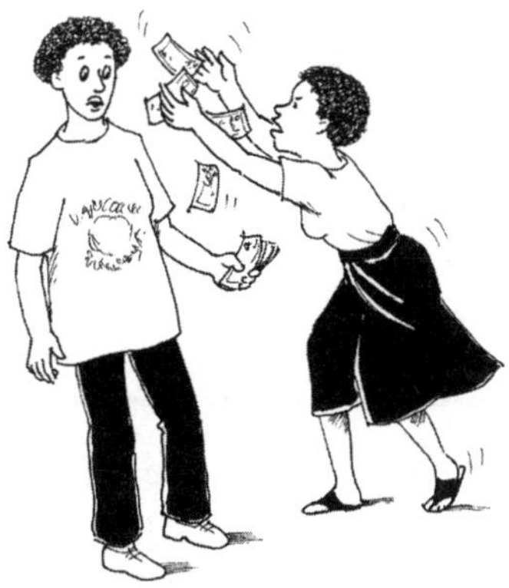

3. Turn on the DVD at the point where it says '10. Saying 'No'?'.

4. Turn off the DVD at the point where the screen goes black.

5. Ask participants to summarise what they saw and heard in the clip.

6. Then ask participants what they thought of the young woman's response to the sugar daddy.

7. Point out that young women often find themselves approached by teachers, male relatives, young men, bosses, or other men in the work place, not just by sugar daddies. Young men are also sometimes propositioned by older women and may find it difficult to refuse them. This technique can work in any crisis. For instance, shouting 'No!' very fiercely can also be a very powerful way of stopping a thief from snatching your money! So building up confidence to say no can be useful to all of us.[1]

☞ Some people may say that the young woman was behaving too aggressively towards the sugar daddy. Point out that women often find it very hard to make it clear when they really mean 'no' and so the young women's group were practising saying it in as clear a manner as they possibly could. Once they had achieved this, they then had more confidence in themselves and could learn next how to say it in a way which was still very clear but less aggressive and, perhaps, more appropriate for this kind of situation. Your own participants will have a chance to practise this themselves in a later exercise. Nevertheless, if a woman is being **attacked** she needs to be confident that she can say 'No!' as fiercely and in as determined a manner as possible. This kind of exercise is very good at giving women this confidence.

NB: At this stage there are two different sets of instructions. For facilitators working with men, follow 7a. For facilitators working with women, follow 7b.

7a. **(Older Men or Younger Men.)** Ask your participants to divide into pairs. Each pair should consider:

- When a woman says 'no', how does a man know whether she **really** means 'no' or whether she might mean 'yes'?
- What could the man and the woman do to change their behaviour to each other so that the man can understand that when a woman **says** 'no', she **means** 'no'?

After this, bring all the men back to the full circle and review what has been discussed. Try to encourage participants to produce some **specific** ideas of how they could behave differently.

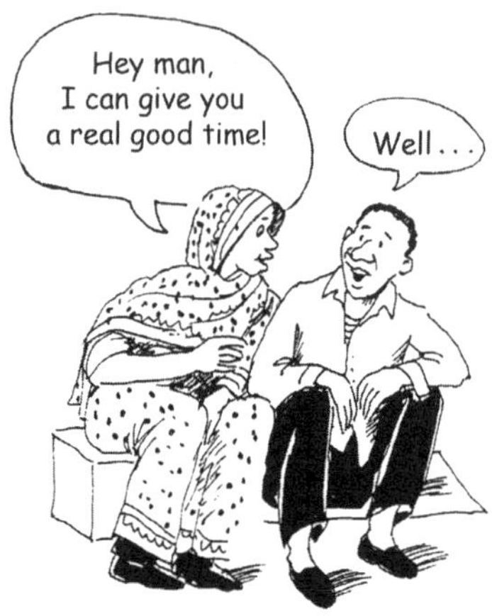
Hey man, I can give you a real good time!
Well...

Then encourage two of them to stand up and role-play this in the middle of your circle: one can pretend to be the man, the other the woman. Their interaction should include spoken language as well as body language.

If someone else from the group thinks they could manage better, get them to replace one of the two in the middle. Go on finding others to have a go until everyone is satisfied that what they see and hear from the man and the 'woman' are both good examples of responsible behaviour.

Then encourage role-play of a young man saying 'no' to an older woman, or of an older man saying 'no' to a woman of his age or younger. (For instance, you could challenge your participants by saying that many men have said they were seduced into having sex by a young attractive woman. Is this really true? How could they say 'no', if they wanted to?) Role-play whatever situation your participants would like to practise.

> ☞ This is, of course, a very sensitive issue. It would be good for you to emphasise that, if we are to take responsibility for our own actions, we should not be trying to blame others but should be trying to behave as responsibly as we can ourselves. This means that you should ensure that your participants don't just say that this is all women's responsibility: they should challenge one another to think of different ways of behaving themselves.

7b. **(Older Women or Younger Women.)** Ask your participants to sit in a circle. Ask them to describe ways in which they themselves have successfully turned down an unwanted advance from a man – even from their husband. Encourage participants to share their experiences with the other participants in the peer group.

Next, ask two volunteers to stand up in the middle. Say that this exercise is called 'standing your ground' and that everyone is now going to learn how to say 'No!' like the young woman in the DVD. Explain that this young woman had never done this before, but had learnt how to do it during the workshop. Say that this form of rejecting an advance can be very effective if a woman is being attacked and now is the opportunity for your participants to practise.

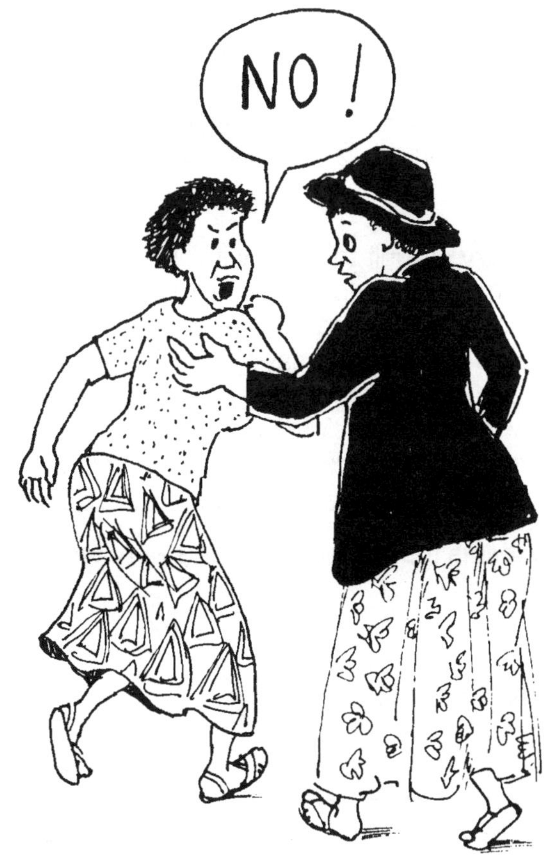

In Buwenda*, to begin with, the young women felt very nervous about raising their voices in this way. But after a couple of tries they began to gain confidence, and even the quietest young woman managed to speak and move clearly and assertively. They felt that this was a real skill which they had learnt: one that would help them to protect themselves.*

Explain that, in most societies, women are taught to obey men. Therefore, it is often very difficult for a woman to resist someone in this way. But with the use of our bodies, our eyes, our faces and our voices, we can make it very clear when we want to say 'no'.

Start off by demonstrating this to your participants. Stand up and ask one of the volunteers to walk up to you and stroke your shoulder. Turn round quickly and shout 'No!' at her, very loudly, before moving off, fast.

Then ask the same volunteer to approach the other volunteer who is standing. It is then the turn of the latter to practise saying **'No!'** When she has done this to everyone's satisfaction, she should go to sit down. Then a new volunteer should stand up and approach the participant who was just acting as the man. The new volunteer plays the man and the first volunteer acts as the woman.

Carry on round the group, so that everyone has a chance first to be the man and then the woman shouting **'No!'** Each of them should go on practising **'No!'** until the rest of the group agrees that they have done it well.

This is an immensely powerful exercise. Women should use all of their body to say 'no'. She should stand tall and firm, 'standing her ground' and feeling that her weight is centred and not unbalanced; she should look the 'man' right in his eyes and she should look forthright, not scared. She should use her voice as a weapon and should **shout**, not whisper, **'No!'**

Participants may find this **very** difficult to begin with. There may be a lot of giggles and women saying they can't do it. You need to give them a lot of praise and encouragement. In your area, the problem for a woman may not be so much saying 'no' fiercely, but what to do at times when she actually **wants** to say 'yes'. If so, how can she react so that she feels in control of the situation? Could she say, 'Yes – with a condom!' safely? You may want to discuss this with your participants, then encourage them to try out which alternative answers best meet their needs through further role-play.

8. Finally, explain to all participants that we are going to see how good we are at persuading others to do what we ask.

EXERCISE K.3: OPENING A FIST

AIM: A quick game to change the pace and provide a challenge!

DESCRIPTION: Pairs work on persuasion.

DIRECTIONS

1. Explain the following to participants, acting it out as you say it:

All these things create a more measured response in the aggressor!

We have seen how our body language can influence other people's response to us. For instance, if someone is acting aggressively towards us, they may be leaning forward with clenched fists. By changing our body language we can improve the situation. For instance, if we are sitting down, we can relax our shoulders, uncross our arms, open our palms upwards, uncross our legs, hold our heads straight, look straight at the aggressor ...

2. Now ask participants to divide into pairs. One will act as the aggressor and the other will act as the persuader, then they will swap roles. The aggressor must hold his/her hand up in a very tight fist and feel very angry. The persuader has to try to persuade the aggressor to undo his/her fist.

The persuader should use all his/her skills to persuade the aggressor to calm down and to open his/her fist. The persuader and aggressor must not touch each other, but the persuader can say or do anything which s/he thinks will work to calm the aggressor down and persuade him/her to open his/her fist. If the aggressor thinks that the persuader has done a good enough job, s/he can agree to open his/her fist. But s/he mustn't give in too easily!

Give the pairs five minutes each way to try out their persuasion on each other.

3. See by a show of hands how many people managed to persuade their partners to open their fists! Praise and encourage everyone end explain that this gets easier with practice.

EXERCISE K.4: DVD Clip 11: 'COMING HOME'

AIM: To discuss how hard it can be to say some important things.

DESCRIPTION: Watching DVD, followed by discussion.

MATERIALS NEEDED: DVD, laptop with DVD player, projector.

DIRECTIONS

1. Explain to participants that we are now going to watch the next DVD clip. This one is called 'Coming Home'. It is acted by the older women's group, who were, as usual, drawing on their own experiences. Ask participants to stand up, have a good stretch, and move around to a new position so that they can all see the screen.

2. Say that, while watching the clip, you would like them to think about the relationship of the couple they see and about how well – or badly – they think the couple are communicating.

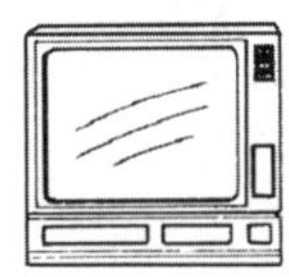

Make sure that everyone can see and hear the DVD clearly.

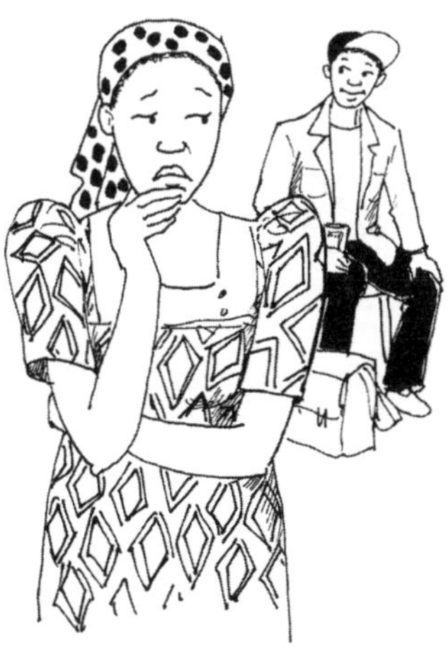

3. Turn on the DVD at the point where it says '11. Coming Home'.

4. Turn off the DVD at the point where the screen goes black.

5. Ask participants to explain what they have just seen, to make sure that everyone understands it.[1]

6. Ask participants to divide into pairs and discuss the following:

- Of the couple, who was expressing their needs effectively?
- Who was acting responsibly?
- Who was acting assertively?
- What do you think of the woman's request?
- What do you think was the likely response of the man to his wife's request?
- What do you think could have been a good response from him to her?
- How do you think the woman could have handled the situation better?

(You may need to repeat the questions one by one as pairs discuss them.)

7. Bring participants back to the large circle and review the questions above with the whole group.

8. Finally, explain that the next exercise will give us all a chance to think of ways in which we can express our own needs in an assertive way.

> This exercise may well raise different opinions in the group. This does not matter: the important thing is that there is a debate, and that the possibility is raised in the minds of all participants that the husband may not have been behaving as responsibly as he could have done here.

A QUESTION OF BALANCE: SUPPORT NOTES FOR ASSERTIVENESS

We can look upon aggression, assertiveness, and passiveness as different points along a line:

AGGRESSIVENESS	ASSERTIVENESS	PASSIVENESS
Expressing your feelings, opinions or desires in a way that threatens or punishes the other person – you are insisting on your rights while denying their rights.	Telling someone exactly what you want in a way that does not seem rude or threatening to them – you are standing up for your rights while not endangering the rights of others.	Giving in to the will of others – hoping to get what you want without actually having to say it – leaving it to others to guess or letting them decide for you.

DOMINATING, for instance: shouting – demanding – not listening to others – saying others are wrong – leaning forward – looking down on others – wagging finger or pointing at others – threatening – fighting

BALANCED, 'for instance: knowing what you want to say – saying 'I feel …', not 'I think …' – being specific – using 'I' statements – looking the person in the eye – not whining or being sarcastic – using your body language too (standing your ground, being centred)

SUBMISSIVE, for instance: talking quietly – giggling nervously – looking down or away – sagging shoulders – avoiding disagreement – hiding face with hands

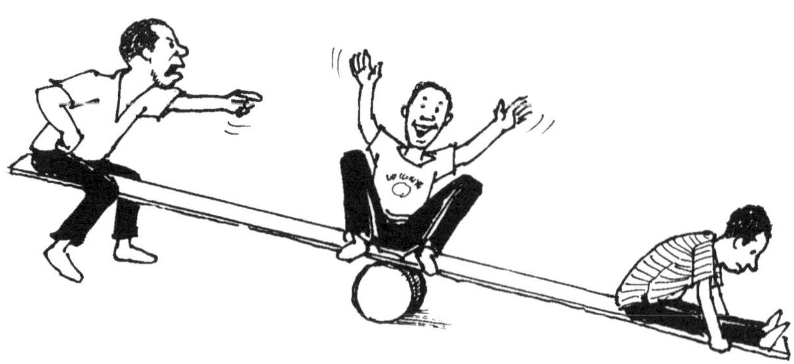

EXERCISE K.5: 'I' STATEMENTS

AIMS: To show how it is possible to face someone with whom you have a problem without either antagonising them or withdrawing from the problem. To practise making non-judgemental statements, and using a structure which can open rather than close discussion of a difficulty.

DESCRIPTION: An exercise which explains and demonstrates an assertive but non-aggressive way of expressing feelings about a problem.

DIRECTIONS

1. Introduce the idea of 'I' statements to the participants, including clear and clean 'I' statements that have worked. See the following pages for details of what needs to be said.

2. With the participants working in pairs, ask them to prepare one 'I' statement each, relating to a current or recurring difficulty in their lives. Partners can help each other to make their statements clear and clean.

3. Ask for a few examples from the participants, giving people an opportunity to comment on them and to offer suggestions as to how they might be improved.

4. In what ways could the 'I' statement formula be useful to participants? What do they think about it?

5. Ask all participants to commit themselves to making one 'I' statement to somebody before the next session.

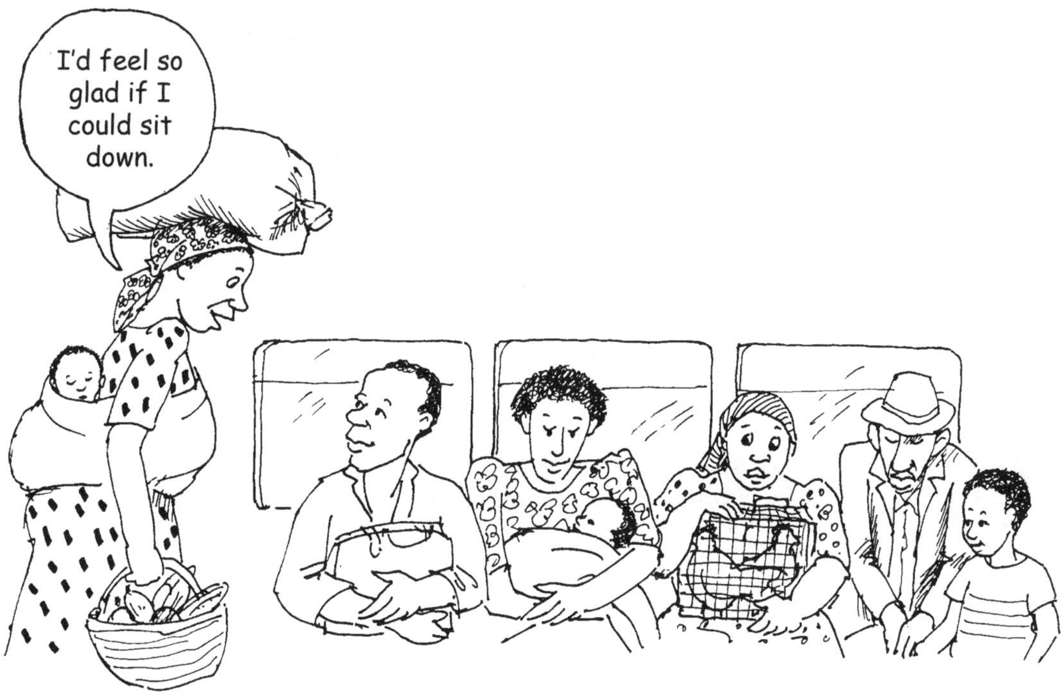

> ☞ This is a useful way of separating feelings and facts in order to clarify what a problem really is. The formula may seem strange and unfamiliar, but with practice it can become an unconscious reaction rather than a laboured response. It is a tough discipline and needs practice.
>
> It is worth pointing out that it can be used at work, at the market, in shops, with friends, on public transport, or at any time when you feel that your needs are not being met. It is not just for use with a partner!
>
> Groups, as well as individuals, can use the formula to help them make a statement about something they feel strongly about. Group statements will be explored in a later session.

INFORMATION FOR 'I' STATEMENTS EXERCISE

An 'I' statement is a way of clearly expressing your point of view about a situation. It includes an expression of how the situation is affecting you, and how you would like to see it change. The best 'I' statement is free of specific demands and blame. It opens up space for discussion and leaves the next move to the other person.

We should aim for our 'I' statements to be **clear** (that is, to the point) and **clean** (that is, free of blame and judgment).

We should beware of 'you' statements which place blame on someone else, hold them responsible, demand change from them, or hold a threat.

Two examples of a 'you' statement:

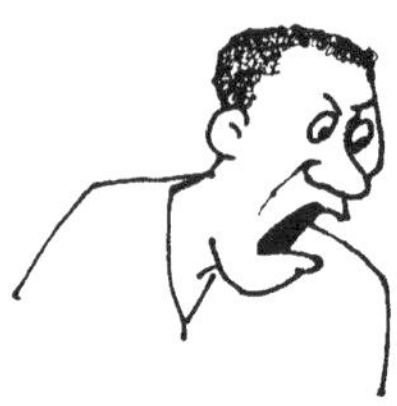

'You are so lazy, you never keep the house cleanly swept, you are always late with my food, and the children are always crying. I don't know why I married you. You must start to work harder from now on!'

'You are always so drunk when you crash into the house at night. And you never give me any money to buy any food. I don't know why I ever married you. You must stop going to that bar from now on!'

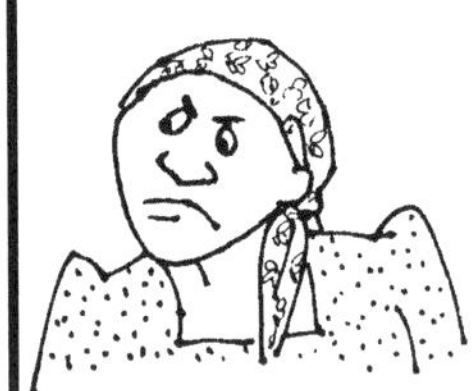

These statements are very judgemental and make the listener feel hemmed-in and thus defensive.

Two examples of an 'I' statement:

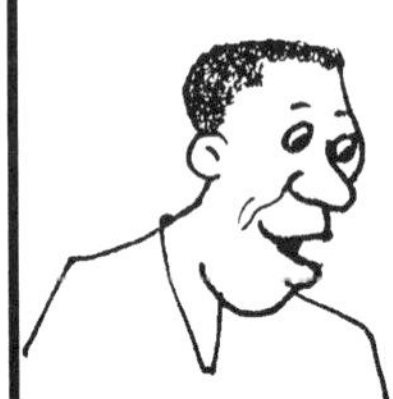

'When I come home I feel disappointed if the food is not ready and the house not swept. I would like us to discuss how we can arrange things better so that this would be possible.'

'When you come home at night from the bar, I feel disappointed because I would like to see more of you, and I would like some money for food for the children. I would like us to discuss how we can arrange things better together.'

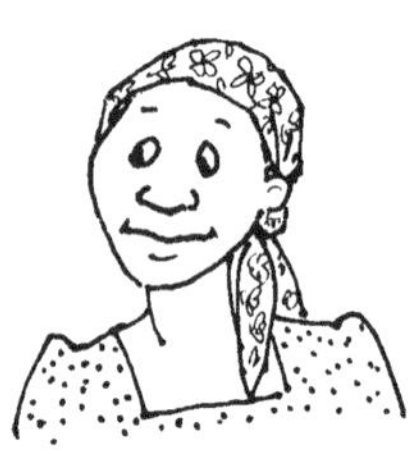

These statements carry no blame and are phrased not to annoy the listener. The expectations within them are presented in a non-judgemental manner (there is no 'you must ...') and are not accusing the listener. They state the speaker's expectations or hopes, but they do not demand that they be met.

'I' statement formula

The action: 'When ...'	Make it as specific and non-judgemental as possible, e.g. 'When you come home at night ...'
My response: 'I feel ...'	Say 'I feel ...' rather than 'I think ...' and keep it to your **own** feelings: 'I feel hurt/sad/happy/disappointed/ ignored ...', for instance. **Not:** 'I feel that you are being mean!'

Reason: '... because ...' — If you think an explanation helps, you can add one here. But make sure it is still non-blaming: e.g. '... because I like to spend time with you.'

Suggestions: 'What I'd like is ...' — A statement of the change you would like. It is OK to **say** what you want, but **not to demand** it of the other person: e.g. 'What I'd like is for us to discuss this' or 'What I'd like is to make arrangements that we can both keep', **not** 'You must stop being so lazy!'

This is a structured format and may seem strange to start with. It takes time to absorb new skills and begin to use them unconsciously. Adapt the language to suit your situation.

- Try to use it first in an easy context, with a friend over a small problem. You can begin just by saying 'I feel happy when ...' and see how that works.
- Then as you gain practice in using it, you can try it with a friend in harder situations. You can start to try out 'I feel unhappy when ...'
- When you feel OK with that, you could try out 'I feel happy when ...' with your partner.
- Finally, you can try out 'I feel unhappy/sad/frustrated when ...' with your partner. This sounds very daunting but, as the women of Buwenda found, it is possible to learn.

The women of Buwenda first said it was impossible for a woman to say such a thing. But after a while they began to try it out and found that it worked for them. They decided to call the formula 'magic medicine' because they were so impressed with the difference that it had made to them. A few months after the workshop had finished, one woman managed to say something to her husband which she had wanted to say for a long time. They had been together for 12 years and had children, but he had never visited her parents. This felt to her like he did not really value their relationship. So she decided to say 'I feel hurt that you haven't visited my parents after these years together.' Whereupon, her husband started buying cloth to take as a present to her mother, and started preparing for the first visit.

One of the young women in Buwenda who attended the workshop is a teacher. She managed to use an 'I' statement with her headmaster, when she was dissatisfied with the way he was speaking to her.

One of the young men in Buwenda who attended the workshop was with a group of his friends. They were having an argument amongst themselves and he said 'I would feel happy if you could settle this problem calmly.' It worked.

Through these and other examples, people in Buwenda have found that everyone can benefit from speaking assertively. It is an effective way of speaking non-aggressively, and without wounding the other person's feelings.

EXERCISE K.6: CLOSING CIRCLE

1. Thank everyone again for coming. Ask each member of the group in turn to mention one thing that they have learnt today and one thing that they are looking forward to doing before the next meeting.

2. Ask if there are any more questions about today's session.

3. Remind everyone of their role as guardian angel.

4. Encourage participants to talk in general about the kinds of issues they have been discussing in these sessions with their friends and neighbours, if they like, but not to share any confidential information from the peer group with others.

5. Remind everyone of the time and place for the next meeting and say you look forward to seeing them all again there. Remember to ask for three volunteers to stay behind for a quick instant review of this session. (See Annex 4 for details.)

FACILITATORS' TEAM FEEDBACK

After the end of Session K, meet again with your co-facilitators, to compare notes on how your sessions went and the information which you learnt from them. Your co-facilitators could have found useful information that could help you to structure your next session more effectively. Remember however not to share individual confidentialities between groups. This is the easiest way to ruin the trust that you have built and to wreck the whole workshop!

ENDNOTE

1. Participants may want to view the clip again. If so, it is usually best for them to have some discussion about it first, then to have a further discussion after the second viewing.

YOUR NOTES ...

SESSION L LET'S CHANGE OURSELVES

PURPOSE

To put these new skills into practice.

CONTENTS	TIME NEEDED
Introduction	
L.1	**DVD Clip 12:** ' 'I' Statements'
L.2	Three to One
L.3	Skills to handle manipulation
L.4	'Exploring Why' Revisited
L.5	Rhythm Clap

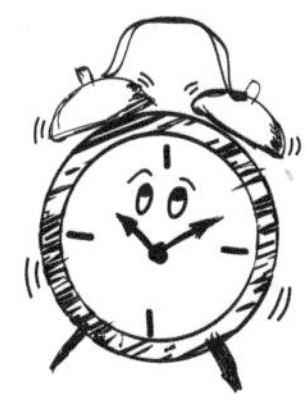

3–4 hours

MATERIALS NEEDED: DVD, laptop with DVD player, projector.

PARTICIPANTS: Four separate peer groups.

SPECIAL INFORMATION

- Don't forget to read 'Before You Begin ...!' before using this section of the manual.
- You need to make sure that, at the end of this session, all four peer groups arrange a mutually agreeable time for the following meeting. This will be the second full workshop meeting.
- Remember to make sure that all four peer groups have had time to complete all sessions, including this one, before a time for the second full workshop meeting is set. Please refer back to the section on workshop duration, under 'When' in 'Before You Begin ...!', for more details.

INTRODUCTION

1. Sit in a circle with the group, preferably on the ground. Everyone should be at the same level, including yourself.

2. Welcome everyone to the new session. Thank everyone for coming. Enquire about late-comers or non-attenders.

3. Ask each participant to recount briefly how they have managed to use an 'I' statement since the last session and how it felt for them to use it. Give a lot of praise to those who succeeded. If someone has not managed to do so, encourage them to try to do so soon – but don't be cross with them. It's hard for some people to summon up the courage the first time! Has anyone found another way of handling conflict which they find effective?

4. Explain that in this session everyone is going to have a chance to practise their new-found skills. First though, another DVD clip from Buwenda.

EXERCISE L.1: DVD Clip 12: ' 'I' STATEMENTS'

AIM: To help participants see how 'I' statements could be used.

DESCRIPTION: Watching DVD, followed by discussion.

MATERIALS NEEDED: DVD, laptop with DVD player, projector.

DIRECTIONS

1. Explain to participants that we are now going to watch another DVD clip of the younger women of Buwenda village. Here they are role-playing one example of how they think 'I' statements could make a difference to them. Ask participants to stand up, have a good stretch, and move around to a new position so that they can all see the screen.

2. Say that, while they are watching the clip, you would like them to think about how they could use the 'I' statement in their own lives.

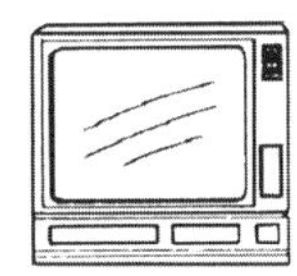

Make sure that everyone can see and hear the DVD clearly.

3. Turn on the DVD at the point where it says '12. 'I' Statements'.

4. Turn off the DVD at the point where the screen goes black.[1]

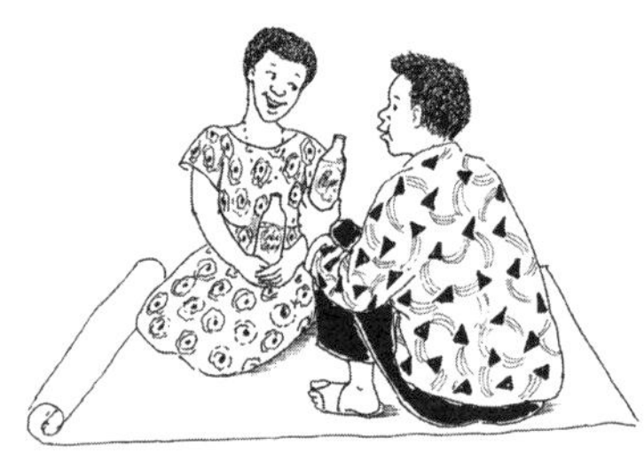

5. Ask participants to summarise what they have seen. (For a synopsis, see Annex 3.)

6. Ask participants to work in pairs. Each person should think of two new real situations where they possibly could use an 'I' statement before the next session. They could discuss these situations with their partner and try them out with their partner's help and using their suggestions.

After a few minutes, call out, so that the members of each pair can swap roles.

7. Finally, call everyone back to the full circle and ask everyone to make a commitment to try out at least one – and preferably both – of the new 'I' statements that they have thought of, before the next session.

EXERCISE L.2: THREE TO ONE

AIMS: To explore different responses to difficult situations. To recognise the tactics and skills we currently use in handling such situations and to learn from the tactics and skills of others. To find appropriate responses to situations that we are involved in. To anticipate difficulties and prepare responses.

DESCRIPTION: Interactive work in small groups looking at difficult situations.

DIRECTIONS

1. Ask participants to think of an incident or situation they faced recently, at home, at work, or socially, which they feel they did not deal with effectively.

2. Divide participants into small groups, and each group agrees to work on one person's situation. They explore the following in relation to this situation: the most likely response, the most provocative response (that is, the one likely to produce the worst reaction) and a 'successful' response (that is, a response which is likely to work for that person at that time – not necessarily an approach that would be successful for **everyone**). The groups role-play the three options. If the most likely response corresponds with the most provocative one, there will be only two options to act out.

3. Either join up as a whole group to see some of the role plays, or join pairs of groups together to show their options to one another.

4. Ask participants what differences were made by the different approaches. What worked and why? In what ways were they familiar or unfamiliar? How often is the likely response the provocative one or the successful one? What skills or tactics, such as body language, are we already using to avoid the provocative response?

> ☞ The most likely response will often be a response which is not successful. If the group feel that, in their example, the most likely response is actually the successful response, you could explore the factors which contribute to making this possible.

> *In Buwenda, the young women's group performed three different role plays of a woman asking her husband if she could go to visit her parents. In the first role play, she talked rather submissively and he replied that there was too much work around the house for her to have time away. In the second role play, she sounded rather demanding and he replied in an annoyed way. She answered him back and she became angry. In the third role play, she said 'I would feel really happy if I could ...'. At this, her husband replied: 'Good, do go. Give my greetings – oh, and here is some money for the journey!' This caused general laughter among the participants and was, perhaps, a little over-optimistic. But practising different styles of speech in this kind of role play can help participants enormously by giving them skills to analyse and change their own styles of behaviour.*

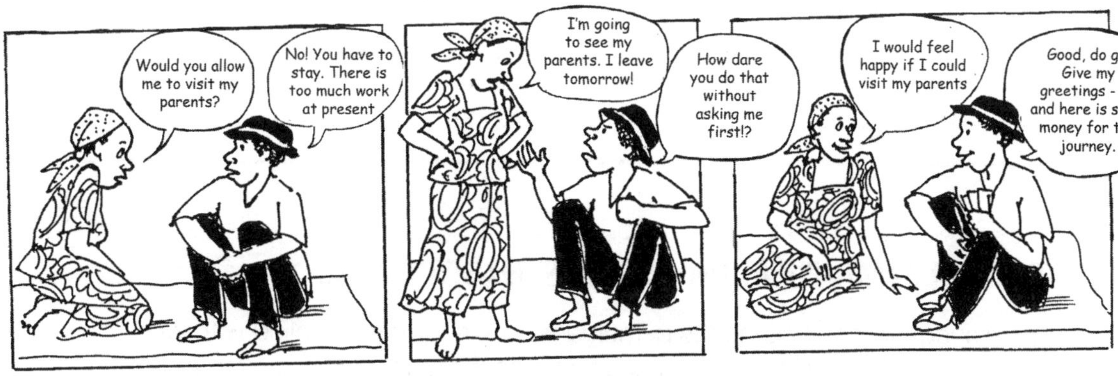

Would you allow me to visit my parents?
No! You have to stay. There is too much work at present
I'm going to see my parents. I leave tomorrow!
How dare you do that without asking me first!?
I would feel happy if I could visit my parents
Good, do go. Give my greetings - oh and here is some money for the journey.

EXERCISE L.3: SKILLS TO HANDLE MANIPULATION

AIMS: To practise facing manipulation and finding assertive responses. To apply skills from the previous exercises.

DESCRIPTION: An interactive group exercise exploring how to give assertive responses under pressure.

DIRECTIONS

1. Explain to the group that we often find ourselves in situations where we have to think very quickly about what we want to say and we often don't think of a good response until it is too late. Like the couple in the previous sketch, what we say – or don't say – can often be very important. This exercise will give us a chance to practise thinking fast!

2. Divide participants into groups of three. Each group will be told about a different situation in which they have to pretend to be a person who is trying to manipulate someone else into doing something they don't want to do. (See the list of suggested situations below.) Each group member should decide **entirely by her/himself** what her/his opening manipulative line will be. For instance, in the younger women's group, if I am told that I am supposed to be an older man chatting up a schoolgirl my opening line might be: 'Did you know you are very beautiful? Would you like a ride in my car?'

3. Participants return to the circle and, one by one, each turns to the person on their left and states very briefly the relationship and the situation – for example, 'I am a sugar daddy and you are a young girl and I want to seduce you.' S/he then states the opening line that s/he has just thought up and the person on her/his left has to make an **immediate** response, trying to state her/his position without rising to the bait. For example, a response to the statement above might be: 'Thank you for the compliment, but I do not want a ride in your car.' Give everyone the chance to use their own line and to respond to someone else's.

4. Ask participants which responses are most effective and why. How did people deal with the bait they were offered? How do they usually respond to similar situations? What could they do differently?

> This exercise draws on work done in previous exercises. The response people are aiming for is one which does not compromise them, and which allows them to state their position without resentment or inappropriate anger. They should face the problem without either attacking or avoiding being assertive. It is hard to start off with but gets easier as participants practise and gain confidence.

SKILLS TO HANDLE MANIPULATION – SUGGESTED SITUATIONS

Here are some suggestions of situations participants could practise dealing with with one another. Choose three that are relevant for your own peer group. However, you may well know of specific situations that your participants have already found themselves in. If so, use those examples as well as, or instead of, the ones listed below.

Younger and Older Women's Groups

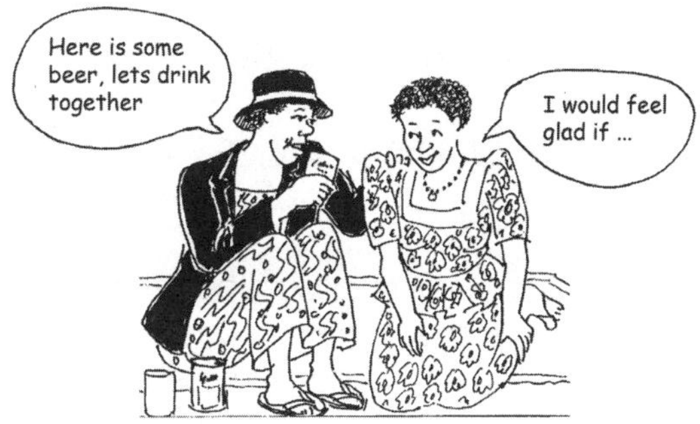
Here is some beer, lets drink together
I would feel glad if ...

- sugar daddy
- partner wanting to have sex with you when you know he has another lover
- boyfriend, husband, or new partner wanting you to have sex with him without a condom, when you want to use one
- school teacher bribing student with higher grades in return for sexual favours
- man at market suggesting sex in return for groceries
- boyfriend putting pressure on you to have sex with him
- husband or boyfriend wanting you to have sex with him when it is late and you are tired
- being laughed at for not wanting to have a boyfriend or to get married yet
- being laughed at for wanting to study, instead of relaxing with your friends
- uncle wanting you to have sex with him, in return for money
- boss saying you will get promoted if you have sex with him
- wanting to have sex with someone when there are no condoms available.

Younger and Older Men's Groups

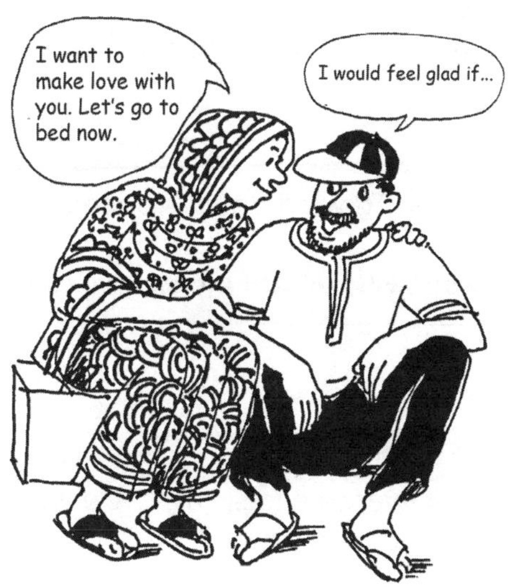
I want to make love with you. Let's go to bed now.
I would feel glad if...

- being encouraged by your friends to drink too much
- being laughed at for not having sex with your girlfriend
- being laughed at for wanting to use a condom
- being ridiculed for not having several girlfriends
- being laughed at for sticking with one woman, or for not wanting a girlfriend
- being ridiculed for wanting to study
- being propositioned by an older woman, maybe in return for money or alcohol
- being propositioned by an attractive young woman
- young woman not wanting to use a condom because she thinks it means you think she's a sex worker.

EXERCISE L.4: 'EXPLORING WHY' REVISITED

AIM: To review a previous exercise in the light of what we have learnt.

DESCRIPTION: Role play, followed by analysis.

DIRECTIONS

1. Remind participants that in Session H we did an exercise called 'Exploring Why', where we performed role plays of situations where someone like them could end up having sex.

2. Explain that now you are asking them to re-enact those situations, but this time the person like them in the role play is taking much more responsibility for their actions and acting in an assertive (but not aggressive) manner.

3. Ask participants to re-form the four smaller groups in which they worked on this exercise in Session H.

4. Ask participants to discuss how they can re-work their scene so that the character like them feels able to handle the situation assertively and responsibly and then practise it. Encourage them to bear in mind all that you have been discussing during the last few sessions: spoken language, body language, eye contact, alcohol use, location, local traditions, and so on. Their new scenes could involve safer sex, unsafe sex, or no sex at all – it is up to participants to re-enact the scene in the way they like.

5. Ask each small group to perform their new scene for the rest of the peer group and encourage a few questions for discussion from the audience at the end of each one.

> During the course of this discussion, encourage participants to recognise that the changes in their role plays can be broken down into **changes in the characters' own personal behaviour** and **changes in what their community expects or accepts of them**.

EXERCISE L.5: RHYTHM CLAP

AIMS: To wind down. To create a feeling of unity.

DESCRIPTION: Full group exercise, with everyone clapping.

DIRECTIONS

1. Ask everyone to sit in a circle and close their eyes. They should each begin to beat or clap a rhythm. Join in yourself.

2. At first this sounds disjointed and chaotic, but gradually people try to change in order to create a rhythmical sound.

3. Explain that this session has now finished and that the second half of the next one is going to be another full workshop meeting for all four peer groups together.

4. Explain that, at the start of the next meeting, each peer group will choose one of the situations which they have just acted out for the other groups to see. Then, after some rehearsal, all four peer groups will come together. Each will perform both its original scene and then its revised scene for all the participants from the other peer groups to see and discuss.

5. Arrange a time and place for your next meeting. Point out that you need to double-check this with the other three peer groups, since all four peer groups will be meeting together.

6. Remind everyone to try again to use one or two of the new 'I' statements that they have practised today.

7. Remind everyone of their role as guardian angel.

8. Encourage participants to talk in general about the kinds of issues they have been discussing in these sessions with their friends and neighbours, if they like, but not to share any confidential information from the peer group with others.

9. Thank everyone for coming today. Remember to ask for three new people to stay behind for an instant review of the session. (See Annex 4 for details.)

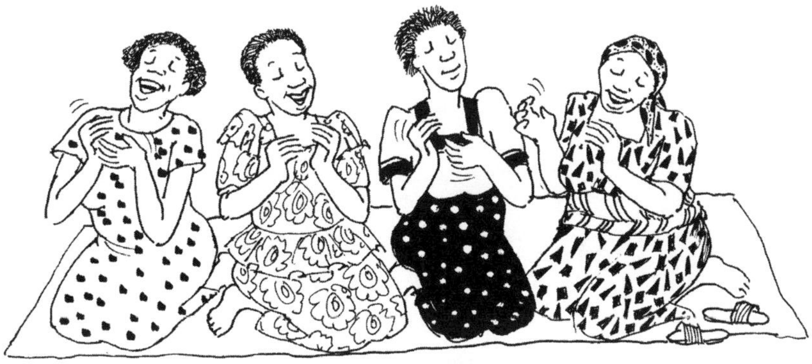

FACILITATORS' TEAM FEEDBACK

After the end of Session L, meet again with your co-facilitators, to compare notes on how your sessions went and the information which you learnt from them. Your co-facilitators could have found useful information that will help you to structure your next session more effectively. Remember, however, not to share individual confidentialities between groups! The next session is going to be the second full workshop meeting. It should last for a maximum of three hours. The first 60 minutes will be spent in four separate peer groups, giving each peer group time to rehearse their two scenes. Their first scene should be one of those from the 'Exploring Why' exercise in Session H. Their second scene should be the corresponding scene from 'Exploring Why Revisited', which the participants have just done. After each peer group has rehearsed its two scenes for performance to the other three peer groups, you will bring them all together again to share their scenes with the other peer groups. NB: This meeting is for workshop participants only. Make sure that all four peer groups have agreed on a common time for your next meeting.

ENDNOTE

1. Participants may want to view the clip again. If so, it is usually best for them to have some discussion about it first, then to have a further discussion after the second viewing.

YOUR NOTES ...

SECOND FULL WORKSHOP MEETING

PURPOSE

To share new ideas further.

TIME NEEDED: Maximum 3 hours.

MATERIALS NEEDED: None.

PARTICIPANTS: Members of the four peer groups, all meeting separately for the first hour, then together. (No general public.)

SPECIAL INFORMATION

Don't forget to read "Before You Begin ...!" before using this section of the manual.

AIMS: To enable all members of the four peer groups to meet together and share their ideas. To help participants realise once again that they do share some similar concerns with other peer groups.

DESCRIPTION: After some initial rehearsals, members of all four peer groups meet together. Each peer group shows the others a set of two role plays, one from the 'Exploring Why' exercise in Session H, and the second from the 'Exploring Why Revisited' exercise in Session L. Each role play is followed by discussion.

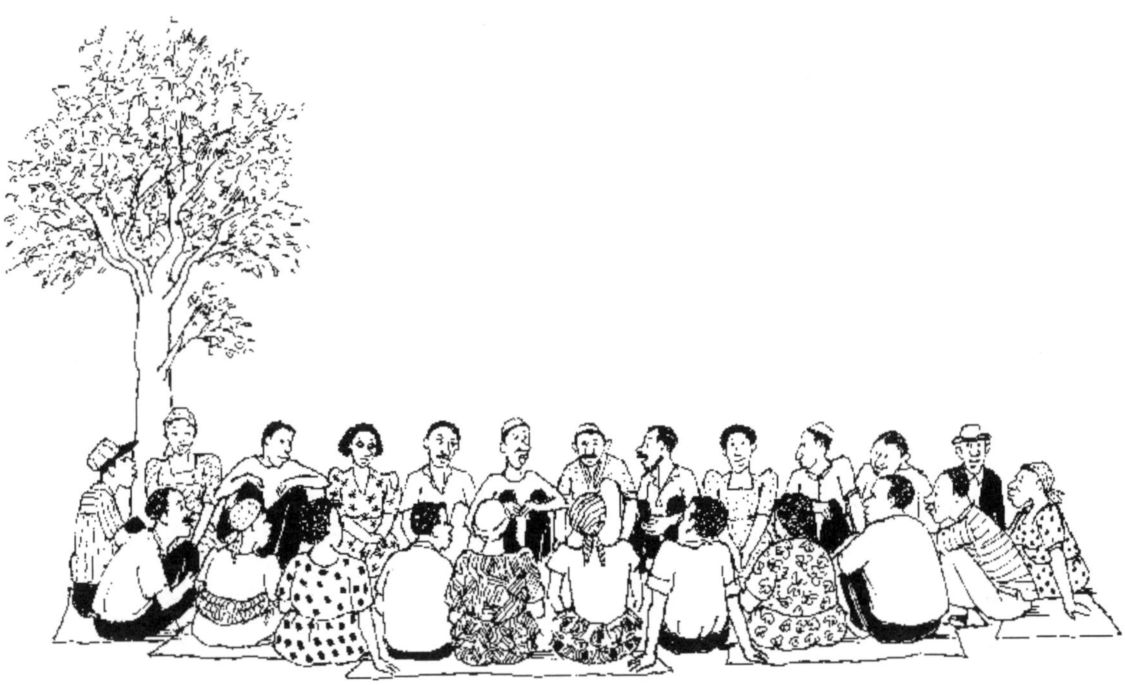

DIRECTIONS

The lead facilitator and/or one other facilitator should:

1. Thank everyone for sparing the time to come to the meeting. Explain that all peer groups have been working on similar exercises and that they have produced some fine ideas and acting. Now they have a chance to see each other's work and to present their own ideas to the full assembly. Explain that this is not a competition, but an opportunity to share ideas. Explain that you know some groups are feeling nervous about presenting their ideas to the others, but encourage them to be brave and encourage the whole audience to support each presentation. Also remind them how well the last full workshop meeting went.

2. Peer groups should then split up.

3. During the first thirty minutes, encourage participants to share their latest experiences of using an 'I' statement. Give praise and encouragement to everyone. The ones who find it more difficult will gain courage from hearing from those who have seen that it has worked for them.

4. During the second thirty minutes, they should decide which situation they want to present to the other peer groups. This should be one of the situations which they have already explored in 'Exploring Why' and 'Exploring Why Revisited'. Since there is not enough time for each peer group to present all four situations, they should choose the situation in which a character like someone in their own peer group is most likely to find her or himself. The first role play will show their character as they portrayed him/her in Session H. The second role play will show the same character as they portrayed him/her in Session L. Your participants should remind themselves of the situation and the two role plays, ready for presentation to the other peer groups.

5. When all the peer groups are ready, and at most after 60 minutes altogether, all four peer groups should be asked to come together again. As at the first full workshop meeting, the peer groups should be asked to decide amongst themselves the order in which they will present their role plays.

6. Give each peer group a maximum of 30 minutes to complete the following (make sure each peer group has the **same** amount of time):

- Role play from Session H.
- Audience discussion.
- Role play from Session L.
- Audience discussion.

During the discussions, the audience should be encouraged by the facilitators to ask questions of the actors in the role plays.

For instance:

- **Who** is each main character?
- **What** are they doing?
- **How** have they come to this situation?
- **Why** has this situation developed?
- **What** traditions, alcohol use, social expectations, or other factors influenced the situation?

The actors in the role play should be encouraged to answer the questions themselves, whilst continuing to 'be' their character in the role play.

7. Next, ask participants whether they noticed any similar themes across all the peer group presentations. What differences emerged between the peer groups?

8. Finally, thank all participants for their fine acting and explain that next time you will go on to Session M. Each facilitator should arrange a mutually agreeable time and place for Session M with his/her own peer group. Also, remind everyone of their role as guardian angel.

9. Encourage participants to talk in general about the kinds of issues they have been discussing in these sessions with their friends and neighbours, if they like, but not to share any confidential information from the peer group with others.

10. Each facilitator should then remember to ask for three new people from their own peer group to stay behind for an instant review of the session. (See Annex 4.)

> ☞ This meeting is important because it is the first time participants have the opportunity to express to other community members their ideas about how they think they could make changes to improve their situation. In this meeting, participants also tend to realise that they share more hopes and fears than they knew with other members of their community. This is more valuable groundwork for developing greater trust and cooperation between different sections of the community. But it is also important for participants to go back to working once more in their peer groups for the final few sessions. Don't be tempted to abandon this principle now!

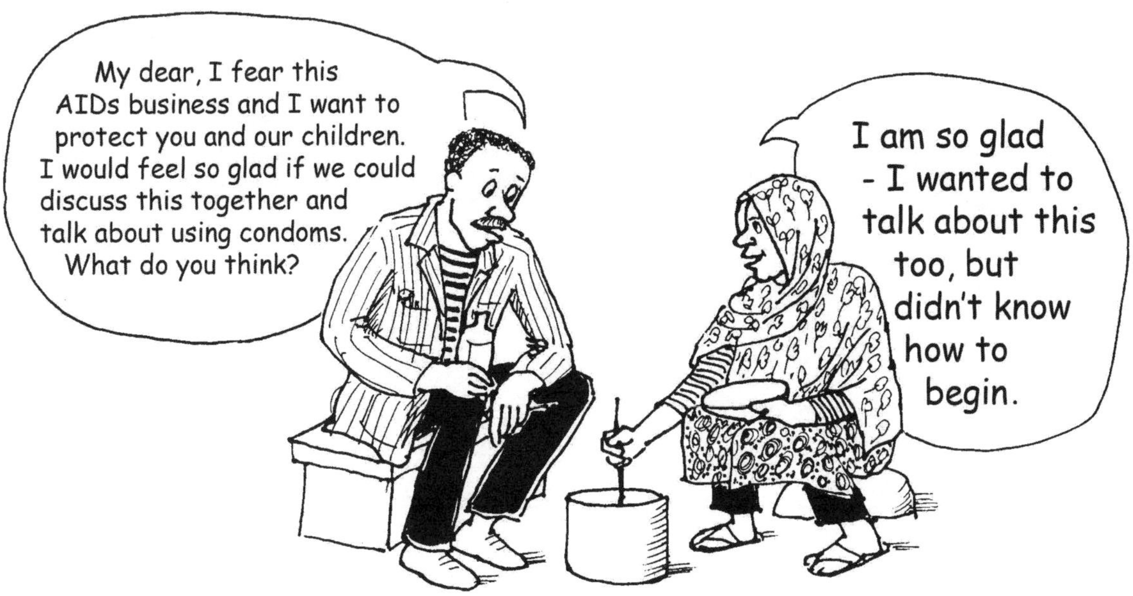
My dear, I fear this AIDs business and I want to protect you and our children. I would feel so glad if we could discuss this together and talk about using condoms. What do you think?
I am so glad - I wanted to talk about this too, but didn't know how to begin.

FACILITATORS' TEAM FEEDBACK

Don't forget to have another feedback session now! Some interesting similarities and differences will emerge in the role play presentations. You may well be able to build on these in the remaining workshop sessions.

YOUR NOTES ...

SESSION M LET'S WORK TOGETHER

PURPOSE

To develop understanding between partners.

CONTENTS	**TIME NEEDED**
Introduction	
M.1	I'm Going on a Trip
M.2	**DVD Clip 13:** 'Trust'
M.3	The Long Journey
M.4	**DVD Clip 14:** 'The Long Journey'
M.5	The Trust Game
M.6	Closing Circle

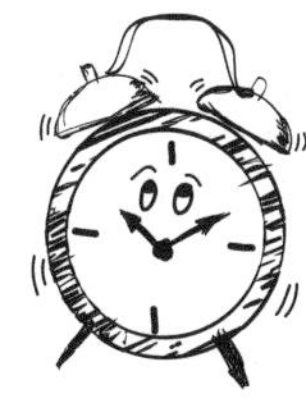

3–4 hours

MATERIALS NEEDED: DVD, laptop with DVD player, projector, and a scarf for a blindfold.

PARTICIPANTS: Four separate peer groups.

SPECIAL INFORMATION

- Don't forget to read 'Before You Begin ...!' before using this section of the manual. The exercises in this session can be very upsetting. Therefore it is essential that you have prepared participants properly, by completing the exercises in the previous sessions with them.
- This may be a particularly difficult session for some since, in 'The Long Journey', participants will be reflecting on the reality of our mortality. Participants who are themselves suffering from an incurable terminal illness, or who are caring for people who may die soon, may feel especially moved by this exercise.
- You may like to discuss with the other facilitators what kind of support you could give, should any participants be particularly distressed. It may well be that all they need is someone to listen to them at the end of the session. Alternatively, if there are trained counsellors nearby, it would be better for you to suggest they go to talk to them. Make sure you know who the counsellors are and where they can be found.
- Despite the possible effects on some people, this is a very important part of the whole workshop and can be a very empowering and uplifting process, so the session should not be dropped unless the participants themselves refuse to do it. See the notes in exercise M.3 for more on this.

INTRODUCTION

1. Sit in a circle with the group, preferably on the ground. Everyone should sit at the same level, including yourself.

2. Welcome everyone to the new session. Thank everyone for coming. Enquire about late-comers or non-attenders.

3. Ask everyone what they thought of the second full workshop meeting. What were their impressions of the role plays performed by the other peer groups? Did any surprise them at all? Were they pleased or disappointed by what they saw? How did they think that other peer groups responded to their presentation? Encourage a few minutes' discussion of these points.

4. Explain that in this session you are going to explore issues of trust and that, as usual, you will begin with a game.

EXERCISE M.1: I'M GOING ON A TRIP

AIMS: Warm-up exercise. Fun. Laughter.

DESCRIPTION: A memory game, with actions.

DIRECTIONS

1. Ask the participants to stand in a circle. Start by saying 'I'm going on a trip and I'm taking a hug.' Hug the person to your right.

2. S/he then has to say: 'I'm going on a trip and I'm taking a hug and a pat on the back'. S/he then has to give the next person a hug and a pat on the back.

3. Go on round the circle, with each person repeating what was said and done before, and adding one new action to the list until everyone has had a go. If someone forgets the sequence, encourage the others to help him or her to do it right.

EXERCISE M.2: DVD Clip 13: 'TRUST'

AIM: To look at how a younger couple have decided to work together.

DESCRIPTION: Watching DVD, followed by pair work and general discussion.

MATERIALS NEEDED: DVD, laptop with DVD player, projector.

DIRECTIONS

1. Explain to participants that we are now going to watch a DVD clip about a young married couple. Ask them to move to a good position where they can all see the screen.

2. Say that while they are watching the clip, you would like them to think about the relationship between the husband and wife, Mr and Mrs Ssimbwa, in the light of what you have discussed in previous sessions.

Make sure that everyone can see and hear the DVD clearly.

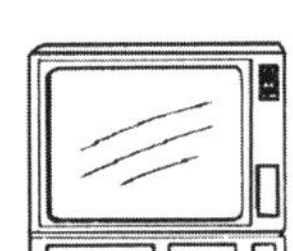

3. Turn on the DVD at the point where it says '13. Trust'.

4. Turn off the DVD at the point where the screen goes black.[1]

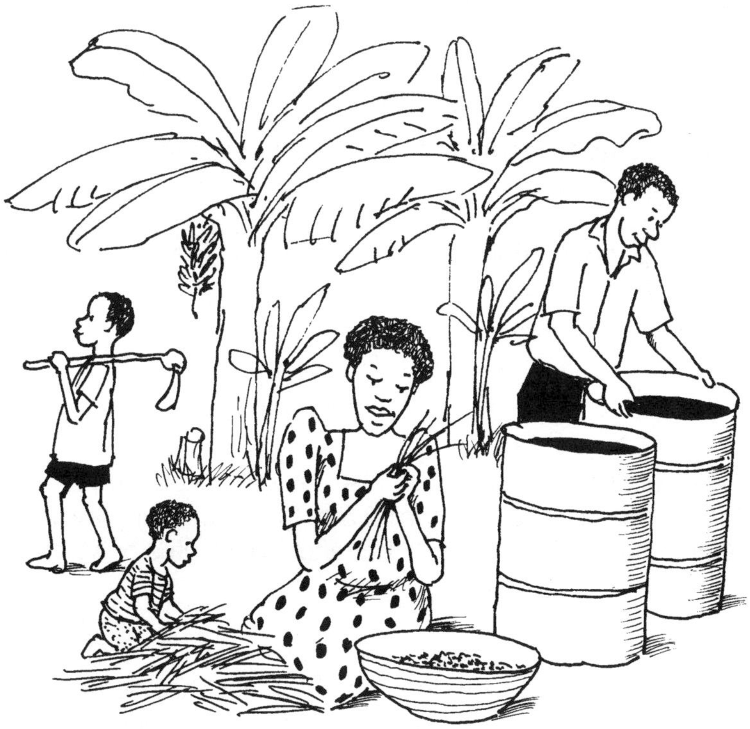

5. Ask participants to describe who they saw in the DVD, and what the couple do for a living. Keep the discussion descriptive at present: it is just to make sure that everyone has understood what they have seen.

6. Then ask participants to divide into pairs and discuss the following:

- What words can you think of to describe the **quality** of the relationship between the husband and his wife?
- What are the **good** things about their relationship?
- What are the **bad** things about it?
- Was the husband right or wrong to let his wife go out to work?
- If the couple lived in the participants' own community, what would be other people's attitudes to them? Would they be the same as those in Buwenda or different? In what ways might local attitudes differ?

7. Finally, ask participants to rejoin the large circle. Go over the questions which they have discussed in pairs, spending more time discussing areas of disagreement.

> Qualities which appear to be present in this relationship include trust, respect, cooperation, planning ahead, and shared support and responsibility. The husband points out that his friends laughed at him for letting his wife work, but he withstood these taunts. Encourage participants to mention and discuss these points for themselves, and to consider whether this kind of mutually supportive relationship could work in their own community. In some parts of Africa, the idea of both partners having paid employment is seen as a very good thing, so the trust Andrea shows Sylivia may seem natural rather than strange. If this is so for your participants, ask them in what additional ways can a man and woman show their trust and support for each other?

EXERCISE M.3: THE LONG JOURNEY

AIMS: To help people come to terms with their own death in a non-threatening way. To help us prepare for our deaths.

DESCRIPTION: Participants work in pairs to share their ideas with each other, followed by feedback and discussion.

DIRECTIONS

1. Do not mention death at this point in the exercise. Start by explaining to participants that, in a minute, you would like them to divide into pairs. Say that you would like first one participant to be the talker and the other the listener and, that after 10 minutes or so, you will ask them to swap roles.

2. Explain that you would like them to consider the following situation. They should imagine that they are going to go on a very long journey in a month's time. They do not know when they will come back to their homes – if ever. Ask them to answer the following questions:

- **Who** would you like to speak to before you go?
- **What** would you like to say to each of them?
- **What** would you like to do before you go?
- **Who** would you trust to look after your land and possessions well, while you are gone?
- **How** would you ensure that your wishes were fulfilled in your absence?

3. Ask participants to repeat the five questions back to you, to make sure that they have remembered them all. Say that you will tell them when 10 minutes have passed, so that they can swap roles with one another. Then ask them to divide into pairs and begin.

4. After both people in each pair have had a chance to talk (about 20 minutes), call everyone back into a big circle. Ask participants:

- What did they learn from this exercise?
- In what way does it relate to real life?

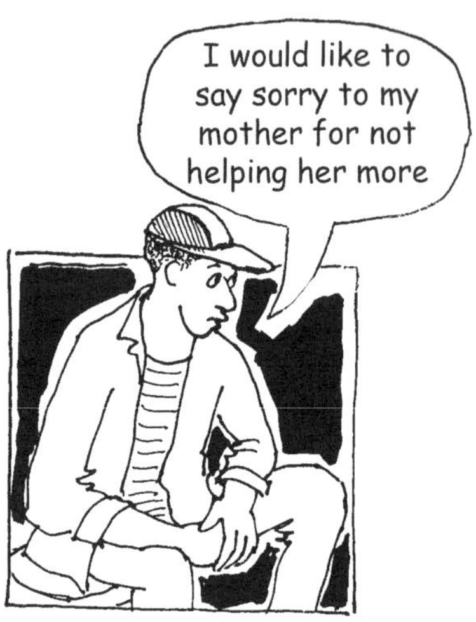
I would like to say sorry to my mother for not helping her more

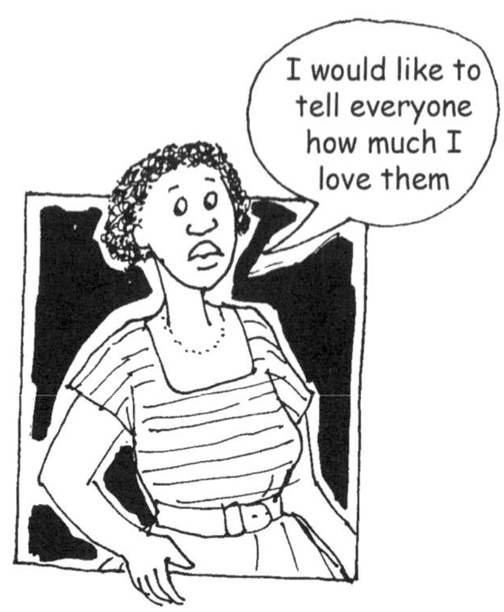
I would like to tell everyone how much I love them

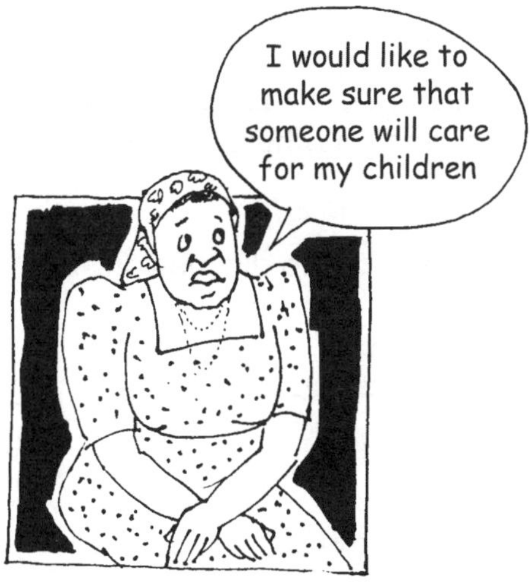
I would like to make sure that someone will care for my children

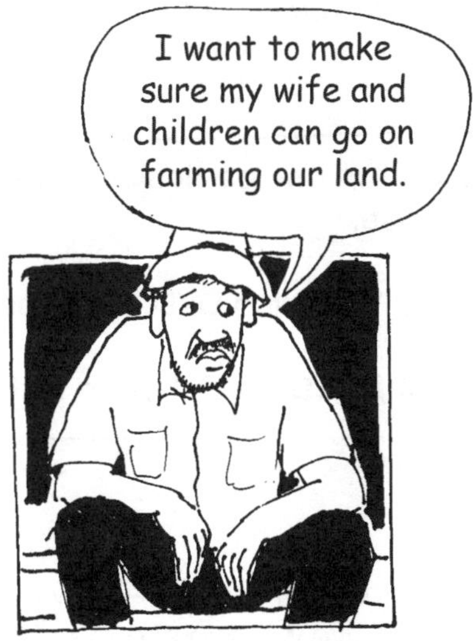
I want to make sure my wife and children can go on farming our land.

- Did they find the exercise scary? helpful? encouraging? difficult? Probably all of these emotions and others too will be mentioned!
- How would they have felt if they had to go on the journey tomorrow, without being given any notice?

Participants will probably have worked out for themselves that they can relate this exercise to our own deaths. But if they have not mentioned it by now, you should gently do so. Explain that we all have to die one day. This can be very frightening for many of us, but to be able to plan for a journey can often be much less terrifying than having to go with nothing prepared.

> The idea of this exercise is to help us to come to terms with the reality of our own death. In many societies it is virtually impossible to talk about death. People often believe that talking about death will make someone die. So the exercise has to be approached sensitively. You could encourage participants to have courage and explain that this exercise is a way of helping us to face death more calmly, by preparing ourselves for it in some way.
>
> Point out that none of us knows when we are going to die. We may be ill and expect to die in a month or two, or we may be struck by lightning, or hit by a car, or bitten by a snake today. None of us knows how much longer we have to live. Therefore perhaps it is better for all of us to prepare for our deaths ahead of time, instead of going on hoping that we won't die this week – or month or year.
>
> This can be a very difficult exercise. Some participants may feel very upset by doing it. It is often easier for us to believe that death won't happen to us! This denial is a normal human reaction to something which is frightening and should not be laughed at. On the other hand, experience has shown that helping people to overcome denial and accept the future can bring them enormous relief and can make them feel much stronger and more prepared to face whatever happens. Therefore a lot of empathy and support from you is needed, as well as a lot of warmth from the whole group. This exercise is a very important step in this whole workshop and should not be missed out, unless your participants completely refuse to do it.

EXERCISE M.4: DVD Clip 14: 'THE LONG JOURNEY'

AIMS: To reflect on one particular couple's decisions, and on others' views of the previous exercise.

DESCRIPTION: Watching DVD, followed by pair work and group discussion.

MATERIALS NEEDED: DVD, laptop with DVD player, projector.

DIRECTIONS

1. Explain to participants that we are now going to watch a DVD clip about a couple in which the husband is sick. We will also see the older men's group from Buwenda discussing what the previous exercise meant for them. Ask everyone to stand up, and have a good stretch, then to move to a good position so that they can all see the screen.

2. Say that, while they are watching the clip, you would like them to think about the relationship between this husband and wife, who are called Mr and Mrs Mulumba, in the light of what we have discussed in previous sessions. Also, they should think about the views of the older men in Buwenda. How similar or different are these views to their own?

Make sure that everyone can see and hear the DVD clearly.

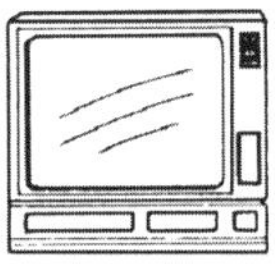

3. Turn on the DVD at the point where it says '14. The Long Journey'.

4. Turn off the DVD at the point where the screen goes black.[1]

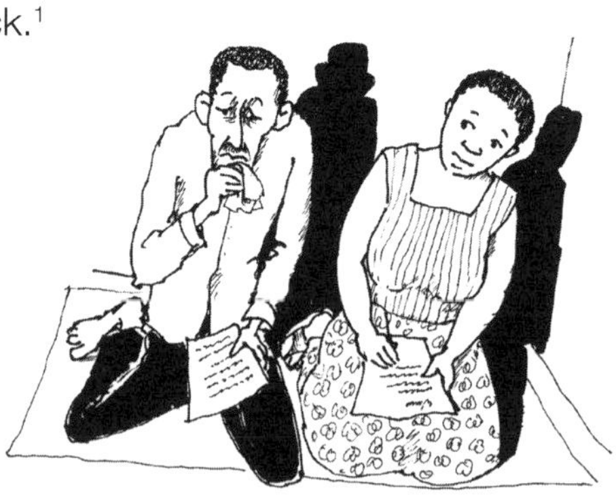

5. Ask participants to describe who they saw in the DVD and what was going on. In what practical ways were Mr and Mrs Mulumba preparing for his death? (See the synopsis in Annex 3 for some help.)

6. Then ask participants what struck them most strongly about the qualities of Mr and Mrs Mulumba's relationship.

- What were the **good** things about their relationship?
- What were the **bad** things about their relationship?
- How was the quality of their relationship affecting the quality of their lives?

7. Now ask participants their views on the discussion amongst the older men in Buwenda.

- In what way do the views on the DVD differ from those held by your participants?
- In what ways are they similar?
- What happens to surviving dependents and to property when someone in your participants' community dies?
- What would be the reaction of others to someone in your participants' community making a will, in the way that Mr Mulumba did? Would anyone respect it?
- If your participants feel there could be improvements to the current system in their own community, what specific steps could they think of taking to change it?

Your participants may want to discuss the fact that Mr Mulumba had AIDS, and whether or not Mrs Mulumba also had HIV. If so, please point out that it **doesn't matter.** The point of this clip, and the previous exercise, is to make it clear that we will all die sometime, whether we have AIDS or not. Like Mr Mulumba, we can all die with dignity, especially if we have made plans to care for our dependents after our deaths.

Mr Mulumba died shortly after this DVD was made, safe in the knowledge that he had made what plans and provision he could for his wife and children. Mrs Mulumba has been able to stay in their house with the children, thanks to Mr Mulumba's will.

It is particularly important to press the older men's group and the younger men's group in the discussion about will-making, since it is usually men who are responsible for the disposal of property and arranging care of dependents when someone dies. Encourage them to explore any ideas they may have to improve the current system. The more specific, practical suggestions they can think of, the better. Ask them what they could do about getting these ideas discussed further in the community, or being put into practice. Of course, if women are also involved in these discussions in your community, press them on these issues too.

EXERCISE M.5: THE TRUST GAME

AIMS: A fun exercise, involving trust between participants. To re-focus.

DESCRIPTION: Participants take it in turns to fall blindfold and be caught by their colleagues.

DIRECTIONS

1. Ask all participants to stand together in a small circle in the middle of the training area.

2. Each participant in turn should stand in the middle of the circle and then close their eyes or put on a blindfold. S/he then falls backwards, sideways, or forwards, keeping their eyes closed, and will be caught in the safety of the arms of the other participants.

3. Each participant needs to have five or six quick goes at this before someone else goes in the middle and puts the blindfold on. It can feel quite scary at first, but should be perfectly safe provided the group work together.

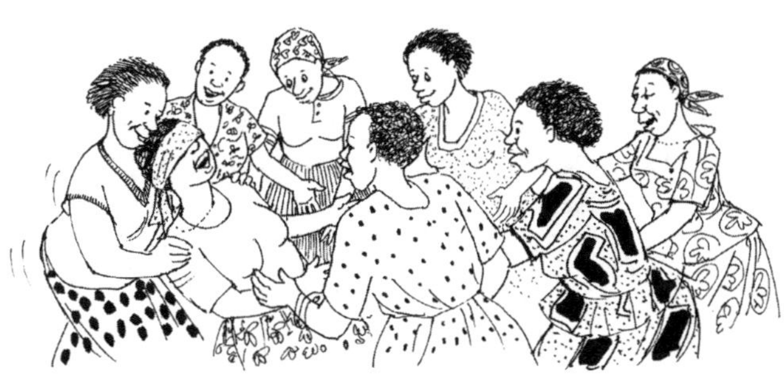

EXERCISE M.6: CLOSING CIRCLE

1. Ask everyone to sit in a circle. Tell them that this session is now at an end.

2. Ask each person to mention one thing which they found good about today's session and one thing which they found hard. Go round the circle until everyone has had a go.

3. Thank everyone for working so well together in such a hard session. Explain that some may have found this the hardest session of all but subsequent sessions are easier. There is only one more session now before the second open community meeting, and there will be a few more optional peer group sessions, if they would like to continue to meet after that. They will all be much easier than this session, so you look forward to seeing everyone at the next one, where we will be preparing for the second open community meeting.

4. Arrange a mutually convenient time and place for the next peer group session.

5. It would also be good to start to find out now which day and time would be most convenient for this peer group to have the second open community meeting. This meeting will be for **the whole community** again, not just for peer group members. Ask your participants for two or three possible dates, so that you can cross-check with the other facilitators and find a date suitable for all the community.

6. Remind everyone of their role as guardian angel. This role may be especially important after this session.

7. Encourage participants to talk in general about the kinds of issues they have been discussing in these sessions with their friends and neighbours, if they like, but not to share any confidential information from the peer group with others.

8. Remember to ask for three new people to stay behind for an instant review of the session. (See Annex 4.)

> You may find that some people felt this session particularly tough. They may wish to stay behind and talk to you. Be prepared: know what kind of things you might say to them, or whom you could encourage them to go to see. All they may need is someone to listen to them ... You need to be sensitive to how stressful some may have found this session. Finally, remember that you too might need some support from someone after this session.

FACILITATORS' TEAM FEEDBACK

After the end of Session M, meet again with your co-facilitators, to compare notes on how your sessions went and the information which you learnt from them. If some good suggestions came up about how people could plan better for their deaths, you need to start thinking about how to keep these ideas alive in the community. See Annex 5 for some ideas on how you could do this. Remember again not to share any confidentialities between groups. The next peer group session, Session N, is very much a preparation for the second open community meeting which will be a time for each peer group to present its own plans for the future to other peer groups and to the wider community. You and your co-facilitators may want to talk amongst yourselves about this in advance, since the peer groups will need your continued time and effort, especially if they wish to continue with further optional sessions (O–R and another open meeting) afterwards. Again, see Annex 5 for more on this.

ENDNOTE

1. Participants may want to view the clip again. If so, it is usually best for them to have some discussion about it first, then to have a further discussion after the second viewing.

YOUR NOTES ...

SESSION N LET'S PREPARE FOR THE FUTURE

PURPOSE

To think of possible decisions and changes. To evaluate the workshop and make plans for the future of the peer group.

CONTENTS	**TIME NEEDED**
Introduction	
N.1	The Special Request
N.2	The Great Debate
N.3	**DVD Clip 15:** 'The Community Challenge'
N.4	Rehearsal of the Special Request
N.5	Workshop Expectations Review
N.6	Preparations for Post-Workshop Review
N.7	Plans for the Future
N.8	Mental Gifts

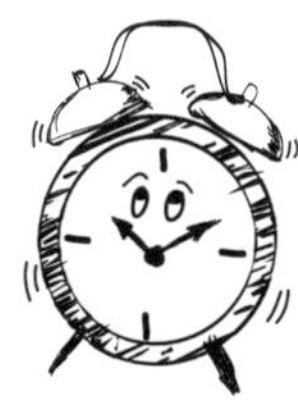

3–4 hours

MATERIALS NEEDED: DVD, laptop with DVD player, projector, flipchart paper, strongly coloured marker pens, one notebook and pen (for you).

PARTICIPANTS: Four separate peer groups.

SPECIAL INFORMATION

Don't forget to read 'Before You Begin ...!' before using this section of the manual. This is the last peer group session before the second open community meeting. All four facilitators need to have agreed a suitable time, date, and location for this meeting, so that you can finalise it with your participants at the end of this session. Remember that the second open community meeting is for as many members of the community as possible to attend.

INTRODUCTION

1. Sit in a circle with the group, preferably on the ground. Everyone should sit at the same level, including yourself.

2. Welcome everyone to the new session. Thank everyone for coming. Enquire about late-comers or non-attenders.

3. Ask everyone what they thought of the last session. Encourage a few minutes' discussion of their thoughts.

4. Explain how in this session you are going to prepare for the second open community meeting, which will be an opportunity for all the peer groups to present to the whole community the work which they have done so far.

EXERCISE N.1: THE SPECIAL REQUEST

AIM: For participants to think of and decide upon one special request concerning their own lives and HIV, which they would like to ask the whole of their community to accept.

DESCRIPTION: Brainstorm of possible requests, followed by deciding on one request to take to the community.

DIRECTIONS

1. Explain to participants that, at the second open community meeting, each peer group will make a special request of the rest of the community. This request will be of direct relevance to their concerns and also relate to HIV in some way. Public support of their request will help them feel more confident in handling their individual lives.

2. Ask participants to divide into groups of four or five and think about what they might ask of their community. They should think of as many ideas as possible before deciding on one to bring back to the rest of the group in ten minutes time.

3. After each small group has chosen a special request, bring all participants back to the big circle. Compare everyone's proposals and ask the group to decide on one special request to present to the rest of the community. This may be difficult, but there will probably be similar requests from different groups, or requests which are connected or overlap with one another in some way. If there are two totally separate requests which have no connection with each other at all, ask the group to accept them both. However, this situation is unlikely.

4. The arguments for and against the chosen special request are going to be rehearsed in the next exercise using a debating game.

In Buwenda, the four peer groups chose special requests relevant to their experiences as follows: ***older women*** *wanted to ask their community to accept that it is good for their husbands to share their money with them during life, and to include them in their wills on their death;* ***younger women*** *wanted to ask their community to accept that it is wrong for older men to entice younger women to have extra-marital sex;* ***older men*** *wanted to ask their community to accept that it is wrong for men or women to drink too much alcohol, and that it is wrong for older men to have sex with younger women;* ***younger men*** *wanted to ask their community to accept that using condoms while 'playing sex' with girlfriends is a good thing.*

Each request was directly relevant to the experiences of the peer group who made it, as well as being connected to the control of HIV. But remember: these requests chosen by the peer groups in Buwenda may have little or no relevance to the needs of your participants. What will your participants decide to request?

EXERCISE N.2: THE GREAT DEBATE

AIM: To prepare participants for presenting their special request to the community in the second open community meeting.

DESCRIPTION: The participants role-play a debate on their special request and analyse the effectiveness of their debating strategies.

DIRECTIONS

1. Ask participants to divide into two groups of equal size. The two groups should sit in semi-circles facing each other. Explain that each group is going to take it in turns to argue for or against the special request that they have decided upon. So, for example, in the older women's group, if they were requesting that their husbands share money with them, half the participants, representing themselves, would be arguing in favour of this request. The other half of the participants would pretend to be their husbands, arguing against this request!

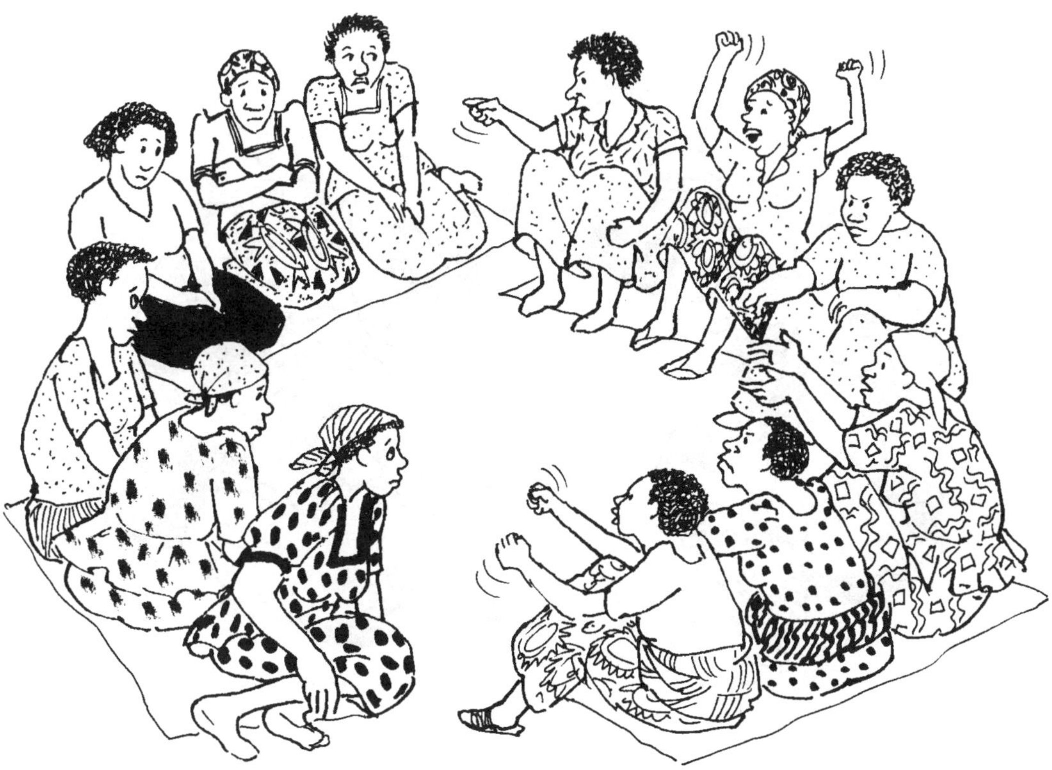

2. Remind the participants about what they have learnt about assertiveness and good persuasive argument. Encourage them to think of all the reasons why their husbands should do what they ask – and all the reasons why their husbands should not do this! The idea of this role play is to help participants think of all the possible arguments on both sides. Encourage everyone to be as realistic as possible.

3. Encourage the participants to argue as one group against the other for 10 minutes or so. Then bring everyone back into one circle.

If they become stuck during the debate, help by quietly giving suggestions to one or two people on each side. But don't take an active, public part in the debate.

4. Next, ask participants to **review** the process of the argument.

- If you are facilitating a women's group, did the women propose their arguments well or did the 'men' get angry? How did the women handle the anger of the 'men'?
- If you are facilitating a men's group, are the 'women' **really** accepting what the men are saying, or are they just saying 'yes' to please the men? Which would be better? How can the men improve their persuasion skills?
- Did they use the assertiveness skills they have learnt, such as using 'I' statements instead of 'you' statements? Were they too aggressive or too submissive?
- What about body language, eye contact, eye levels, and so on?

5. Next, ask participants to return to the two semicircles facing each other. This time they will argue in opposite roles. So those who argued in favour of the special request before will now argue against, and vice-versa. Encourage participants to think of reasons for or against the request, which may not have been mentioned earlier. Again, allow 10 minutes or so, if necessary.

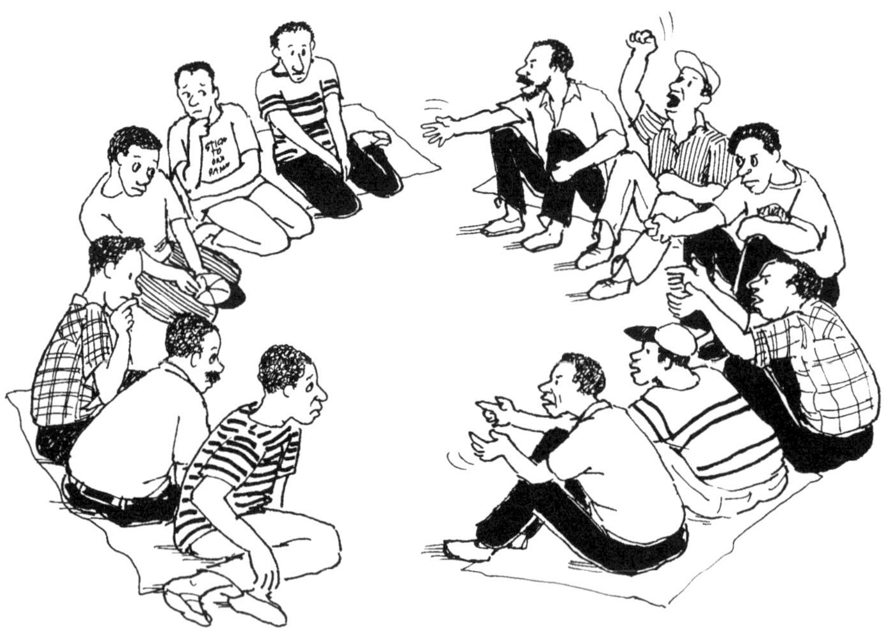

6. Then call everyone back to the full circle and review the process again.

- Have their techniques improved? If so, how? If not, why not?
- What was the effect of their arguments on their audience? Was it better or worse than before?

7. If anyone would like to have another go at rehearsing certain points of the discussion, or at the whole exercise, encourage them to come forward to role-play better ways of presenting the arguments. They need to feel really confident that they can produce a coherent, persuasive, assertive, and well-balanced argument in favour of their special request.

8. Congratulate everyone on the progress which they have made with their presentations in this exercise. Soon they will create and practise a dramatic presentation of this special request. First, however, participants will have a chance to see how the people of Buwenda staged their special requests.

EXERCISE N.3: DVD Clip 15: 'THE COMMUNITY CHALLENGE'

AIM: To show how the second open community meeting can be staged.

DESCRIPTION: Watching DVD, followed by review.

MATERIALS NEEDED: DVD, laptop with DVD player, projector.

DIRECTIONS

1. Explain to participants that we are now going to watch a DVD clip showing how the people of Buwenda staged their second open community meeting. The aim of watching it is not to copy the special requests of the people of Buwenda – every group needs to decide on their own special request – but it will give participants a chance to see how effective a public presentation can be in giving people confidence to speak out to one another publicly about their concerns.

2. Say that, while they are watching the DVD, you would like them to think about ideas for their own presentation. What could they do to make their own second open community meeting special?

3. Ask everyone to have a good stretch, and to move round to a new position so that they can all see the screen.

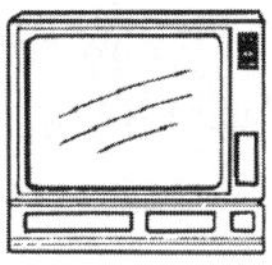

Make sure that everyone can see and hear the DVD clearly.

4. Turn on the DVD at the point where it says: '15. The Community Challenge'.

5. Turn off the DVD where the screen goes black.[1]

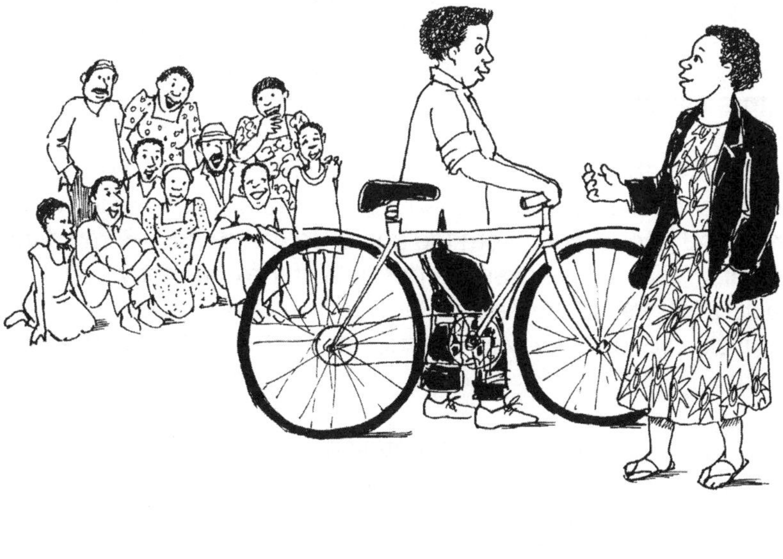

6. Ask your participants:

- What they liked about the presentations.
- What they didn't like about the presentations.
- What they thought of the questions which the onlookers asked?
- What they thought of the answers which the participants gave?
- What they thought of the comments made by Mrs Senyondo and Julius about the whole workshop process?

7. Explain to your participants that it is now time for them to plan their own presentations. This DVD may have given them a few ideas. But the important thing is that they plan their own presentation in their own way and using their own special request: they **don't** need to take any ideas from the Buwenda example. Add also that, in Buwenda, they had to have this last presentation indoors, because of a big rainstorm. But it would be better for your participants to be outdoors together, if possible, so that the actors can be surrounded by onlookers more easily.

EXERCISE N.4: REHEARSAL OF THE SPECIAL REQUEST

AIMS: To rehearse and finalise a role play presentation for the second open community meeting.

DESCRIPTION: Discussion, preparation and rehearsal.

DIRECTIONS

1. Explain to participants that they have now reviewed all the arguments for and against their special request. The next step is for them to illustrate the importance of their special request through a role play and a concluding 'we' statement which presents their special request to the whole community. (For instance: 'We feel happy when ...')

2. In the second open community meeting, each peer group will have a maximum of, say, 20 minutes to present their special request (through a role play and 'we' statement) and to respond to follow-up questions from their audience. Therefore it is recommended that they perform for a maximum of five minutes and allow 15 minutes for discussion. During the discussion time, they will see how 'The Great Debate' exercise helps them to think through good responses to questions and to arguments against their special request.

3. Ask your participants to think up a plot for the role play. Encourage as many members of the peer group as possible to take part. They should also ensure that as many of them as possible are prepared to respond to questions from the audience afterwards. Remind them to keep the plot as straightforward, clear, and relevant as possible. If they like, they could start off or finish with a dance or a song on the same theme. Remind them that, the end of the role play, they should state the special request clearly to the audience in the form of a 'we' statement (i.e. a plural 'I' statement).

4. Ask your participants to rehearse their presentation a few times. Help by praising them and by making constructive comments, suggesting improvements on the positioning of the actors and the clarity of what they are saying, as you see fit.

EXERCISE N.5: WORKSHOP EXPECTATIONS REVIEW

AIM: To review participants' original expectations.

DESCRIPTION: Discussions and assessment.

DIRECTIONS

1. Explain to participants that, as you draw near to the end of the main workshop, it would be helpful for you as facilitator to learn from participants what they think of your guidance. It is also always good practice to review the workshop process, so that everyone has a chance to reflect on what they have learnt.

2. Say that you would like to begin this process by reviewing the expectations which everyone had of the workshop when they first began it. Remind participants that each of them mentioned one hope and one fear about the workshop in Session A. Go round the circle now, asking each participant to be honest and open and to:

- Say again the hope and fear they had.
- Comment on whether or not their hope was fulfilled.
- Comment on whether or not what they had feared actually happened.
- Make one comment about what they thought of the workshop overall.

3. Discuss any negative points which are raised by the participants so that you understand clearly why they felt disappointed or let down. Make sure that you take note of these so that you can improve the way in which you run future workshops. Make sure that you accept criticism of yourself without being defensive. We often find it very hard to listen to and accept criticism!

EXERCISE N.6: PREPARATIONS FOR POST-WORKSHOP REVIEW

AIM: To discuss with participants ways in which the effectiveness of this workshop can be assessed.

DESCRIPTION: Discussion, followed by drawing of suggestions.

MATERIALS NEEDED: Flip-chart paper, felt tip marker pens, one notebook and pen.

DIRECTIONS

1. Explain to participants that they have all been involved in quick reviews of one session or another. You would now like to ask them to review the effectiveness of the whole workshop. A good way of doing this is to think of changes that they would like to see in their community in six months' time.

2. Of course, it is hoped that the community will **accept** each peer group's special request. But there may be other, more general, changes that each peer group may hope to see in the ways people in their community behave. If they think of these now, in six months' time you can have a review meeting together, to see whether these changes – or other, unexpected ones – have taken place or not.

3. Ask the participants to think quickly of five to ten things which they hope will change over the next six months.

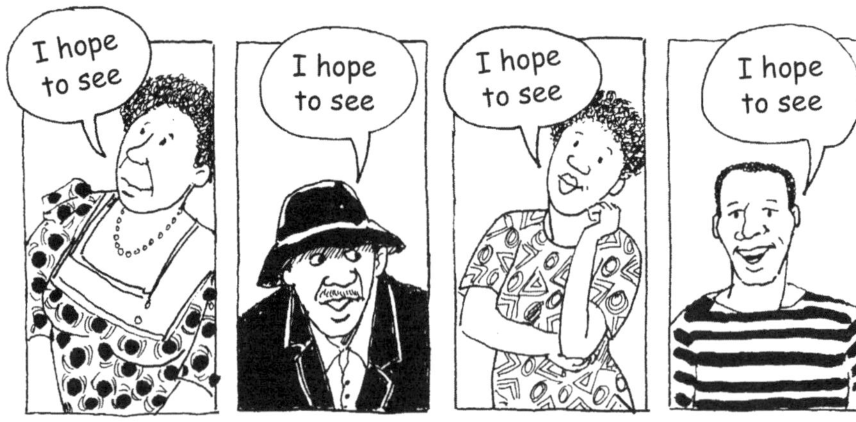

4. Once they have some ideas, ask participants to think of a different symbol for each of the changes they hope to see. They can then draw all the symbols on a piece of flip-chart paper. In this way the peer group will have a record of their expectations that they will be able to review in six months' time.

5. Make a quick note in your notebook of the changes which participants expect to see and have drawn. Ask for one member of the group to volunteer to keep the flip-chart paper. in a safe place.

In Buwenda, six months after the workshop, participants described how there was less quarrelling, less wife-beating, and more cooperation between couples. They said that, at funeral ceremonies, older men were encouraging other community members to accept the use of condoms, and that general demand for condoms had increased. The local Ministry of Health dispensary was now distributing condoms to anyone who asked for them, not only to people living with HIV. One couple in particular were delighted with how the use of an 'I' statement had helped them to talk about something which neither of them had dared to discuss for several years. Mr. Mulumba's will had been respected. Finally, all four peer groups were still meeting regularly, sometimes on their own and sometimes with the help of all four facilitators. There were also plans for each peer group to develop some income-generation activities.

☞ In Buwenda, the exercise described here was not conducted, so all these developments were only reported six months later; there was no prediction of possible results beforehand. However, we recommend strongly that you do this exercise in this session, so that you have some kind of 'base-line' for possible indicators of change, against which to review what **actually** happens in six months' time. In this way, you will also be able to see and compare the priorities of each different peer group in terms of the changes that would be of most help and relevance to them.

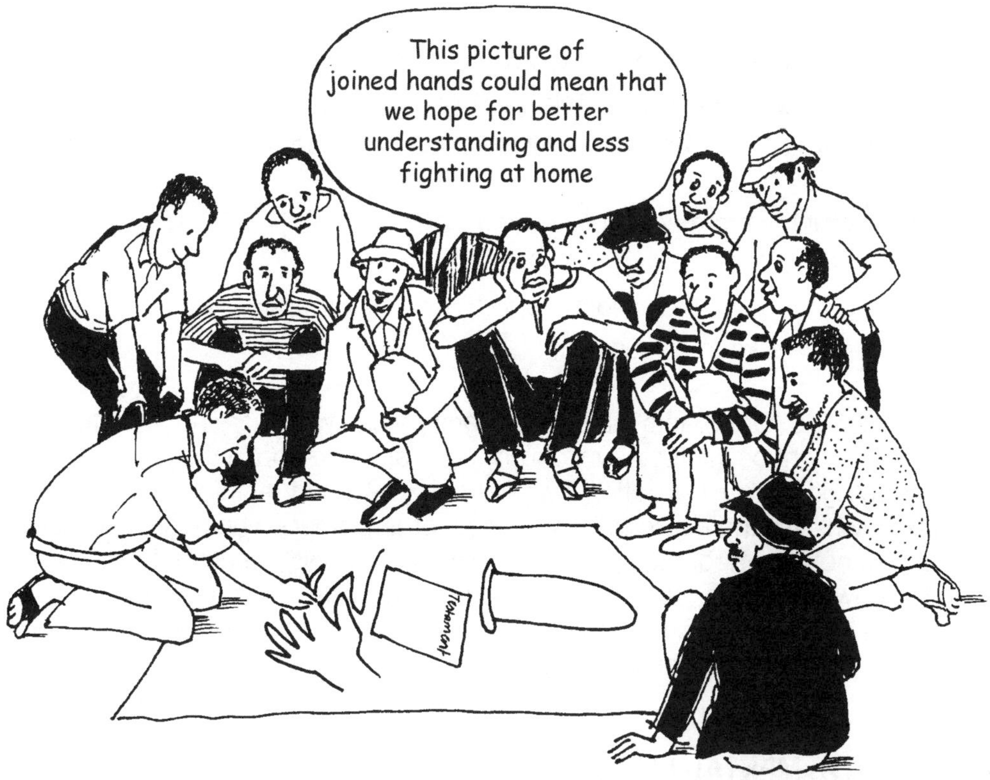
This picture of joined hands could mean that we hope for better understanding and less fighting at home

EXERCISE N.7: PLANS FOR THE FUTURE

AIM: To make future plans for the continued existence – or otherwise – of this peer group.

DESCRIPTION: An open discussion.

DIRECTIONS

1. Remind the participants that this is the last workshop session before the second open community meeting. Therefore you would like to ask them if they would be interested in continuing to meet as a peer group for future discussions of these kinds of issues. Explain that there are four more sessions (O–R), which are optional and lead to another open community meeting. You could facilitate these if they would like you to, but this is for them to decide.

2. If they say no, do not try to persuade them to change their minds. No group will work unless those in it want to meet. Instead, try to find out why not. Perhaps they already belong to other groups, such as income-generating groups, which they would rather stick with. Perhaps they do not have enough time to join more than one group. Perhaps they found these meetings boring or too difficult ...

3. If they **are** interested in continuing, find out from them:

- Why they think that continued meetings would be good.
- What kind of things they would like to discuss or do.
- When they would like to start meeting (maybe a short break before you start the optional sessions would be good).
- How often they would like to meet (weekly, etc.).
- Where they could meet.
- How many weeks or months they might like to try out the group for.
- Anything else they may like to discuss.

4. Find out also from the participants if they know any people who were not able to join this workshop, but who might be interested in joining a similar workshop in the future, starting from the beginning again, after the optional workshops (O–R) end. Ask for their names, which you could write down. Ask them also to bring names of any others who might be interested but whom they are not sure about to the second open community meeting. Explain that this will help you to know whether or not there is enough demand to plan ahead for a repeat of this workshop, starting it again from the beginning with new participants. If there is, you or a community leader could contact those new people.

EXERCISE N.8: MENTAL GIFTS

AIMS: **Closing exercise. To give a sense of sharing and appreciation.**

DESCRIPTION: **Each participant receives a 'gift'.**

DIRECTIONS

1. Sit in a big circle. Start off by pretending to hand a big present to the person on your left. Say his or her name, then say that you would like to give them a present – something which you know they would really like. For instance, if your neighbour is called Margaret and you know she likes chocolate, you could say, 'Margaret, I would like to give you a year's supply of chocolate!' Meanwhile pretend to pass her this with your hands.

2. Next your neighbour turns to his/her neighbour, offering him/her an imaginary gift of something s/he really likes. This goes on round the circle, until you end up being given a 'present' by the neighbour on your right.

3. Finish by thanking everyone for attending this session. Check with everyone that they all know the time and location of the second open community meeting and can come to it. Remind them that this meeting is going to be for anyone in the community who wants to come – it is **not** just for the workshop participants so encourage them to bring their neighbours and anyone else who would like to come.

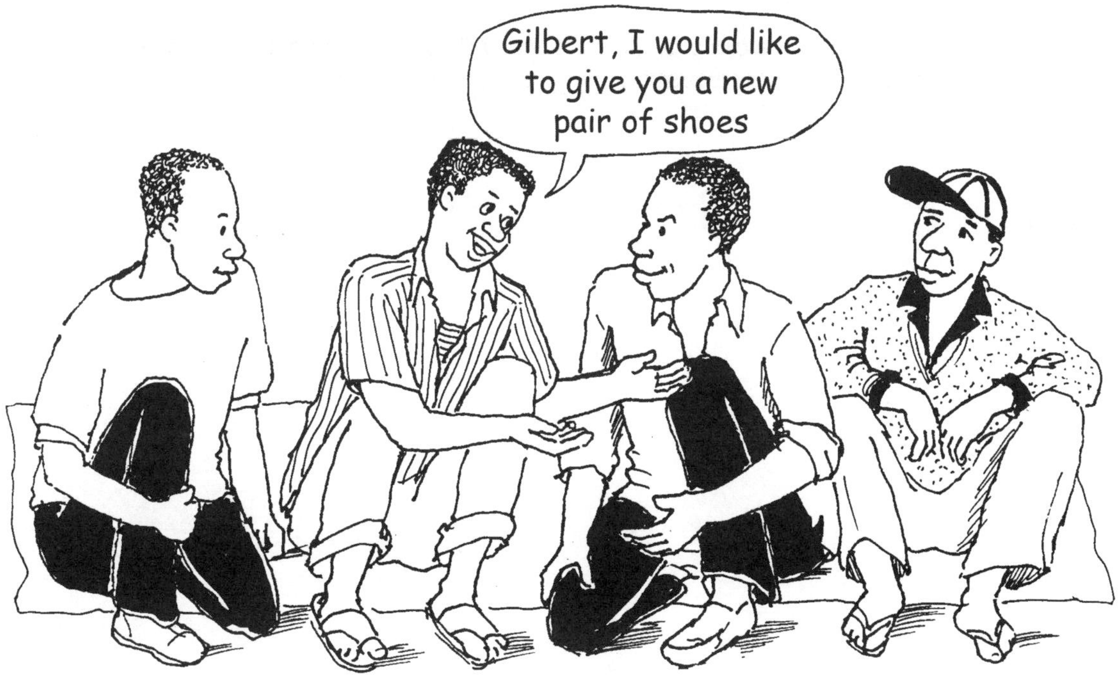
Gilbert, I would like to give you a new pair of shoes

4. Remind everyone of their role as guardian angel.

5. Encourage participants to talk in general about the kinds of issues they have been discussing in these sessions with their friends and neighbours, if they like, but not to share any confidential information from the peer group with others.

6. Remember to ask for three people to stay behind for an instant review of the session, making sure to include anyone who has not already been involved in an instant review. (See Annex 4.)

FACILITATORS' TEAM FEEDBACK

After the end of Session N, meet once more with your co-facilitators to review this session and the special request of each peer group. Discuss the suggestions participants made about how to improve the workshop when you run it in future with other groups. Talk through plans for the second open community meeting, in the light of your discussions. Compare also the changes that each peer group would hope to see in six months' time. It is really important that you make a note of all these as soon as possible, so you can use them for evaluation. It should be interesting to see the different priorities of each peer group. See Annex 4 for details of what to do with this information when the six months are up.

ENDNOTE

1. Participants may want to view the clip again. If so, it is usually best for them to have some discussion about it first, then to have a further discussion after the second viewing.

YOUR NOTES...

SECOND OPEN COMMUNITY MEETING

PURPOSE

To enable all four peer groups to share their special requests with the rest of their community.

TIME NEEDED: Maximum 3 hours.

MATERIALS NEEDED: A long, **strong** rope. Musical instruments? Special clothes for dancing? Refreshments? Food? (The materials with question marks are not essential, but would be good to have if participants would like a general public celebration of the achievements of the workshop so far. See more details below.)

PARTICIPANTS: All workshop participants and **any other community members who want to attend**.

SPECIAL INFORMATION

- Don't forget to read 'Before You Begin ...!' before using this section of the manual.
- Your participants may like to turn this second open community meeting into a bit of a celebration. Would it be possible for them or for you to find money to pay for some light refreshments for everybody? Could a meal be provided for all the workshop participants to share, before or after the meeting? Can some of the participants do some singing or dancing to entertain everyone at the start and the end of the meeting?
- You will also need to think through how the special requests which are to be presented can be taken up seriously by community leaders and others. Read through the notes for this meeting carefully and talk with your colleagues and others about how best you could begin the process during the meeting.

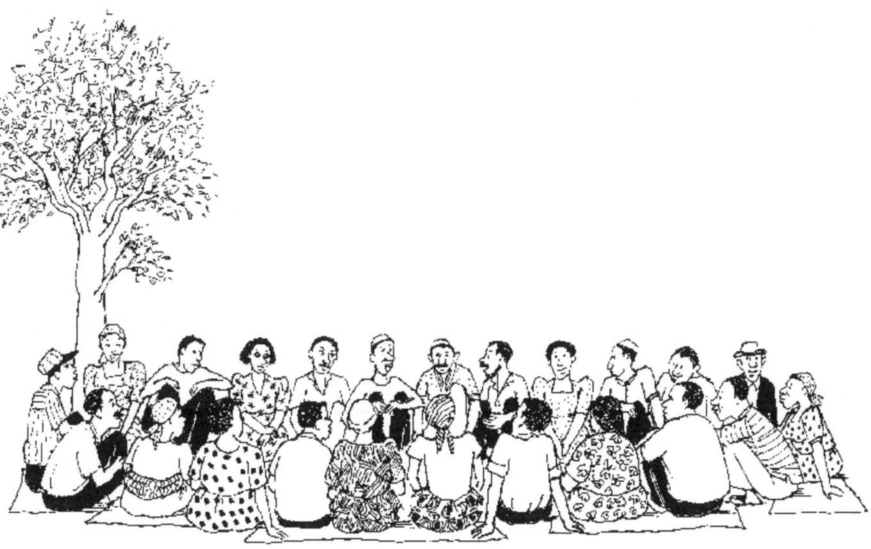

INTRODUCTION

AIMS: To complete the workshop and to present some of its findings to the community in the form of special requests.

DESCRIPTION: Presentation of role plays, each followed by public discussion.

DIRECTIONS

As in the previous public meetings, one or two lead facilitators should do any talking required. The following points need to be made to the audience:

1. Thank everyone for sparing the time to come to the meeting. Give a special welcome to any community leaders or other officials who may have turned up.

2. Reintroduce yourself and let each of your co-facilitators reintroduce themselves to the audience.

3. Explain that, as everyone is probably aware, there has been a workshop running in the community in recent weeks. This meeting today will provide everyone with an opportunity to see and hear a bit about what the participants have done in the sessions so far. The participants will also present some special requests that they would like to make of one another and the whole of the community.

4. At this stage, perhaps, some of the participants could sing or dance for everybody.

5. Next, say that you have often used games during the workshop to lighten the proceedings and to illustrate some of the issues which you have been discussing. Say that you would now like to ask the participants to come forward to play one of the games for everyone to see.

EXERCISE 1: TUGS OF WAR AND PEACE

AIMS: Warm-up exercise to illustrate to everyone benefits of working together.

DESCRIPTION: All workshop participants pull together on a rope, whilst others watch.

MATERIALS NEEDED: A long, strong rope.

DIRECTIONS

1. Divide all the workshop participants into two teams, one of all the women and the other of all the men. Ask these two teams to stand up and hold opposite ends of a long strong rope. Mark a line across the middle of your training area, over which each team must try to pull the other.

2. When you have said 'One, two, three, go!', the teams should start pulling against each other. Let them go on until one team has ended up falling over the dividing line.

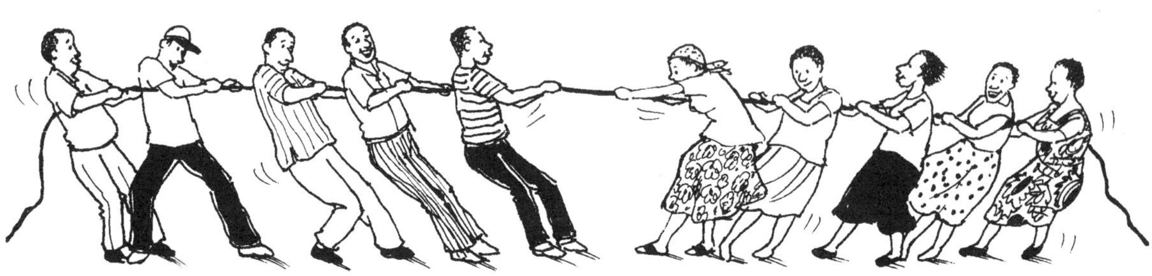

3. Next, ask everyone to divide into two different teams to repeat the exercise: this time the older men and women can pull together against the younger men and women.

4. Next, ask everyone to sit in a circle. Now tie the same strong rope in a large circle and hand it to them, so that they are sitting round the edge of it. (See illustration in Session K.)

5. Ask all the participants to pull together on the rope so that they can all stand up.

6. Now ask the onlookers, i.e. the people who were **not** involved in the original session, what this game illustrates.

> The idea is to give the onlookers an idea of what the workshop was all about: i.e. how, instead of pulling on opposite ends – a tug of war, where only one team wins – we can respond to situations in a way that benefits everyone. True, the tug of war might feel more fun for the victors – but how do the losers feel?

EXERCISE 2: PRESENTATION OF SPECIAL REQUESTS

1. Each peer group has about 20 minutes to present its piece and respond to questions from the onlookers. Participants should decide for themselves the order in which they want to make their presentations.

2. One of you should act as time keeper, to ensure that every peer group has the **same** amount of time. Another of you should chair the discussion, to ensure that a number of different people in the audience have a chance to ask questions of the participants.

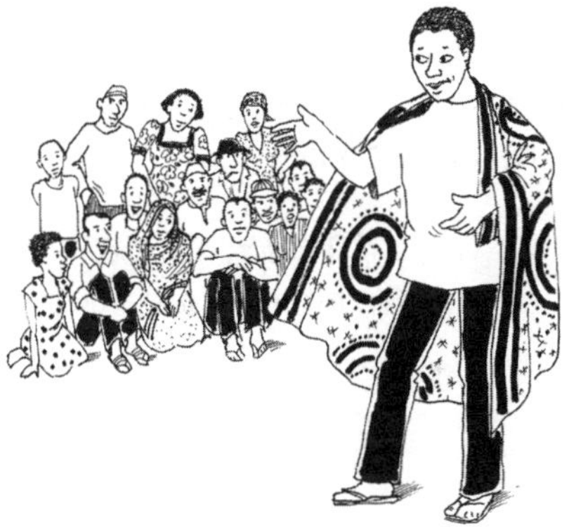

EXERCISE 3: FINAL COMMENTS FOR THIS SESSION

1. You could ask any of the community leaders who have come to the meeting whether they would like to make any comments. If there are community leaders amongst the participants, they should, of course, also be asked to say something.

2. Try to encourage community leaders to adopt the special requests, or have them considered by the community, or at least to discuss them further at the next community council meeting or other appropriate time.

> You may well need to do some background work on this in advance. It might be too easy for everyone to agree to adopt a special request in public, but for nothing to happen about it afterwards. Discuss with your co-facilitators and any community leaders who are attending your workshop, what the best line to adopt might be.

3. If any of the peer groups have stated a wish to go on meeting, for the optional sessions (O–R), you could announce this publicly now.

4. If there seems to be enough interest in starting up a repeat workshop for **new** participants, you could also make an announcement about this now.

5. Ask once more for three participants from each peer group to meet for a few minutes with their own facilitator, after you have finished, in order to conduct a quick review of this second open community meeting **and to decide with them how you can best arrange to meet again with your peer group for the optional sessions (O–R)**. (See Annex 4.)

6. Finish the proceedings by thanking all the participants for their great support and hard work in the workshop so far, and thanking the community leaders for their support. You could then ask everyone to join in more singing and dancing.

FACILITATORS' TEAM FEEDBACK

Don't forget to share your views of this second open community meeting. Again some interesting similarities and differences will emerge from the role plays and special requests. You may well be able to build on these in the later sessions. Talk through plans for the optional sessions O–R (and the further open community meeting), in the light of your discussions. Annex 4 gives you ideas about how you can conduct a full evaluation of the workshop so far. You could make plans now about when and how you can do this.

This is the end of the original *Stepping Stones* workshop. Congratulations to YOU for all you have done so far!

Next you will find instructions for the four extra optional sessions, O–R, and a further community meeting. We hope your participants will find these sessions helpful too.

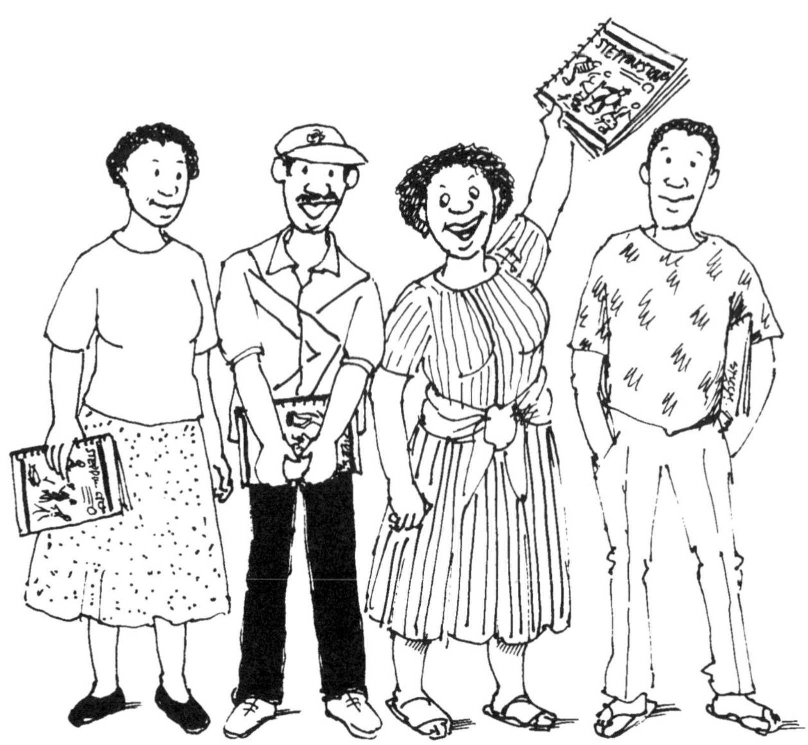

THEME FIVE – MOVING FORWARD TOGETHER

☞ Theme 5 is a new theme, developed originally as a supplement to the original *Stepping Stones* programme and published initially as *Stepping Stones Plus*. Here it is presented as an *optional* follow-on from the original programme. You and your participants may want to have a short break between the second open community meeting and these further sessions.

In Buwenda, after the second open community meeting, the young men's peer group were keen to develop their livelihoods. They were supported with income generation grants by Redd Barna, who had already been working with the community before the Stepping Stones programme. You can see what happened in the community over the following 12 years by viewing the film Stepping Stones Revisited.[1]

LIST OF EXERCISES AND DRAWINGS TO BE PRODUCED BY PARTICIPANTS FROM SESSIONS O–R

Here is a list of exercises and outputs from optional Sessions O–R. The drawings from some of the exercises are to be shared with the other peer groups and the whole community in the further open community meeting, which follows these four extra sessions. They can also form a key part of the record of what has happened in the sessions, which will be needed later for evaluation purposes. So it is very important that, after each session, you and the participants write (small) notes on each flip chart, to remind yourselves about the topic and what each individual drawing on the chart means. Otherwise, this important information might be forgotten.

Exercise title	Description	Outputs
O.1 Knotty Problem Revisited	People tie themselves in a knot	Reminder about who is best at working out problems
O.2 Risk Assessment: Drawing the Line	People move along a line	Reminder of HIV transmission issues
O.3 What Happened Next	Role plays and statues	Understanding of social dynamics of transmission. (1a) Timeline of positive outcome for woman living with HIV and her baby
O.4a Supporting Health Staff to Support Us: Perinatal Care	Discussion and role plays and drawing of action points	(1b) Drawings of suggestions for improved health services
O.4b Accessing Young People's Health Services	Discussion and role plays drawing of action points	(1c) Drawings of suggestions for improved teenage health services
O.5 Closing Circle - If I Were a Tree	Closing game	Back to reality

Exercise title	Description	Outputs
P.1 Interconnecting Circles	Discussion and drawing of groups' influences	(2) Drawing of interconnecting circles of groups' influences
P.2 Body Maps and Special Requests	Discussion of drawings	Greater understanding of issues facing people with HIV and their special requests to others around them
P.3 Working with Faith Leaders	Watch DVD and discuss its contents, role plays, followed by drawing of action points	(3) Drawing of action points to promote care, support and full involvement of positive people in faith communities
P.4 Promoting a Supportive Network Among Neighbours	Discussion and role plays and table of solutions	(4) Table of problem analysis and solutions for neighbours to act on
P.5 Four Things	Discussion and drawings of change	Personal drawings of change
P.6 Closing Circle - If I Were a Bird	Closing game	Back to reality
Q.1 Spider's Web Revisited	Network creation through ball of string	Mental awareness of importance of self as part of group and of the wider community
Q.2 Our Memories from Childhood	Discussion and drawing action points for improving children's lives	(5) Drawing of action points to improve children's lives
Q.3 Supporting our Mothers to Nourish their Children Safely	Discussion and drawing of practical steps to supporting mothers to feed their infants most safely	(6) Drawing of practical steps for community to support mothers to feed their infants most safely
Q.4 The Voices of Orphans	Watch DVD, discussion, drawing of table of analysis and solutions	(7) Drawing of table of analysis and solutions
Q.5 One Thing I Remember	Discussion of past memories of childhood stories, songs etc.	Good thoughts to go home with
R.1 Sharing Information With Sexual Partners: Challenges and Positive Possibilities	Discussions of challenges and benefits, followed by drawing of ways of supporting people	(8) Drawing of ways of support
R2 Sharing Information With Wider Family Members: Challenges and Positive Possibilities	Discussions of challenges and benefits, followed by drawing of ways of supporting people	(9) Drawing of ways of support

Exercise title	Description	Outputs
R.3 Looking After Yourself If You are living with HIV: Challenges and Positive Possibilities	Discussions of advantages, disadvantages and solutions and drawings	(10) Drawing of advantages, disadvantages and solutions
R.4 Review of all Drawings from Sessions O–R and Preparation for the Further Open Community Meeting	Preparing for the public meeting	Everyone knows what they are going to be saying and doing
R.5 Closing Circle	Finishing the session	To draw everyone together to go back to daily life
Further Open Community Meeting: Tugs of War and Peace Walk-Round Exhibition of Drawings Presentation of Special Requests Final Comments and Community Procession	Presentation to the wider community of all the activities of the four peer groups during these new workshop sessions	To share with the community, and seek community approval and support, for planned follow-up activities

Here is an example of one drawing with a key beside it, so that you can see the original drawing and what it means. It would be good for your peer group to do the same with all their drawings in the following sessions.

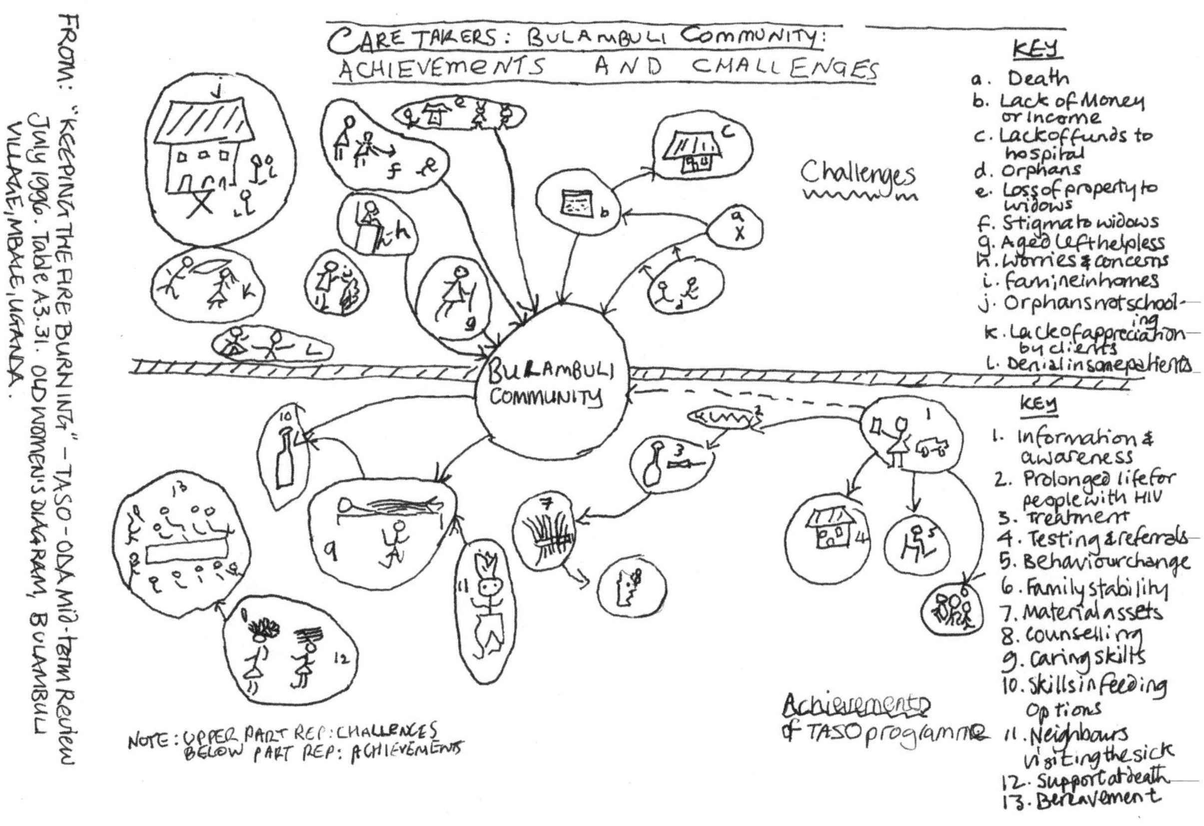

SESSION O WHAT HAPPENED NEXT?

PURPOSE

To address and overcome negative and challenging issues facing people around HIV in their communities and healthcare settings.

CONTENTS	TIME NEEDED
Introduction	
O.1	Opening Game: Knotty Problem Revisited
O.2	Risk Assessment: 'Drawing the Line'
O.3	What Happened Next?
O.4	Supporting Health Staff to Help Us: a) Perinatal Care b) Accessing Young People's Health Services
O.5	Closing circle – If I Were a Tree

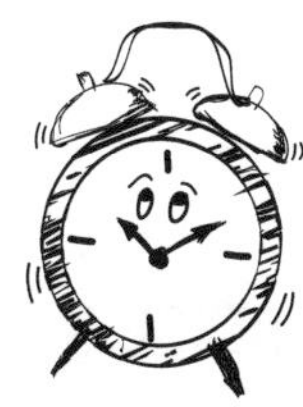

3–4 hours

MATERIALS NEEDED: Chalk, ball of string or length of rope, sticky tape, Flip-Chart paper and marker pens.

PARTICIPANTS: Four separate peer groups.

SPECIAL INFORMATION

Don't forget to read 'Before you Begin ...!' before using this section of the manual.

This is the first of four new sessions in which we introduce some optional exercises that will help participants to explore further why we all tend to stigmatise people who are somehow different from us. These exercises also aim to encourage participants to be more supportive of others different from ourselves.

> ☞ It would be good if you can support community leaders to make contact with the director(s) of any local health services before this session, in order to find out from the health staff how open or not they are to hearing the views of community members about their services. Health staff may or may not be aware of or prepared to respond to some of the issues which participants raise in exercises O.4a and O.4b. So it would be good to try to develop some kind of contact with local healthcare providers in advance. It would also be great if the director could be invited to come to the final community meeting, after these four new sessions, so that she or he can hear for themselves what participants think about the services on offer, and participants' suggestions for improving them.

INTRODUCTION

1. Sit in a circle with the group, preferably on the ground. Everyone should be at the same level, including yourself.

2. Welcome everyone to the new session. Thank everyone for coming. Enquire about latecomers or non-attenders.

3. Ask each participant to recount quickly something good which has happened to them since the last session.

4. Review the last session. Ask participants to remind us what we learnt together at the last session – the final open community meeting – and what it means to us. Remind them if they have forgotten.

5. Explain that we are going on to discuss new topics in this session, but will start with a game.

EXERCISE 0.1: KNOTTY PROBLEM REVISITED

Play the Knotty Problem game, from Session A.6, again. Remind participants who is best at working out for them what their problems are and how to solve them.

EXERCISE 0.2: RISK ASSESSMENT: DRAWING THE LINE

AIMS: For participants to understand risks and facts about HIV transmission.

DESCRIPTION: Checking again the facts about risks of transmission of HIV. This is meant to be quite a fast, dynamic game. By now participants should quickly be able to make their decisions about HIV risks.

MATERIALS NEEDED: A long piece of rope to stretch diagonally across the workshop area, or a piece of chalk.

DIRECTIONS

1. Draw a diagonal line on the ground across the floor of the workshop area, e.g. in chalk, or place a long string or rope across the workshop area. Explain that one end of the rope is going

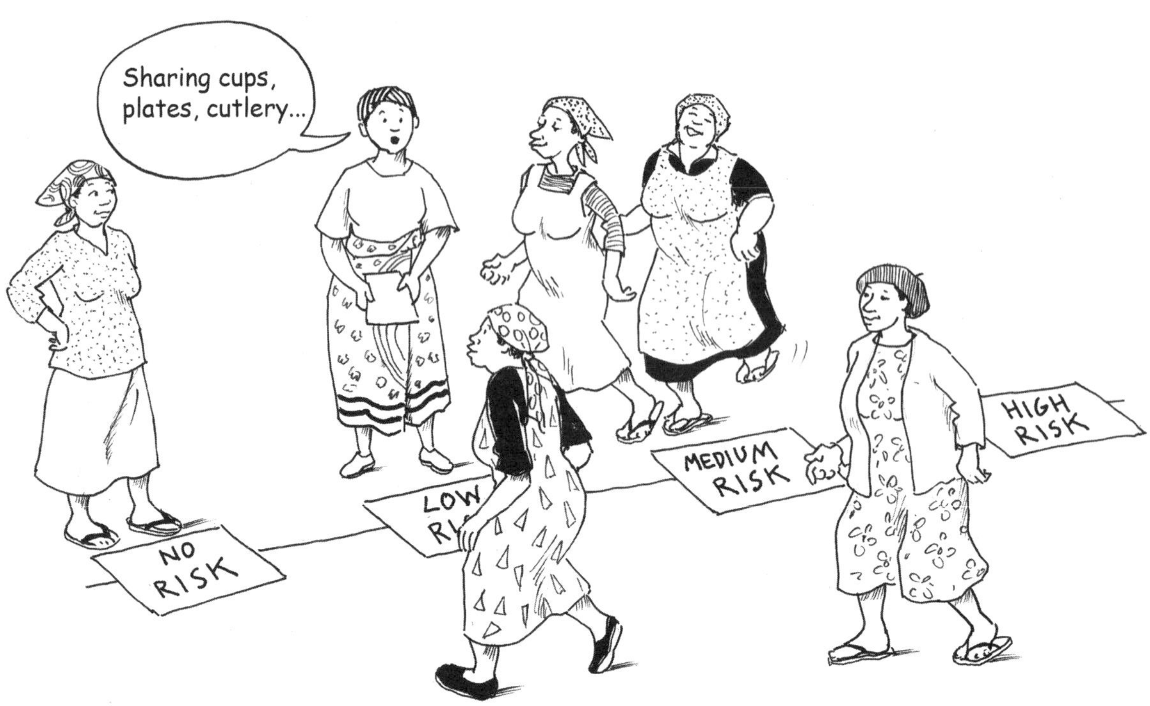
Sharing cups, plates, cutlery...
NO RISK
MEDIUM RISK
HIGH RISK

to mean 'high risk', and the opposite end is going to mean 'no risk'. Between them the rope runs through areas of 'medium' and 'low risk'. In another part of the workshop area, away from the rope, is an area which you are going to call the 'don't know island'.

2. Read the statements from the chart below to the participants.

3. Ask participants to decide for themselves whether they think that each action produces a high, medium, low, or no risk of acquiring HIV, or whether they don't know. Ask them, once they have decided, to run or move quickly and stand either on the rope or away from the rope, depending on their own personal thoughts about the statement. Participants need to be encouraged to think and move quickly in this game, to make it more like real life.

4. For each statement, once participants have spread themselves out along the rope, or placed themselves in the 'don't know' area of the workshop, ask them to look around to see where their peers are. If there are major areas of disagreement, ask two or three participants to stay in their places and defend their positions to the others. After a few minutes' discussion of the statement, encourage participants to move, changing their place if they have changed their mind.

5. In the table below there are some points to consider about each action which you may need to raise with participants if they don't raise them themselves. These statements may at first look quite straightforward, but they are not necessarily as easy to respond to as participants might think. Encourage participants to think through their reactions to the statements each time.

Statements to read	Points to consider
1. Having many sexual partners	This is not necessarily as high-risk for someone who always uses a condom (provided it never breaks) as for someone who never uses a condom, or doesn't use one properly.
2. Holding or shaking hands with a person with HIV	Normal social contact carries absolutely no risk of acquiring HIV.
3. Cleaning up spilled blood	There are other blood-borne conditions around that are more easily transmitted than HIV, so it is best whenever possible to wear protective gloves, or to remove spilled blood with water, or antiseptic, or mild bleach, and a cloth or broom, rather than with bare hands.
4. Unscreened blood transfusion	This can carry high risk of acquiring HIV and other conditions.
5. One man having several wives	If he only ever has sex with those wives, and they only ever have sex with him, they are not at risk of acquiring HIV. If the man or any of his wives has ever had unprotected sex with someone else, then the risk for all of them will rise considerably.
6. Needlestick injuries or using unsterilised needles, razors or knife blades	People should always use sterilised new needles, razors and knife blades. However once blood has dried out, the HIV virus cannot survive. Ideally, needles and blades should never be re-used, but if people really need to re-use them they should clean them well, by washing them through with bleach and clean water, to remove any possible risk of acquiring HIV (or hepatitis).

7. Dry sex (using herbs to make vagina dry)	This is high-risk because it can increase the chances of the vagina walls being torn, so enabling the virus to enter the body.
8. Parent-to-child transmission	There is a one in three chance of a baby being born with HIV if its mother has HIV and is not given the right care, support, and ARV medication. With the right support and treatment from all around her, this risk can be very greatly reduced. We are going on to look at this in more detail in the coming sessions.
9. Breastfeeding	Again, there is a risk of a baby receiving HIV from its mother's milk if she has HIV and is not given the right care, support and ARV medication. With the right care, support, ARV medication, and understanding, this risk can be very greatly reduced. We will also look at this in more detail in the coming sessions.
10. Using condoms	If they are used every time and the instructions for use are followed carefully, especially holding the tip of a male condom when it is first put on the penis to avoid an air bubble, condoms and female condoms both offer a high rate of protection.
11. Sex without condom	This leads to a high risk of acquiring HIV, and/or other STIs, and/or unplanned pregnancy.
12. Non-penetrative sex	This is low-risk, if no body fluids are exchanged.
13. Kissing	If no cuts or ulcers are present, kissing is a low-risk activity.
14. Cleaning or bathing a person with HIV	This is a low-risk activity and provides much support for the person with HIV, if done with love and care.
15. Sharing cups, plates, cutlery, food, sheets, towels and clothing	There is no risk involved in sharing any of these items, provided normal hygiene rules are followed.
16. Using toilets or latrines	Again, there is no risk involved in sharing toilets. Faeces and urine do not carry enough HIV to be risky.
17. Sleeping in the room of a person with HIV	There is absolutely no risk connected to this. In fact sharing a bed or room with a person with HIV, if he or she wants this, can demonstrate respect and provide a lot of care, love, and support.
18. Bites from mosquitoes or fleas	Transmission through insects has never been proven. If transmission took place through insect bites, there would be far many more people with HIV than there already are.
19. Meeting and chatting with visitors to the house	This can be a good way of supporting people with HIV so they feel loved, cared for, and supported, and it can help them to feel happier and more relaxed. There is absolutely no risk of acquiring HIV through normal social contact.

20. Playing with other children	Children with HIV love to run and play with other children. There is no risk whatsoever of acquiring HIV through normal social contact.
21. Inclusion in family events, discussions, decisions	It is highly important for people with HIV to continue to be valued as full family members. There is no risk whatsoever of acquiring HIV through normal social contact. Excluding people with HIV from family life can add greatly to depression and other possible psychological strains of having HIV.
22. Cooking for family and friends	Many women and men with HIV continue to cook for their families or in the workplace. There is no danger whatsoever of HIV being transmitted through food.
23. Cutting meat	Provided nobody is cut, and no human blood is spilt, there is no risk whatsoever of HIV transmission through preparing meat.
24. Road traffic or other accidents	Provided the person caring for others has no cuts or wounds, there is no danger of HIV transmission. In any case, if someone does have a cut, their blood will be flowing out of their body, therefore making it very difficult for HIV or anything else to enter that wound. Nonetheless, because of other blood-borne conditions, it is good medical practice to protect against all blood spills, irrespective of the HIV status of the injured person or the rescue worker.
25. Other situations which participants may like to raise	Use the principles of 'quality, quantity and route of transmission' (QQR) as shown in the fact sheet below and used above to assess the risk of any other situations which participants describe.

QQR FACT SHEET[2]

For HIV transmission to take place, the quality of the virus must be strong, a large quantity must be present and there must be a route of transmission.

QUALITY

For transmission to take place, the quality of the virus must be high. HIV cannot survive outside the human body – it starts to die as soon as it is exposed to the air. If it is exposed to heat (for example if someone bleeds into a cooking pot) it will die. HIV does not live on the surface of your skin – it lives inside the body. The only place the virus can survive outside the body (except for unscreened blood from someone with HIV stored for blood transfusions) is in a vacuum (like a syringe) where it is not exposed to air. Nowadays if people with HIV are able to take ARV medication regularly and have an 'undetectable viral load', then the quality of the virus is very weak and it is almost impossible for them to pass HIV to someone else. Explain that we will discuss this in more detail in in Exercises O.4 and Q.3.

QUANTITY

For transmission to take place there must be enough of the virus to pose a risk. HIV is found in large quantities in blood, semen and vaginal fluids, and breastmilk. It is not found in sweat or tears. It is found in tiny amounts in saliva, vomit, faeces, and urine but there is not enough for there to be any risk of transmission, unless blood is present.

ROUTE OF TRANSMISSION

For HIV transmission to take place, the virus must get inside your bloodstream. Our body is a closed system. HIV cannot pass through unbroken skin and it cannot even pass through broken skin very easily. If you cut yourself, the blood flows outwards, away from the bloodstream. If you touch someone else's cut, blood will not swim into your bloodstream.

Common sense and everyday hygiene mean that many situations that people worry about would not really happen in everyday life. For example: you wouldn't share a toothbrush if it was covered in blood, you would wash if you cut yourself, you could wear gloves if you were cleaning up someone's diarrhoea.

Using QQR, you can see why HIV CANNOT be transmitted by:

- kissing
- hugging
- mosquitoes
- sharing cups and plates
- shaking hands
- giving blood
- sharing toilets or latrines
- using the same washing water
- going to school together

EXERCISE 0.3: WHAT HAPPENED NEXT?

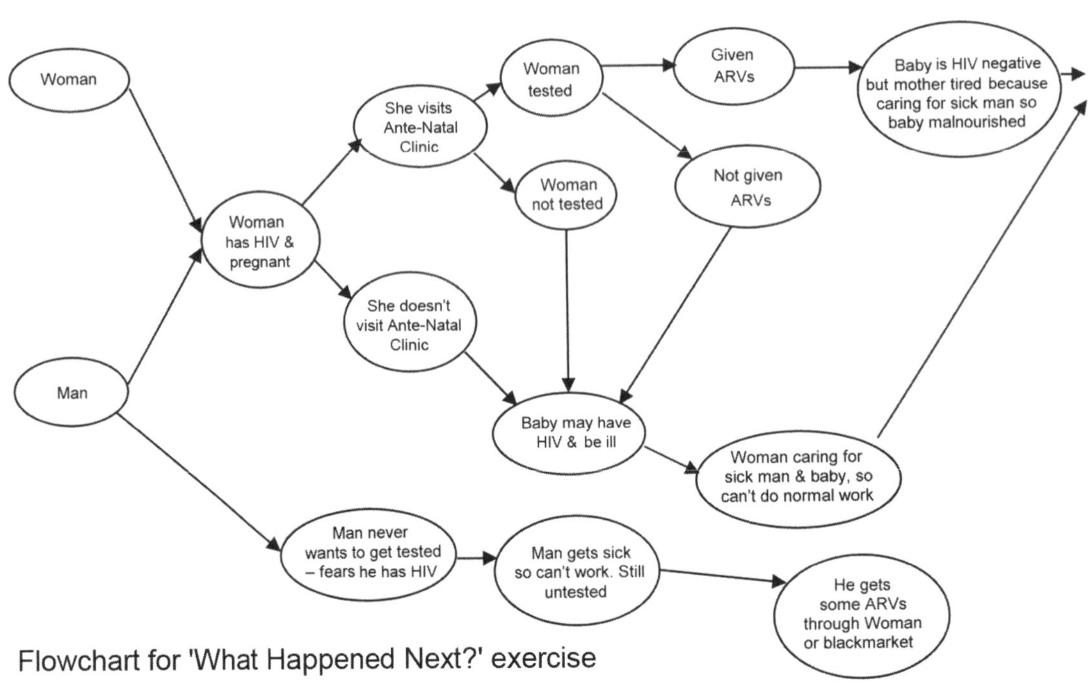

Flowchart for 'What Happened Next?' exercise

AIMS: To help participants to understand how HIV has spread through many communities and what they have done or can do to avoid it.

DESCRIPTION: Participants are asked to form a human 'flow diagram' through role play and statues, and then encouraged to discuss how these situations can be avoided and changed for everyone's benefit.

MATERIALS NEEDED: Flip-chart paper and markers, lengths of string, sticky tape, and scissors.

The flow diagram shows what has happened in many rural families in sub-Saharan Africa and also in other parts of the world. This diagram is designed to help participants understand the pattern usually observed by individuals, communities, and health practitioners.

Your task as facilitator is to support your participants to understand this pattern by drawing it on the ground with them and asking them to place themselves as statues to illustrate the different stages of the diagram. You can then work with participants to change the story into one that is positive for all concerned.

NB: This diagram is *not* designed to raise any discussions about blame. It is designed purely to show participants a pattern which has been seen in many communities, in many different parts of the world. The diagram paints the negative scenario. The final part of the exercise is to enable participants to create the *positive* contrasting scenario.

DIRECTIONS

1. Create this diagram on the ground with people as statues instead of words (see Annex 1 for more help with this), placing an individual participant in each circle and giving them a particular role. (For instance: a man who is untested for HIV could stand with his arms crossed across his chest, a woman whose baby is not well could be pretending to hold a baby and looking at it with a worried expression on her face.) Ask each participant to connect to the previous circle,

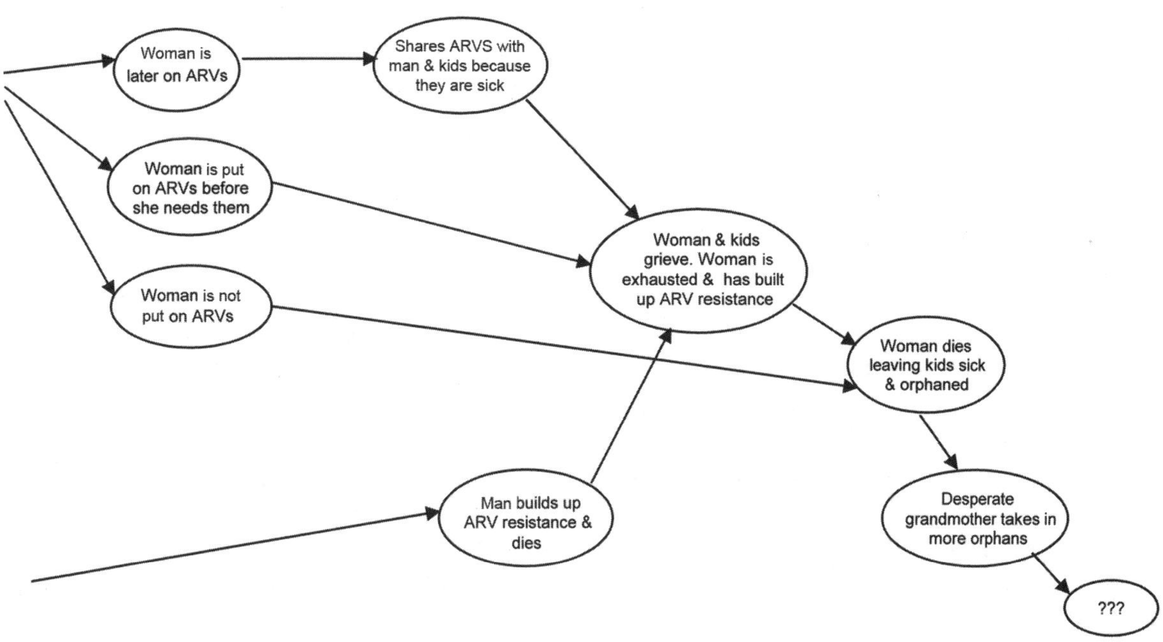

and the next one, by holding one end of a piece of string. Ideally, you need 24 participants in your group to model this diagram – one to represent the man or woman in each circle. But if you have fewer than this you can still do the exercise. Just ask participants to draw a picture to represent the stage of the flowchart on a sheet of flip-chart paper then place the sheet on that circle, with stones to keep it in place.

2. Once you have placed all the flip-chart sheets or participants in their places on the chart, ask participants to continue to stand in their circles and tell, in turn, the stories shown in the flow chart. Each participant should tell his or her part of the story of what is going on, from start to finish.

3. Once you feel confident that all the participants have understood the story, ask them how they can prevent these things from happening in their community, starting at the end of the story and working backwards. Begin, for instance, by asking participants what they could do to help the 'grandmother' with all her orphan grandchildren from feeling so desperate. At each stage, once someone has been helped, he or she can step out of their role in that circle and the string can be wound up and removed from the ground. That person can then join you as the 'audience', supporting other participants by making suggestions about what everyone could do to help the rest of the participants who are still 'stuck' in the story.

4. If participants mention issues to do with VCT, and how it could help prevent the story from happening, remind them of the VCT exercise in Session E (Testing Issues). Explain that we are going to go on to look at 'HIV testing as part of antenatal care'. Testing is usually done by health staff, not by community members on their own. If participants talk about the man not acquiring HIV in the first place, remind participants (if necessary) of what they have learnt about male and female condoms, and explain how these could help everyone to stay healthy.

QUESTIONS TO ASK PARTICIPANTS

Encourage participants to discuss the issues below. As much as possible, try to facilitate it so that it is not judging anyone - just exploring issues and the good things and the difficult things about them.

1. If participants start to argue about who brought HIV into the relationship, ask them this: if some people came home and opened their shopping bags, emptied their homework bags, and changed out of work clothes only to discover later that evening that a scorpion had jumped out from somewhere, would they sit there and argue about how it got into the house while it scuttled around stinging their feet? Or would they all jump up together to look after the person who has been stung and get the scorpion out of the house? Try to help participants to understand that all of us have at times found scorpions or snakes in places where we didn't expect them, no matter how careful we have been. The important thing is that we immediately try to comfort the person who has been stung or bitten, minimise the harm to them, and remove the scorpion or snake – not the injured person – from the house making sure it doesn't harm any more of us; we then take steps to prevent it getting into the house again.

2. In many communities, girls are married at an early age, when the vaginal wall is particularly at risk of damage during sex. This means that they can be at greater risk of acquiring HIV and other conditions than when they are older. Remind participants of the optional session on the female reproductive system, developed in the Gambia, if you have used it (you can contact us for this session).[3]

3. In this community, what tends to be the age difference between girls and boys who are having sex with each other? When are boys expected to start having sex – and when do they start? When are girls expected to start having sex – and when do they start? Has this changed at all over the years? If so, in what ways? Are there issues here which may make girls more vulnerable to HIV and other STIs because of their age?

4. In many parts of the world, men are expected by their peers to have sexual relations with several different women. Men may become sexually experienced, but too often they know little about STIs or HIV and how they can be acquired – or about pregnancy, how the sexual organs of males and females work, and how women experience orgasms. Also, men often feel scared to ask anyone about these things in case they get laughed at for not knowing. This means that in many communities older men are marrying younger women but both the men and their wives know very little about sex because they have never had the chance to learn. Is this true here?

Finally, invite participants to line up again, this time to show a story where all the people in the story – men, women, children, and their carers – remain happy, healthy, and safe. Participants can either draw on success stories from their own community or they can imagine what positive things they would *like* to happen to everyone. If participants have difficulty in shaping this positive story, tell them that this is what these extra sessions will support them to do and thank them for their efforts so far.

As participants relate their new story and line up anew, ask them to draw a diagram with the new story in circles and lines on two or three pieces of flip-chart paper joined together: they can draw new circles then put in each one the positive thing that happens instead of the negative thing shown in the original flowchart. (Drawing 1a.) Ask the participants to act out quickly the positive changes they are showing as they are filling in the circle. This will help them to remember the changes they are describing.

It would help also greatly if you could record which of the positive changes the participants mention have *already* started to take place in the community and which are those that may not have yet happened which *they would like* to happen.

EXERCISE 0.4: SUPPORTING HEALTH STAFF TO HELP US

0.4A: PERINATAL CARE: SUPPORT FOR PREGNANT WOMEN AND PREVENTION OF PARENT-TO-CHILD OR VERTICAL TRANSMISSION[4]

NB: This exercise is for peer groups that already have children or are thinking of having children. In the next section (O.4b) there is a parallel exercise about teenage sexual health service provision for peer groups whose members do not yet want to have children. Peer groups can do both exercises if they want to. You should read through both exercises, and discuss them with your facilitation team, so that you are aware what is being discussed in the other peer groups even if your group doesn't do both exercises.

AIMS: To enable participants to acquire knowledge and explore their attitudes about: (a) care for all pregnant women, whatever their HIV status and (b) support for women living with HIV in the prevention of vertical transmission (PMTCT) of HIV and in overcoming the challenges of stigma and discrimination faced by women living with HIV who are, or wish to be, mothers.

DESCRIPTION: Group discussion and role play, followed by drawing of action points.

MATERIALS NEEDED: Flip-chart paper, marker pens.

DIRECTIONS

Before discussing the information in this section with participants, please work through all of it very carefully with your co-facilitators – and maybe with others too – in order to be really clear about all the details.

1. Explain to participants that everyone in the world has the right to have children, and that it makes no difference if they have a sickness or an illness. Explain that this is in the United Nations Declaration of Human Rights (1948). People have always had the right to have their own children, whoever they are and wherever they live in the world. If they have the right medication and support, people with HIV can live long, happy and productive lives. And they can have children who are HIV-negative.

2. Ask participants whether or not they agree with the above statement. If they don't, find out why they disagree and see what others in the group have to say about it. If some continue to disagree, say that you would like to ask them to do this session and that then we can return to this issue at the end of it.

3. Ask participants whether they think it is better for a man and woman to know their HIV status before they start to have a baby, or wait until the woman is already pregnant. By now, we hope that participants will all agree that it is better for both men and women to know their status beforehand so that, if one of them is living with HIV, they can plan to have a baby with minimum risk of HIV passing from the man to the woman, or from the woman to the man, or from the woman to her baby.

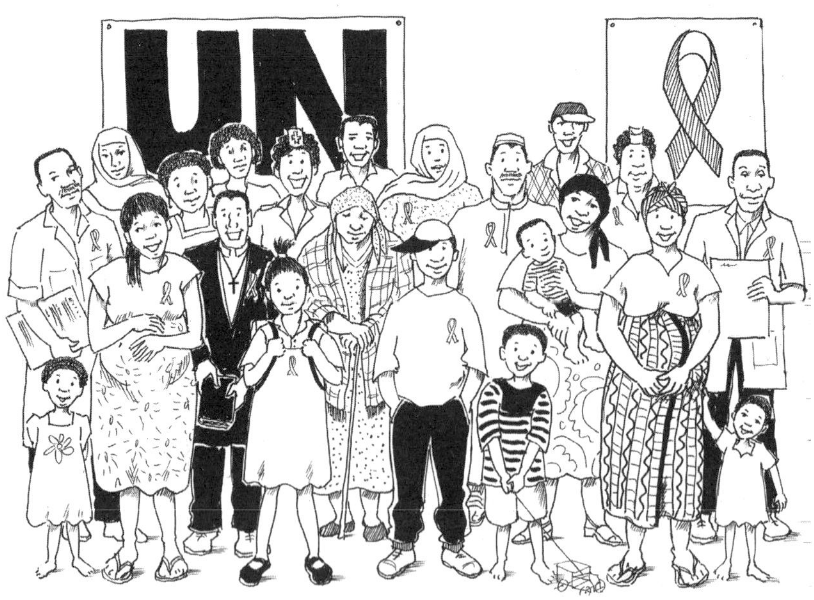

4. Ask if anyone can remember how, if a man is living with HIV and a woman isn't, they can have a baby without him passing the HIV to her and then, possibly, the baby acquiring HIV. First of all explain that if the woman is not living with HIV then the baby can't have HIV either – the HIV can't just jump directly from the man to the baby.

Then remind them that nowadays, scientists have learnt that if a man has HIV, is taking ARVs, **and has an undetectable viral load**, then it is almost impossible for him to pass the HIV to others. An undetectable viral load means that the man is able to take all his ARV medication regularly and that it is working well in his body to keep the HIV at a very low level (see Session E for more on this). This is great news for couples who want to have a baby, because it means that the man's partner can stay HIV-free and she can also get pregnant by them having sex without a condom. On the other hand, it is still a good idea for them to use a male or female condom when they are *not* trying for a baby, to avoid unplanned pregnancies and/or to avoid transmission of any STI the woman or man may have.

It is really important for both the man and the woman to stay in touch with supportive health services. This is firstly so that the man's viral load can be monitored regularly, to make sure it remains undetectable – both before and throughout the pregnancy, to make sure that he is very unlikely to pass HIV to his partner. Secondly, so that she can be tested (again) for HIV by the health staff as soon as she is pregnant – and then, if she does acquire HIV at any time when she is pregnant, the health staff can make sure that she is on the right medication to stop the baby getting HIV too.

Ideally, condoms should be used by the couple throughout the pregnancy to avoid the small risk of the man transmitting HIV to her during the pregnancy – or of any other STI to passing between them. This is the best way to protect the health of both adults – and the health of the unborn baby.

If a man is *not* yet taking ARVs, then condoms should be used for sex at all times. In order for a couple to have a baby, at the time when the woman is most fertile (about 13–15 days after her last period started), the man can ejaculate ('come') into a clean glass or plastic jar or into a condom. He can then immediately draw the sperm into a clean syringe that does not have a needle attached. He could get this from a health centre or pharmacy. The woman can then lie down and use the syringe to insert the sperm carefully into her vagina. She should do this as soon as possible, to make sure the sperm is as fresh as possible, and then stay lying down for 10 minutes or so. Doing this minimises the chances of the woman acquiring HIV in the process of conception. However both people should remain in touch with health services, so that she can continue to be tested for HIV, in case she does acquire it and needs medication.

Explain that there is also research going on about something called 'microbicides' which are in a gel or ring which a woman would be able to use by putting it in the vagina. This would mean that men and women would be able to have babies without passing HIV – or other STIs – between the man and the woman and without having to use condoms or syringes at all. This would keep both partners safe and the baby safe. But the research on microbicides is still going on.

5. Now let's think of another situation. Ask if anyone can remember how, if a woman is living with HIV and a man isn't, they can have a baby without her passing HIV to him or to the baby. Explain that, just as in the case above, a woman with HIV can take ARVs and, if she has an undetectable viral load, it is also almost impossible for her to pass HIV to her partner or her baby. So, again, it is good to keep in touch with health services so that she can continue to check her viral load as she prepares to become pregnant and throughout the pregnancy.

If she is not yet taking medication, then the jar and syringe method described above can also be used by the couple.

Remember to ask participants if they remember when is the best time for a woman to try to get pregnant. The answer is 13–15 days after the woman has started her period.[5]

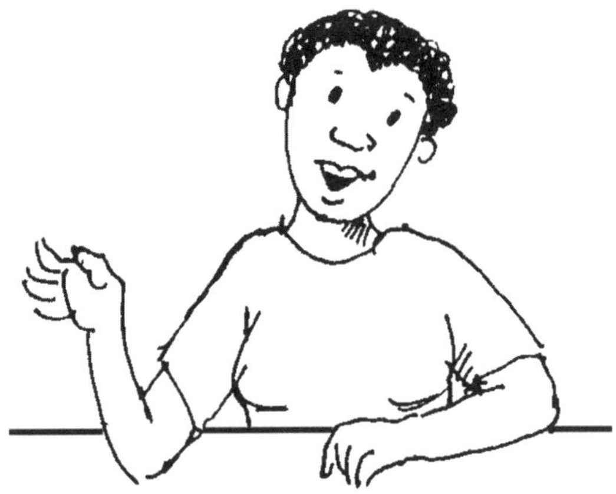

Then explain how, once a woman has become pregnant, with the right support from healthcare staff and her family, she can either start or continue to be given medication to make sure that the virus is not passed on to the baby. Again, remind participants that a condom should be used whenever the couple have sex during the pregnancy so as to continue to minimise any risk of HIV or any other STIs being passed between the couple. In this way they will best protect one another's health – and the health of their unborn baby.

Using medication to avoid passing HIV on to a partner or from a woman to her baby is known as 'treatment as prevention.'

PrEP. Explain to participants that ARVs are now also starting to be used by people who don't have HIV at all, to prevent them acquiring it. This new method is called PrEP, which stands for 'Pre-Exposure Prophylaxis'. However it is not yet clear (September 2015) how safe this is for women who are pregnant and do not have HIV.

In September 2015, WHO said 'Contraception services, safer conception management and links to antenatal care should be available when providing PrEP services for women. The risks, benefits and alternatives of continuing to use PrEP during pregnancy and breastfeeding should be discussed with each person. Further research is needed to fully evaluate PrEP use during pregnancy and breastfeeding'.[6]

6. Explain that what is key to all this is for us to have health staff who are good listeners. Ask participants to remember the exercise we did in Session A, when we talked about good listening skills and trust and confidentiality issues. Explain to participants that these are things which we should expect from health staff, but that sometimes health service providers don't offer this quality of care. Brainstorm with the participants for a short time about any poor experiences of healthcare that they have had.

7. Explain that a pregnant woman is in particular need of care, support and encouragement from healthcare staff – especially during her first pregnancy. So to have an HIV test at this time can be very traumatic, especially if she is not given full back-up and support both by health staff and the community. Encourage participants in the older and younger men's groups to think about situations which might be faced by our wives or girlfriends, sisters or daughters, if they were to test positive for HIV during their pregnancy.

8. Ask participants what concerns there may be about care and support for pregnant women and perinatal services in this community. Divide the participants into three or four smaller groups of five or six people so that, for instance, one can be a pregnant woman who tests positive, two can be health staff, one can be another pregnant woman who tests negative, and one or two others can be a receptionist or a cleaner. Ask at least one group to work on a role play of pregnant women being well-treated at a health centre and ask at least one of the others to work on a role play of pregnant women being badly-treated at a health centre.

9. Each of the three or four groups presents their role play to the rest of the peer group. Show the one or two role plays demonstrating bad treatment first, then have a discussion about the elements which were bad, using the kinds of questions listed below. Then show the one or two role plays that demonstrate good treatment and discuss these.

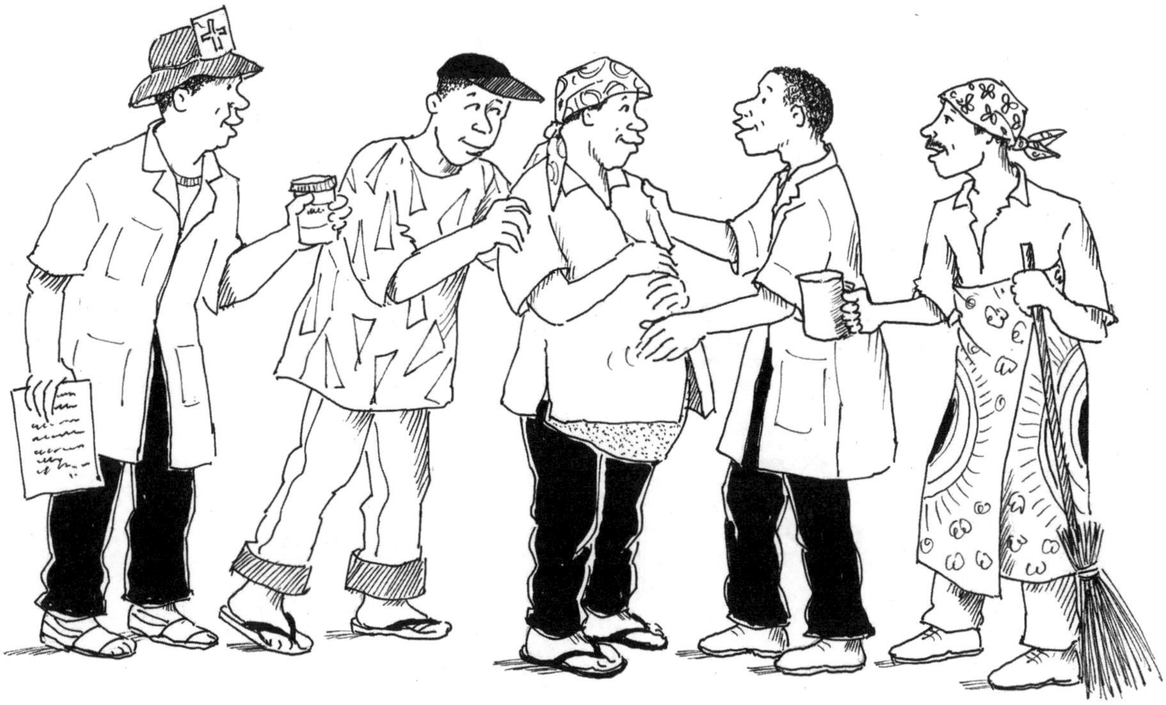

Were there any elements of the 'bad' role plays which have given participants ideas to improve the 'good' role plays even more? Here are some questions you can ask the participants to help get the discussion going:

- What happened in the role play?
- What was each person doing?
- Where was the action taking place?
- What are the possible causes of this kind of action?
- Does this happen in our community?
- What are its effects on the pregnant woman and her family?
- Is the health worker's behaviour good for the pregnant woman?
- Is the health worker's behaviour good for the pregnant woman's older children or unborn child?
- How does this kind of behaviour affect the use of PMTCT services by community members?
- What have we learnt from this exercise?
- **What can we do to improve behaviour in our health facilities?** (The next two paragraphs will help to develop ideas amongst participants in response to this question.)

10. Here are some extra points that it would be good to discuss with participants:

- Many health staff are overworked, underpaid and under-supported by their superiors, so they feel burnt out and take it out on their clients. Is this true of health staff whom participants have met?
- Health staff often need to develop their own coping mechanisms, and perhaps appear unsympathetic if they are overwhelmed with all the sickness they see.

- Health staff are human too and may feel overwhelmed by commitments to their husbands, wives and children at home before they even come to work.
- Many health staff have also acquired HIV through their own relationships, and have felt unsupported by the health systems which employ them. In fact, some health staff experience even more prejudice from their colleagues, who feel that they have somehow let the health profession down.
- Health staff from other regions may feel upset that they have been posted far from home and take out their frustrations on their patients.
- Local health staff may treat clients from a minority ethnic or faith group unsupportively.
- Some health staff may just be in the wrong profession and are not best suited for caring roles.

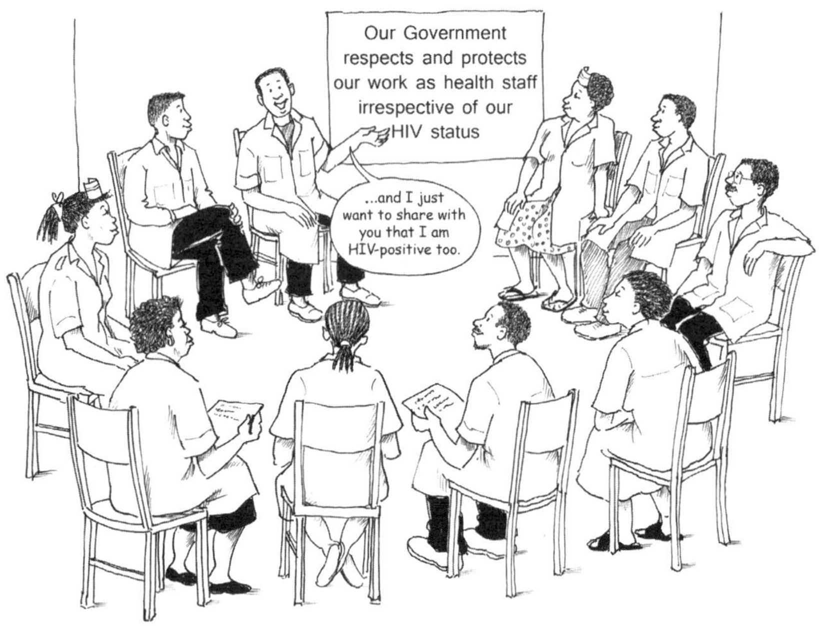
Our Government respects and protects our work as health staff irrespective of our HIV status
...and I just want to share with you that I am HIV-positive too.

11. Another important issue is to do with the pros and cons of men attending an antenatal clinic (ANC) with their partners for testing, or to help their partner and children access treatment. In some countries, Ministry of Health policy now encourages men to attend ANC with their partners at least once during each pregnancy. Is that the case here? What do participants think of this?

Ask participants to brainstorm possible pros and cons of men going with their partners to the antenatal clinic to be tested. If that was available here, would participants think that was a good thing or a bad thing? What issues do they think would need to be considered?

For instance, there may be practical problems such as clinic opening times which mean that if a man goes with his partner he may miss out on working and income that day.

- It may be that the ANC doesn't actually offer testing services for men. If not where can he go to be tested?
- The woman or man might want to go alone, or at least have some time with the health staff to discuss issues which she or he doesn't want to talk about in front of their partner. This should be their right, but the partner or the health staff may not be happy with this.
- The health staff may all be men – or all women.
- The health staff may be local people, which may cause fear of lack of confidentiality.
- The health staff may be rude and abrupt, which may cause unhappiness and lack of trust.
- The health staff may demand too many tests of both partners, requiring too much time or money.

12. **Action Point:** (Drawing 1b) Ask participants to **draw on pieces of flip-chart paper** a list of the issues which they have mentioned. This list, and the lists from the other peer groups, can be used later to present suggestions for improved services to the local health centre, or Ministry of Health official. For example, if they wanted services to be open to men as well as women, they might want to draw a male health worker and a clock to show a good time for that service to be available for them. Make sure to draw up concerns and questions as well as requests.

The flip-chart paper could illustrate the points below – but encourage participants to think of their own issues and drawings for each one.

SUGGESTIONS FOR IMPROVED HEALTH SERVICES		
Questions about local health service provision	**Concerns about local health service provision**	**Requests for services from local health service providers**
Could men be seen separately? Could women be seen separately? Could couples also be seen together? Could male and female health staff be available for separate clinic times? What else?	Session times Costs of tests Confidentiality of tests Waiting times Number of tests needed What else?	VCT for both men and women before conception Free, comprehensive conception services for all women, if wanted Free male and female condoms Aciclovir to avoid repeat herpes attacks Free ARVs for all Paediatric ARVs for children with HIV Comprehensive post-rape services (e.g. post-exposure prophylaxis – ARVs to prevent acquiring HIV, pills to avoid unplanned pregnancy etc.) Free tests TB testing Pap smears[7] Staff to be friendly and respectful to all clients What else?

Suggest to participants that they might like to think about a representative from their peer group joining the local health centre's Community Advisory Board (CAB). WHO guidelines suggest that health workers start these boards up in order to connect more effectively with communities for HIV management. See chapter 4 especially.[8] If a CAB doesn't already exist, maybe you could start one!

EXERCISE 0.4B: ACCESSING YOUNG PEOPLE'S HEALTH SERVICES

NB: This is the same exercise as the one above, except that it focuses on young people's health services. Choose which of these two exercises is more relevant for your peer group (or you can do both exercises if you prefer).

This exercise begins to raise issues about unplanned pregnancy and young people's access to youth-friendly health services. These issues will be raised again in a later session with all four peer groups. This session is designed to help young people particularly to become aware of and think about these issues for themselves.

If you are working with younger children aged 5-14, see also *Stepping Stones with Children* – our new manual specifically designed for this age group.

AIMS: **To enable participants to explore their fears and acquire knowledge about: (a) healthcare for all young men and women, whatever their HIV status, and (b) support for young men and women living with HIV to access good quality healthcare.**

DESCRIPTION: **Group discussion and role play, followed by drawing of action points.**

MATERIALS NEEDED: **Flip-chart paper and marker pens.**

DIRECTIONS

NB: It would be best for you to work through all the information in this section really carefully with your co-facilitators — and maybe with others too – so you are really clear about all the details before you discuss it with participants.

1. Explain to participants that everyone in the world has the right to good quality, non-judgmental health information and services, and that it makes no difference what age they are or if they have a sickness or an illness. Explain about young people's sexual and reproductive rights, as outlined in the IPPF *Exclaim*! document.[9] This applies to all young people, whoever they are, wherever they live in the world, and whether or not they are already living with HIV. If they have the right medication and support, people with HIV can live long, happy and productive lives. And they can grow up to have children who are HIV-negative, if and when they want them.

2. Ask participants whether or not they agree with this statement. If they don't, find out why they disagree and see what others in the group have to say about it. If some continue to disagree, say that you would like to ask them to do this session and that then we can return to this issue at the end of the session.

3. Ask participants how young men and young women might have HIV before they have ever had sex. If they can't think how this could be, remind them to think of the different routes of HIV transmission, and then gently prompt them by asking what happens when a baby born with HIV gets older. Some participants may be surprised to realise that teenagers could be living with HIV without looking ill. Explain that, provided that they were well nourished as they grew up, their HIV may not yet have progressed to illness. They may not even realise they have HIV.

4. Next ask participants what might be the three most important things to try to remember about having sex, to make it feel good and safe, and so they don't feel bad about it in any way afterwards. See what they reply. Suggest the three following answers, if participants don't come up with them, and see what they say about them:

a) ONLY to have sex when both partners feel really ready to become sexually active and not before.
b) ONLY to have sex when both partners fully want to and when their decisions are not influenced by alcohol or other drugs, so they are fully conscious of what they are doing and able to say 'stop' if they change their minds.
c) To be *prepared* to have sex — i.e. to have thought about it and planned for it beforehand, so that you can have a condom (male or female) with you to protect yourself and your partner.

5. Then ask participants whether they think it is better for young people to know their HIV status before they start to get involved in relationships and have sex, or when they have already started to become sexually involved with others. By now, we hope that participants will all agree that it is better for both young men and young women to know their status before they become sexually involved with others so that, if one of them has HIV, they can plan to have sex, if they want it, with minimum risk of either passing HIV to the other person – or of the young woman passing HIV to her baby, if she wants to have one.

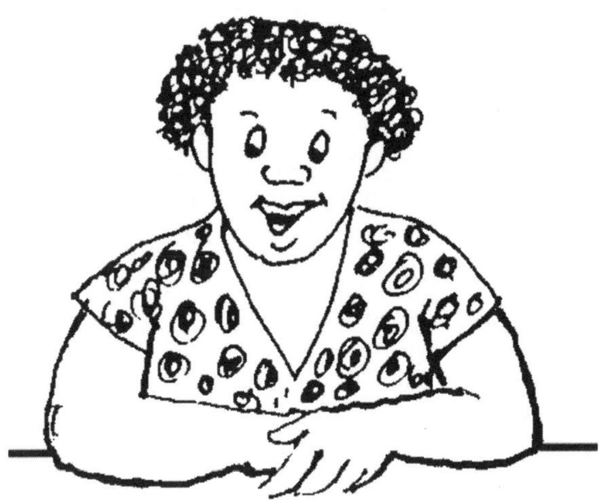

NB: At this stage of their relationship, as ever, one or both of these young people might also decide instead to discontinue the relationship. Either of them has the right to do so – although they also have the responsibility of doing this in a caring and respectful way.

6. Ask participants whose responsibility they think it is to ensure that HIV is not transmitted from a young or older man to a young woman, or vice versa. If participants answer that it is the responsibility of only one and not both partners, ask them if they can think of a more balanced answer than the one they have given. It would be great if participants could agree that the responsibility lies on both sides, but they may not be ready to accept this yet.

7. Ask if anyone knows how, if a young man has HIV and a young woman doesn't, they can have sex without him passing HIV to her. Encourage participants to remember what they have learnt about non-penetrative sex; and also about male and female condoms.[10]

8. Ask if anyone knows how, if a young woman has HIV and a young man doesn't, they can have sex without her passing HIV to him. Encourage participants to remember what they have learnt about non-penetrative sex and male and female condoms.

9. Now repeat questions 6, 7 and 8 with regard to unplanned pregnancy: whose responsibility is it to make sure that an unplanned pregnancy doesn't happen? If participants just blame people of another gender than their own, keep encouraging them to ask themselves why they think this.

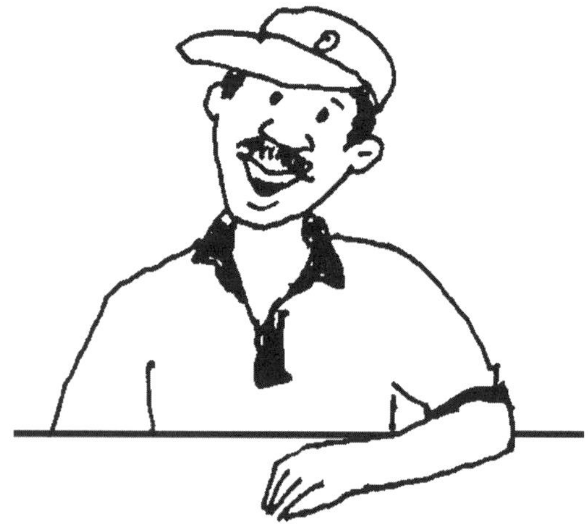

10. Then ask participants to remember the 'Who's Labelling Whom' exercise – and whether they think it is fair for an individual to be blamed for the rest of their lives for something which they have done by mistake, or out of fear of rejection, or without fully realising the consequences.

11. Next, ask participants to remember the exercise we did way back in Session A, when we talked about good listening skills and trust and confidentiality issues. Explain to participants that these are the qualities which we should expect from health staff, but that sometimes health service providers haven't been trained to offer this quality of care. Brainstorm with the participants for a short time a bit about any poor experiences of healthcare that they have experienced.

12. Explain that teenagers who are just beginning to have sexual experiences are in particular need of care, support and encouragement from healthcare staff – especially if they are visiting a health centre for the first time. Young people should expect to receive full back-up and support from health staff, from their schools, and from the wider community. This is their right. Encourage participants, if they are in the older peer groups, to think about situations which we may all have faced when we were young people in need of advice and help from health staff.

13. What fears do we have about care and support in our community for us as young men and women seeking good quality health services related to our sexual and reproductive lives?

14. Divide the participants into three or four smaller groups of five or six for role plays in which, for instance, one person can be a young woman who learns that she is pregnant, one can be a health staff member, one can be the young woman's boyfriend, and two can be the parents of the young woman. Ask at least one of the smaller groups to work on a role play of the young pregnant woman being well-treated at a health centre, and at least two of the smaller groups to work on role plays of a pregnant women being badly treated at a health centre. In one 'bad situation' the young woman could be badly treated because she is unmarried. In the other, she could be badly treated because she has HIV.

Each of the three or four groups presents their role play to the rest of the peer group. Show the two role plays demonstrating bad treatment first, then have a discussion about the elements which were bad, using the kinds of questions listed below. Then show the one or two role plays demonstrating good treatment and discuss these. Were there any elements of the 'bad' role

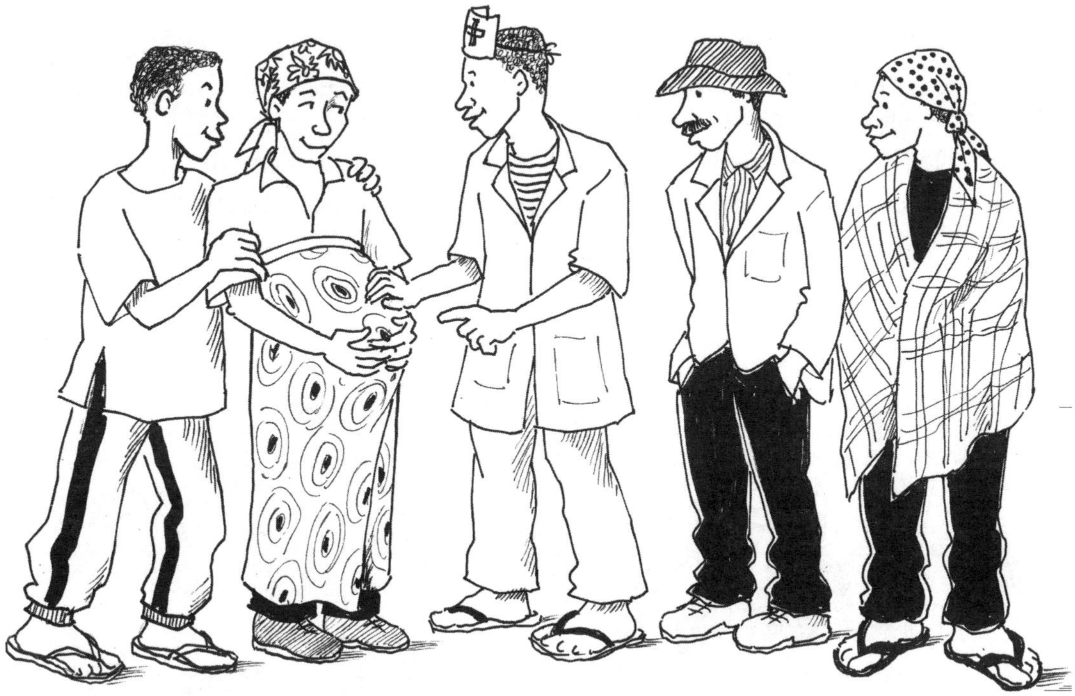

plays which have given participants ideas to improve the 'good' role plays even more? Here are some questions you can ask the participants to help you:

- What happened in the role play?
- What was each person doing?
- Where was the action taking place?
- What are the possible causes of this kind of action?
- Does this happen in our community?
- What are its effects on the young pregnant woman and her family?
- Is the health worker's behaviour good for the young woman?
- Is the boyfriend's behaviour good for the young woman?
- Is the behaviour of the parents of the young woman good for the young woman?
- How does this kind of behaviour affect the use of health services by young community members?
- What have we learnt from this exercise?
- What can we do to improve behaviour in our health facilities?

15. Here are some extra thoughts you may want to share with participants:

- Many health staff are overworked, underpaid, and under-supported by their managers. Often they have not been given specific training in providing services designed for young people, so they feel burnt out and take it out on their clients.
- Health staff often need to develop their own coping mechanisms and perhaps appear unsympathetic if they are overwhelmed with all the sickness they see.
- Health staff are human too and may feel overwhelmed by commitments to their husbands, wives, and other family members – maybe worries about their own teenage children – before they even come to work.
- Many health staff might have acquired HIV through their own relationships, or themselves had an unwanted pregnancy when they were teenagers, and have felt unsupported by the health system

they work for. In fact, some such health staff experience great prejudice from their colleagues, who feel that they have somehow let the health profession down by their actions.

- Health staff from other regions may feel upset that they have been posted far from home and take out their frustrations on their patients.
- Local health staff may treat clients from a minority ethnic group unsupportively.
- Some health staff may just be in the wrong profession and may not be cut out for caring roles.

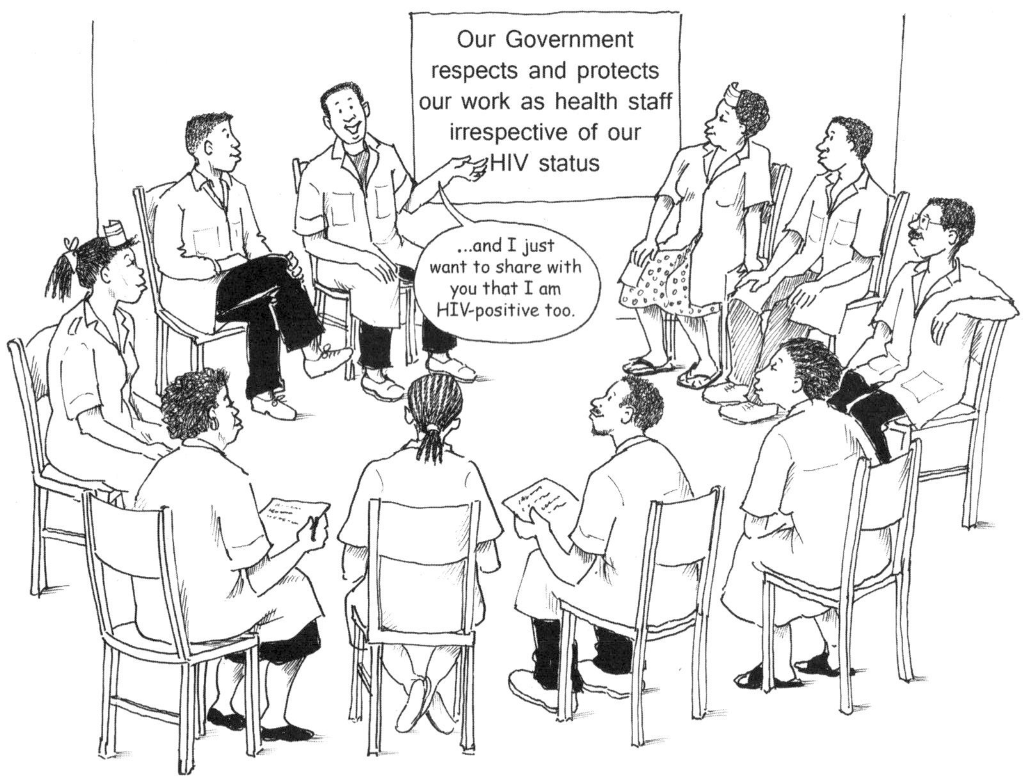
Our Government respects and protects our work as health staff irrespective of our HIV status
...and I just want to share with you that I am HIV-positive too.

16. Ask participants to brainstorm possible pros and cons of young men going to a young men's health clinic, to be tested for HIV, to access condoms, or to ask about their other concerns. For instance:

- There may be practical problems such as clinic opening times which mean that, if a young man goes to school or out to work, he may not be able to get to the health centre during its opening hours.
- A young man might want to go with his girlfriend, but she might want to go alone, or at least have some time with the health staff to discuss issues which she doesn't want to talk about in front of her partner.
- The young man might want to have a private conversation with the health staff as well.
- The health staff may all be men – or all women.
- The health staff might all be too old for the young man to feel he can connect with them.
- The health staff may be local people, which may cause fear of lack of confidentiality and concerns that his peers or his family may find out about his visit.
- The health staff may be rude and abrupt, which may cause unhappiness and lack of trust.
- The health staff may demand too many tests of the young man, needing too much time or money.

17. **Action Point:** (Drawing 1c) Ask participants if they could draw on flip-chart paper a list of the issues which they have mentioned. This list – and those of participants from the other peer groups – can be used later to present suggestions for improved services to the local health centre or Ministry of Health official. For example, if they wanted services to be open to young men as well as young women, they might want to draw a young male health worker and a clock to show a good time for that service to be available for them.

SUGGESTIONS FOR IMPROVED TEENAGE HEALTH SERVICES		
Questions about local health service provision	**Concerns about local health service provision**	**Requests for services from local health service providers**
Could young men be seen separately? Could young women be seen separately? Could couples also be seen together? Could male and female health staff be available for clinics at separate times? Could health staff be younger? What else?	Session times Costs of tests Confidentiality of tests Waiting times Number of tests needed What else?	VCT for both young men and women before conception Free, comprehensive conception services for all young women, if wanted Free male and female condoms Aciclovir to avoid repeat herpes attacks Free ARVs for all Free tests Comprehensive post-rape services TB testing Pap smears[11] Staff to be friendly and respectful to all clients, no matter how young What else?

Suggest to participants that they might like to think about a representative from their peer group joining the local health centre's Community Advisory Board (CAB). Some new guidelines from WHO have suggested that health workers start up these boards in order to connect more effectively with communities for HIV management. Another way in which young people can become involved in healthcare in their community is suggested in Exercise R.4 (point 10).

EXERCISE 0.5: CLOSING CIRCLE – IF I WERE A TREE

This is a fun energiser, to bring participants back to the present. Trees come in all shapes and sizes, some very beautiful, some more useful. All of them have a place in the landscape.

1. Ask each person in turn in the circle to say 'One thing I have learnt from today's session is ...'; and 'If I were a tree, I would like to be a ... because it ...'. Start with yourself.

2. This should be quite a quick game. Encourage participants not to spend too long on their choice.

3. As a going-home exercise, you could ask participants to reflect on their choice of tree, on the basis of what they have learnt at these sessions. Ask them to think at home about whether they would like to be another kind of tree instead of, or as well as, the one each of them has just chosen.

4. Finish off by thanking everyone once more for coming to this session. Remind everyone that the next time you meet there will be some more exercises. Encourage participants to talk in general about the kinds of issues they have been discussing in these sessions with their friends and neighbours, if they like, but not to share any confidential information with others.

5. Remind everyone of their role as guardian angel.

6. Remember to ask for three volunteers to stay behind for ten minutes for a quick review of this session. (See Annex 4 for details.) Make sure that everyone has agreed a mutually convenient time and place for your next session before saying goodbye.

FACILITATORS' TEAM FEEDBACK

After the end of Session O, meet again with your co-facilitators to compare notes on how the sessions went and the information which you all learnt from them. Your co-facilitators could have found useful information that could help you to structure your next session more effectively. Remember, however, not to share individual confidentialities between groups. This is the easiest way to ruin the trust that you have built up, and to wreck the whole workshop! The next meeting is the second optional session. Remember that this is still only for members of the four peer groups (meeting separately) and not for the general public.

ENDNOTES

1. Strategies for Hope (2006) *Stepping Stones Revisited: Stories from the Village of Buwenda, Uganda.*
2. Adapted from Kidd and Clay (2003).
3. See our contact details at the front of this volume.
4. This is also known as PMTCT. However we prefer to call it 'perinatal care' and prevention of parent-to-child (or vertical) transmission or 'prevention of vertical transmission'. See Introduction to this volume for more on this.
5. Optional additional exercises on STIs and the female reproductive system, including information about the woman's reproductive cycle and when she can best get pregnant, if she wants to, are available in *Stepping Stones - Gambia* – please contact us for these if you would like to use them.
6. WHO (2015).
7. Gaym et al. (2007) explain the importance of PAP smears in the context of HIV.

8. WHO (2008). See Chapter 4 especially.
9. This document by IPPF (2008) makes the links between the rights laid out in the UN Convention on the Rights of a Child (CRC) in 1989 and sexual and reproductive rights – traditionally one of the most controversial areas in UN discussions. These rights are the most powerful legal instrument available to all children for the protection and enforcement of their human rights. This UN Convention has been ratified by every country in the world, with the exception of USA and Somalia.
10. Please also see the information earlier in this session about undetectable viral loads and HIV transmission.
11. Gaym et al. (2007). See Endnote 7 above.
12. WHO (2008).

REFERENCES

Gaym, A., Mashego, M., Kharsany, A., Walldorf, J., Frohlich, J. and Abdool Karim, Q. (2007) 'High prevalence of abnormal pap smears among young women co-infected with HIV in rural South Africa – implications for cervical cancer screening policies in high HIV prevalence populations', *South African Medical Journal,* 97:120–4.

IPPF (2011) *Exclaim! Young People's Guide to Sexual Rights: An IPPF declaration*, IPPF, London, <http://www.ippf.org/sites/default/files/ippf_exclaim_lores.pdf> [accessed 23 January 2016].

Kidd, R. and Clay, S. (2003) *Understanding and Challenging HIV Stigma: Toolkit for Action* Change add [location], <http://www.icrw.org/publications/understanding-and-challenging-hiv-stigma-toolkit-action> [accessed 23 January 2016].

Shaw, M. (2002) *Stepping Stones – Gambia,* ActionAid, London.

Strategies for Hope (2006) *Stepping Stones Revisited: Stories from the Village of Buwenda, Uganda* [film on website], Salamander Trust, <https://vimeo.com/album/3419245/video/134751173> [accessed 16 November 2015].

WHO (2008) *Operations Manual for Delivery of HIV Prevention, Care and Treatment at Primary Health Centres in High Prevalence, Resource-Constrained Settings*, WHO HIV/AIDS Department, Geneva, <http://www.who.int/hiv/pub/imai/operations_manual/en/> [accessed 23 January 2016].

WHO (2015) *Guideline on when to start antiretroviral therapy and on pre-exposure prophylaxis for HIV*, WHO, Geneva, <http://apps.who.int/iris/bitstream/10665/186275/1/9789241509565_eng.pdf> [accessed 15 November 2015].

YOUR NOTES ...

SESSION P NURTURING COMMON GROUND: PROMOTING CARE AND SUPPORT AMONGST PARTNERS, FAMILIES AND THE WIDER COMMUNITY

PURPOSE

To promote respect and support for people living with HIV, and their families, across communities.

CONTENTS	**TIME NEEDED**
Introduction	
P.1	Interconnecting Circles
P.2	Body Maps and Special Requests of People Living with HIV
P.3	Working with our Faith Leaders
P.4	Promoting a Supportive Network Among Neighbours
P.5	Four Things
P.6	Closing circle – If I Were a Bird

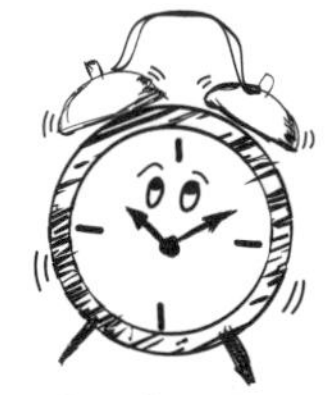

3–4 hours

MATERIALS NEEDED: Ball of string, chalk, flip-chart paper and marker pens, scissors, tape, one candle for each member of your peer group (including yourself) plus one extra, a box of matches, *What Can I Do?* DVD, laptop with DVD player, projector.

NB: You will also need to prepare some materials for one of the exercises in this session. In Exercise P.2 you will see two body maps drawn by men and by women in OPAHA — a self-help support group of people living with HIV in Garissa, northeast Kenya. You will also see two 'special request' drawings by the same members of this group. Before you run this session, please either ask men and women in your local support group of people living with HIV to draw similar body maps and special request drawings for themselves for you to use (with their permission) in this session; or photocopy the body-maps and special requests drawn here, and translate each comment into the language of the community with which you are working writing on the chart next to the English. Then make enough copies of both the body maps and the special request drawings for all members of your peer group to have their own copy of all four drawings.

> ☞ In Kenya, one organisation (ActionAid) arranged a *Stepping Stones* workshop specifically for faith leaders from different religions so that they could come together, share, and discuss what HIV means to them in their own lives. This workshop really helped the faith leaders to understand how HIV can affect us all. It would be good if you could support community leaders to make contact with all the local faith leaders, including traditional healers, before this session, in order to find out from these leaders how open or not they are to hearing the views of community members about their services. Some of the issues which participants raise in Exercise P.3 may or may not be welcomed by the faith leaders. So it would be good to try to develop some kind of contact with them in advance. It would also be great if they could be invited to the further open community meeting, after these four new sessions, so that they can hear for themselves what participants think about attitudes of members of the faith communities towards people with HIV, and participants' suggestions for improving them.

PARTICIPANTS: Four separate peer groups.

SPECIAL INFORMATION

Don't forget to read 'Before you Begin ...!' before using this section of the manual.

INTRODUCTION

1. Sit in a circle with the group, preferably on the ground. Everyone should be at the same level, including yourself.

2. Welcome everyone to the new session. Thank everyone for coming. Enquire about late-comers or non-attenders.

3. Ask each participant to recount quickly something good which has happened to them since the last session.

4. Review the last session. Ask participants to remind us what we learnt then – thoughts about our healthcare services and what these mean for us. Remind them if they have forgotten.

5. Explain that we are going on to discuss other things in this session, but will start with a drawing exercise.

EXERCISE P.1: INTERCONNECTING CIRCLES

AIMS: To help participants to realise how we all belong to many different groups, each of which influence us, and this sometimes make us feel pulled in different directions.

DESCRIPTION: Drawing interconnecting circles in the sand, or on the ground, or on paper.

MATERIALS NEEDED: Chalk for a concrete floor, or a stick for sandy ground, and some flip-chart sheets, tape, scissors and marker pens, to record the drawings afterwards.

DIRECTIONS

1. Ask the peer group members to brainstorm some of the formal and informal groups which they belong to within and beyond their community.

2. After they have named a few – e.g. family members, friends, peers, others at school or who work with them, fellow clan members, fellow well-users, fellow church- or mosque-goers – say that we are going to see if we can represent all these different groups of people by **drawing them in circles** either on the ground, or on pieces of paper cut out with the scissors.

3. Remind participants of the exercise we did earlier on ideal images and personal destroyers, and how we get pulled in different directions by different people and groups in our lives. If you

are using a stick or a piece of chalk, start off by drawing a small circle, about the width of your outstretched hand, in the middle of the area. Then explain to the participants that this circle represents someone like one of them, as an individual person. Explain that we are not identifying or discussing one specific individual but that this circle represents someone like them, so they can draw the circles around this person based on their own experiences.

4. Then hand the chalk or stick over to one participant, so that they do the rest of the drawing. First of all, if most members of the group are already sexually active, they need to draw one (or more) circles which overlap with the original circle, each of which represents their current sexual partner. (For instance, in a men's peer group, a man may have several wives, or one wife and other sexual partners. In a women's group, a woman may have a husband and also have a boyfriend. Women may be reluctant to admit this but nobody has to own up to having a boyfriend – just gently encourage the group by asking whether some women in the community have more than one sexual partner at the same time. Remember to make sure, once more, that this isn't a judgment exercise!) Participants will also need to be reassured that this diagram will not be shown to other peer groups afterwards, unless they are happy for it to be.

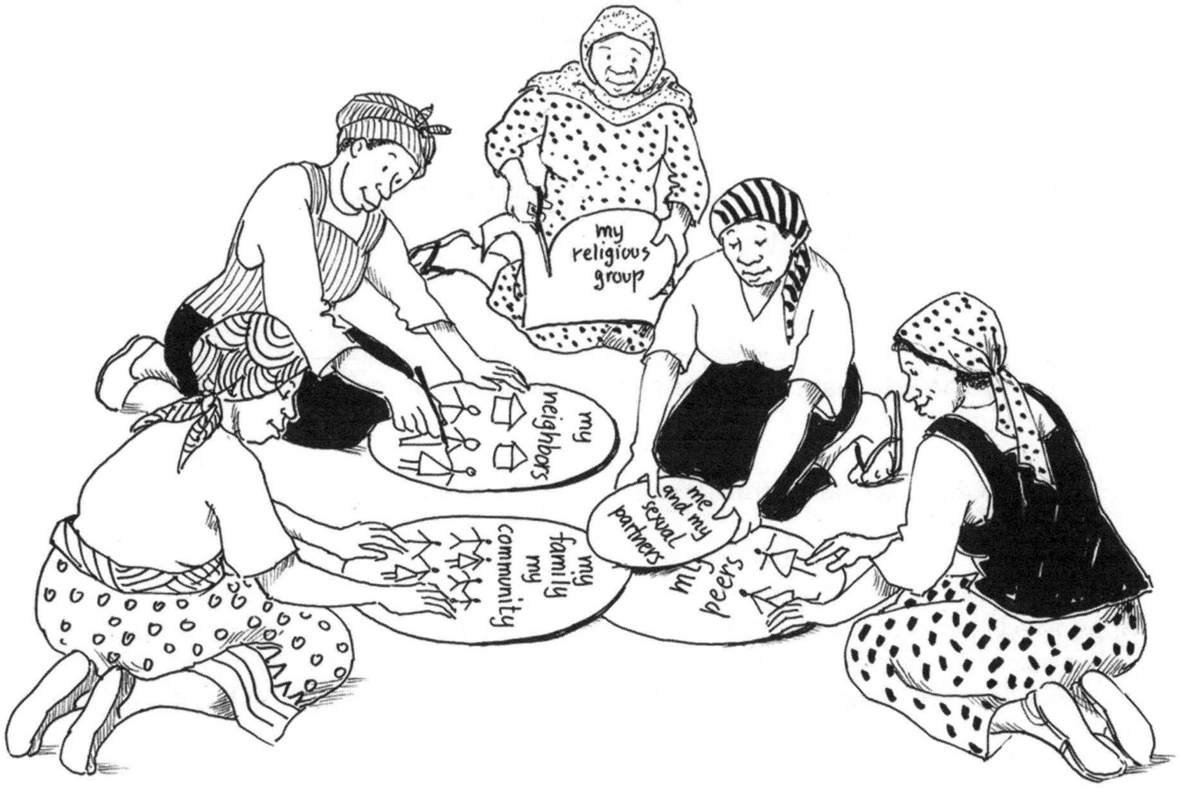

5. Encourage participants to think next about which of the groups to which they belong have the most influence on when and how they have sex. For groups with more influence, encourage them to draw (or cut out) bigger circles; for those with less influence, encourage them to draw (or cut out) smaller circles. All the circles should somehow relate to the original circle, and may also overlap with one another to a greater or lesser extent, depending on how connected or not they are to one another.

Please let your participants decide for themselves how their drawing looks. Don't tell them how big to make each circle, or where to put it, or what each circle should represent. For instance, some peer groups may want to add more circles of different sizes and in different positions. Please let them do this as they want.

6. If the participants have used flip-chart paper and marker pens, and have decided to cut out different sizes of circles with scissors, participants can overlap the full circles on top of each other (with the larger ones beneath the smaller ones) to show different strengths of influence.

7. Explain that this drawing exercise can help us to understand why we often feel torn in different directions by different influences in our lives that tell, force, or enable us to do or not do different things. (The female peer groups in particular may feel that they have very little control over who they have sex with, when, and whether or not they can practise safer sex.) In this session we are going to look at what we think of these influences, before we look at some of the key groups in our communities in turn. Ask the participants to make a copy on flip-chart paper of their final arrangement of circles and to keep this safely (Drawing 2).

EXERCISE P.2: BODY MAPS AND SPECIAL REQUESTS OF PEOPLE LIVING WITH HIV

AIM: To enable participants to understand better the experiences and wishes of people living with HIV.

DESCRIPTION: Analysis of drawings, followed by discussion.

MATERIALS NEEDED: On the following pages you will see two body maps and two special requests drawn by men and by women in OPAHA, a self-help support group of people living with HIV in Garissa, north-east Kenya. Before this exercise, please either ask men and women in your local support group of people living with HIV to draw similar body maps and special requests for themselves for you to use instead in this session; or photocopy the two body maps and special requests drawn here, and translate each comment into the language of the community with which you are working. Then make enough copies of both the body maps and the special requests for all members of your peer group to have a copy.

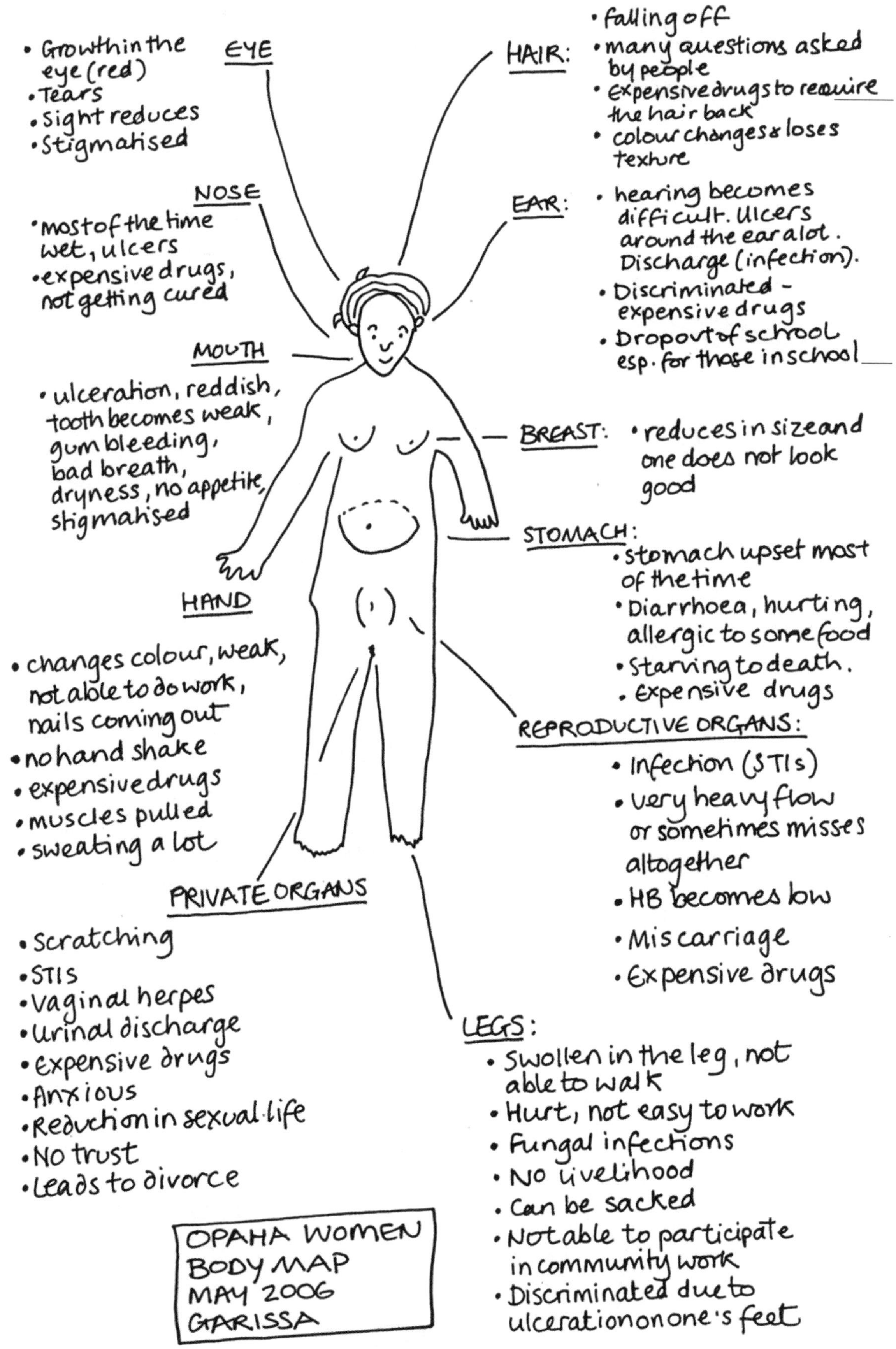
EYE
• Growth in the eye (red)
• Tears
• Sight reduces
• Stigmatised
NOSE
• Most of the time wet, ulcers
• expensive drugs, not getting cured
MOUTH
• ulceration, reddish, tooth becomes weak, gum bleeding, bad breath, dryness, no appetite, stigmatised
HAND
• changes colour, weak, not able to do work, nails coming out
• no hand shake
• expensive drugs
• muscles pulled
• sweating a lot
PRIVATE ORGANS
• Scratching
• STIs
• Vaginal herpes
• Urinal discharge
• Expensive drugs
• Anxious
• Reduction in sexual life
• No trust
• Leads to divorce
OPAHA WOMEN BODY MAP MAY 2006 GARISSA
HAIR:
• falling off
• many questions asked by people
• Expensive drugs to require the hair back
• colour changes & loses texture
EAR:
• hearing becomes difficult. Ulcers around the ear alot. Discharge (infection).
• Discriminated - expensive drugs
• Dropout of school esp. for those in school
BREAST:
• reduces in size and one does not look good
STOMACH:
• stomach upset most of the time
• Diarrhoea, hurting, allergic to some food
• Starving to death.
• Expensive drugs
REPRODUCTIVE ORGANS:
• Infection (STIs)
• very heavy flow or sometimes misses altogether
• HB becomes low
• Miscarriage
• Expensive drugs
LEGS:
• Swollen in the leg, not able to walk
• Hurt, not easy to work
• Fungal infections
• No livelihood
• Can be sacked
• Not able to participate in community work
• Discriminated due to ulceration on one's feet

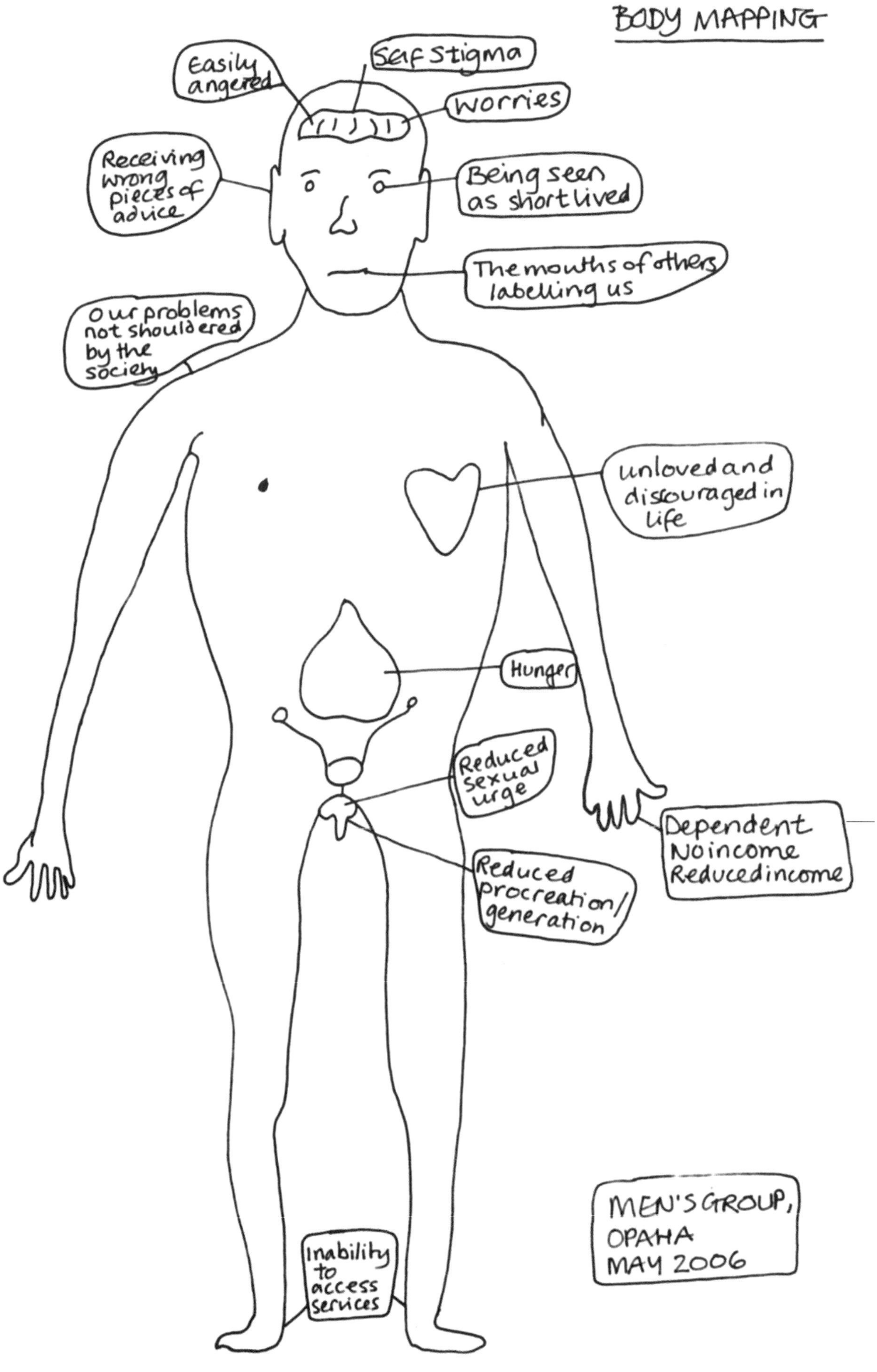
BODY MAPPING
Easily angered
Self Stigma
Worries
Receiving wrong pieces of advice
Being seen as short lived
The mouths of others labelling us
Our problems not shouldered by the society
unloved and discouraged in life
Hunger
Reduced sexual urge
Dependent
No income
Reduced income
Reduced procreation/generation
Inability to access services
MEN'S GROUP, OPAHA MAY 2006

SPECIAL REQUESTS

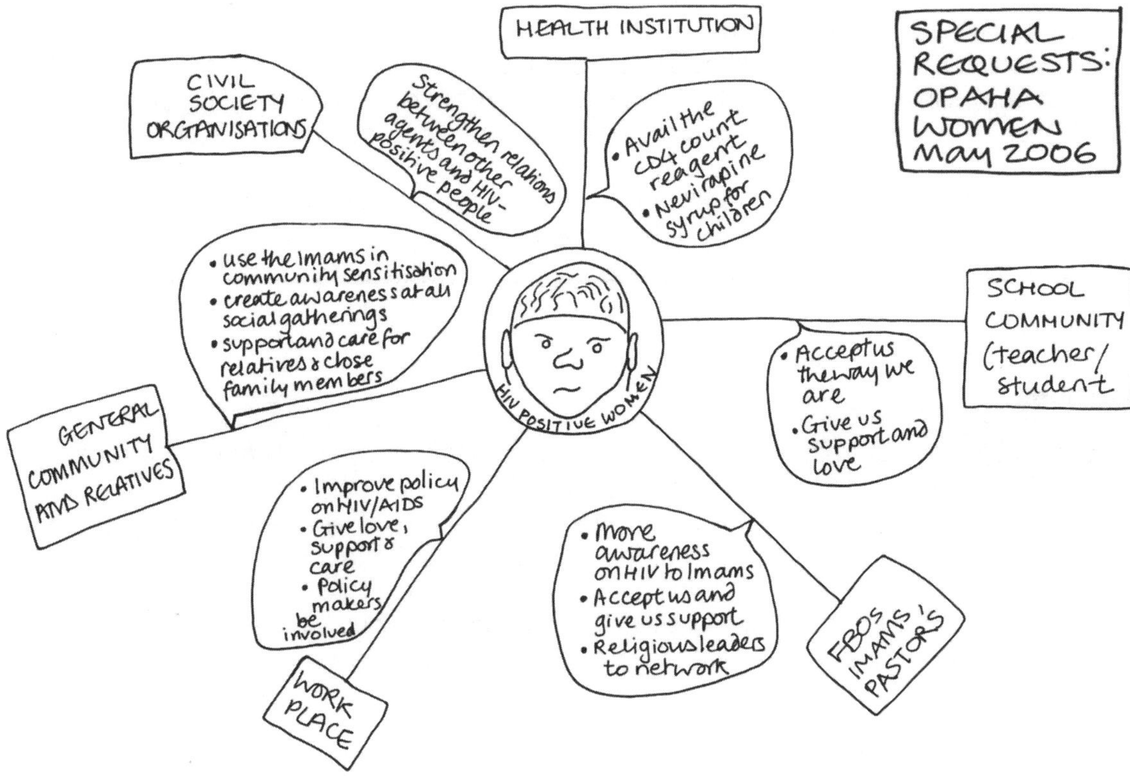

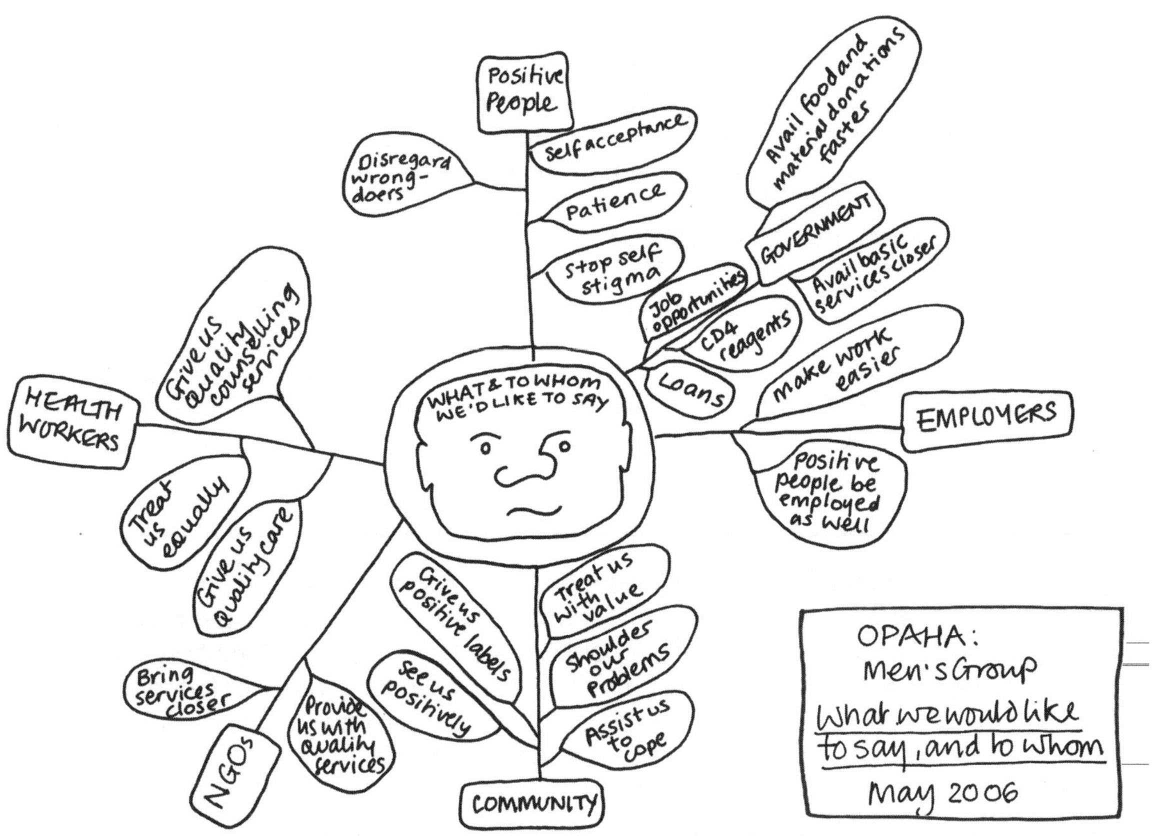

If your local HIV-support group is ready to do this exercise themselves, it would be better to use their drawings and comments than those here, because it would make the information more relevant to your community. They can do this by dividing into separate groups of men and of women (divided also by age if there are enough of them in the group), sticking together some flip-chart sheets and laying them on the ground. Then one group member lies on the ground while others draw around that person with the marker pens. The group then work together to write or draw whatever comments they feel like recording on the body outline, as you see illustrated above. Please note: once they have done this, it is important for them to follow this up with the special request exercise because the body map exercise by itself can feel too negative and distressing.

DIRECTIONS

1. Distribute copies of both the OPAHA body maps (or locally drawn body maps if you have them) to all the members of your peer group so that they can look at them for themselves. If someone from the local group of the same gender (and ideally similar age) is ready to come to present their drawings to your peer group, this would be even better.

2. Ask participants to look first at the body map drawn by the group whose members who are of the same gender as them. Ask what they see on this drawing which doesn't surprise them, and what they see that does surprise them.

3. Then ask participants to compare this body map with that drawn by people of the other gender. Ask participants if they can identify any similarities and any differences in what the two groups have mentioned on their body maps. Ask participants if they can think of any reasons for the differences they have identified.

4. Repeat this exercise with the two special request diagrams – again starting by showing participants the drawing made by the group whose members who are the same gender as they are. Ask what they see on this drawing which doesn't surprise them, and what they see that does surprise them. Then show them the other special request, and ask your participants to compare and contrast the two. Can they think why these might be different from each other?

5. Next, if you have used the OPAHA drawings rather than locally produced ones, ask participants how much they think the OPAHA drawings are likely to reflect the experiences and feelings of people living with HIV in their own community.

6. Finally, explain to participants that the next few exercises are going to look at different groupings within their community in turn, and how these groupings can influence a community's attitudes towards its members living with HIV.

NB: In this volume, we don't have room to look at the influence of more institutionalised groups, such as the workplace or the school, on people's sex lives. *Stepping Stones* has been adapted for both these settings by different organisations and, if you would like to find out more about this, do please contact us for further information. Here we are just going to focus on less structured groupings, including faith groupings, neighbours, and family. Please see the Introduction for more information about adaptation of these materials for other contexts.

EXERCISE P.3: WORKING WITH OUR FAITH LEADERS

AIM: To enable participants to explore attitudes in faith groups.

DESCRIPTION: Watching DVD, followed by role plays, feedback and discussion.

MATERIALS NEEDED: *What Can I Do* DVD[1], laptop with laptop with DVD player, projector, flip-chart paper and marker pens.

DIRECTIONS

1. Explain to participants that faith communities are an extremely important component of our societies. Some faith leaders, however, may believe that HIV is caused by widespread immorality in the world. Yet many faith leaders who have attended training workshops about HIV and AIDS have realised that the story is far more complex.

2. Ask participants to sit in a semi-circle so that they can watch a DVD clip of Canon Gideon Byamugisha talking about how HIV has affected him and what he has learnt about HIV through this. Ideally include what he has to say about attitudes to people living with HIV, and about sexual behaviour and condom use.

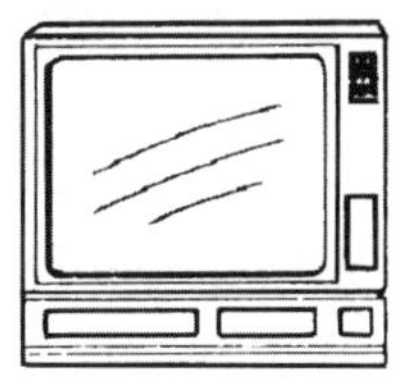

3. Ask participants what they have heard in the DVD clip.

4. Then ask participants what they have learnt from what they heard in the DVD clip.

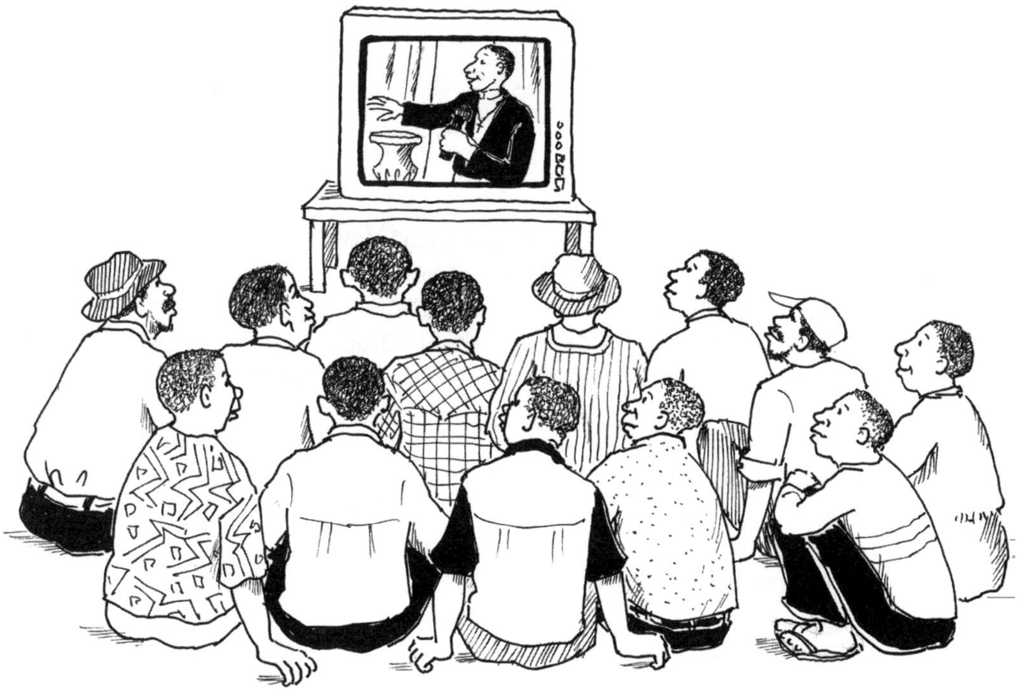

5. Ask the participants to divide into groups and role-play an example of negative attitudes in a faith setting (e.g. a leader in a faith community is prevented from leading faith services because he or she is thought to have HIV, or a faith community denies a couple living with HIV the right to get married or to use condoms).

6. Call the participants back to show their role plays to the rest of the peer group.

7. After each play has been acted out, ask the following questions:

- What was happening in each role play?
- What feelings did each person in the role play experience?
- What are the causes of such behaviours?
- Does this happen in our community?
- What effect does this have on HIV prevention, care, and support in our community?
- What can we do to help challenge negative effects?
- What have we learned?

8. **Action Points:** (Drawing 3) Ask the participants to select three or four of the ideas which they have identified to challenge stigma and promote the care, support, and full involvement of people living with HIV in faith communities and **draw these action points on some flip-chart paper**. Participants may feel nervous about actually criticising their own faith leader. Encourage them to think of ways of expressing things tactfully. You could remind participants that this issue of how to say critical things tactfully, for example using 'I' statements, was covered in Sessions K to L).

EXERCISE P.4: PROMOTING A SUPPORTIVE NETWORK AMONG NEIGHBOURS

AIM: For participants to consider how neighbours can affect attitudes in the community.

DESCRIPTION: Discussion, role play.

DIRECTIONS

1. Explain that we will share our experiences about how HIV and people with HIV are treated by people in communities. Ask for two volunteers to each describe one good and one bad experience which they have heard about attitudes to people living with HIV, or their friends or family members, in other communities. Probe by asking participants if they can identify the usual causes of these experiences and asking if we have also had similar experiences in our community.

2. Divide participants into small groups to do the following:

- Each group member shares one bad and good experience that s/he has had with a neighbour, or heard about in other communities.
- Each group chooses one of the bad experiences and discusses it in detail by answering these questions: What was the context? What was the cause? Who acted badly? What could have been the best possible behaviour?
- Discuss how families with people living with HIV are treated in our community today by neighbours, clan members, and other social groups (women, men, boys, girls). Note: we are not talking here about how faith leaders or health workers behave.
- Ask half the groups to come up with a role play about someone acting badly towards (i.e. stigmatising) a neighbour who has HIV, or talking badly about a him or her to another

neighbour, a friend, relative, faith leader, local leader, landlady/lord or boss. Ask the other small groups to develop a role play showing how people living with HIV and their families can be well supported by their neighbours.

NB: The person living with HIV and any other person or people being badly treated or being well treated should be a part in the role play.

3. Each group presents its role play to the bigger group, starting with the negative and then the positive role plays. The facilitator leads a discussion on the role plays by asking the following questions:

- What have we seen happening in the role plays (who was doing what)?
- Does this happen in our community?
- Why does the neighbour behave this way?
- What fears might the neighbour have about the family of the person living with HIV? And why?
- How does the family of the person with HIV feel about the neighbour's action?
- What is the effect of the neighbour's action on the person living with HIV, their family, and the wider community?
- What can we do to maximise positive neighbourly actions and relationships amongst us?

4. **Action Point:** (Drawing 4) Ask the participants to select three or four of the ideas which they have identified to challenge stigma and promote the care, support, and full involvement of people living with HIV amongst neighbours, and then discuss these ideas to see how they can start putting them into action. Participants could **draw a table** to identify these issues and come up with solutions.

The diagram can be drawn first on the ground or on flip-chart paper – it doesn't need writing. But it is good then to transfer the drawing to flip-chart paper, so that your participants can keep a record of what they have suggested, and can share these ideas with the other peer groups later.

PROMOTING A SUPPORTIVE NETWORK IN THE COMMUNITY				
What is the issue? e.g. picture of an issue	**Issue 1:** e.g. person living with HIV sick and needing care but no-one giving it	**Issue 2:** e.g. people gossiping and laughing behind the back of a person living with HIV	**Issue 3:** e.g. HIV+ children made to sit separately from other children at school	**Issue 4:** e.g. people refusing to buy food or other products from the person with HIV
What's the cause in the community?	A picture of the cause: e.g. people fearful of acquiring HIV through contact			
What are the **effects**?	A picture of the effects: e.g. a mother has to stop weeding fields, to look after sick person; whole household then faces starvation			

Possible solutions				
What we want to do **ourselves?**	Another picture: e.g. to request neighbours to help with care, weeding fields, fetching water and firewood, providing rest breaks for carer etc.			
What do we need?				
Available resources	Another picture: e.g. our own faces and voices, support from our husbands and young men (if this is the older women's group)			
Resources **needed** from outside our group or our community (there may be several)	More pictures: e.g. support from faith leaders, health staff, elders etc. to promote community-wide care			
How to obtain the resources we lack	Pictures showing e.g. community-wide meeting, meetings with faith leaders and health staff to request their public support for these ideas, etc.			
When to implement				
What changes expected and by **when**				

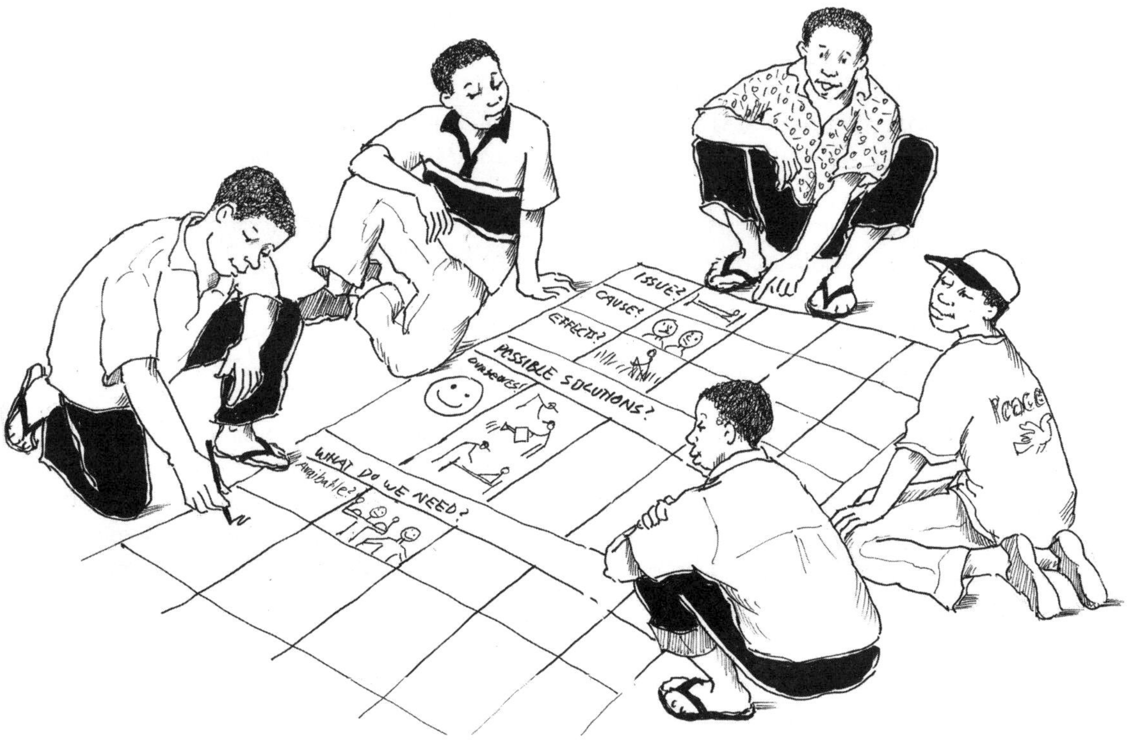

EXERCISE P.5: FOUR THINGS

AIM: **To help participants to realise that we can all do something to improve our response to HIV and to people with HIV, no matter who we are or what we do in life.**

DESCRIPTION: **Drawing action points on flip-chart paper.**

MATERIALS NEEDED: **Some flip-chart paper, tape and marker pens. One candle for each member of the group (including yourself) plus one extra, and a box of matches.**

DIRECTIONS

1. Ask participants to brainstorm things which they think they might be able to do to improve their own response to HIV and to people with HIV. First, they should think on their own for five minutes. Encourage them to think of a time frame for each action. Remember that some people in the group may already know themselves to be living with HIV, or have family members who are. Don't raise this as an issue right now, but do point out that people in the group may find this exercise quite painful if they already know people who are living with HIV. Encourage the whole group to support one another in this exercise. They should think in terms of:

- What can *I* do?
- What can *my immediate family* do?
- What can *my wider family* do?
- What can *one of the other groups I belong to* do?

2. Ask participants to chose a partner, if possible someone with whom they haven't yet worked, and share with that person as much or as little as they would like about the ideas they have just had in these four areas, including the time frame. Remember that some people may be feeling very emotional right now and might not want to share very much with someone else, so reassure everyone that they need to share only what they feel ready to share, and no more.

3. After 10 minutes, ask everyone to join the full circle to discuss the four questions which you have just asked. Explain that anyone can say just what they like.

4. Explain to all participants that change always has to begin with ourselves, and that we can never expect others to change unless we are willing to change ourselves first.

5. Distribute a candle to each member of the peer group, including yourself. Light one extra candle and place it in the middle of the circle. Explain that this candle is lit to represent all the people living with HIV in this community and those whom they love. Ask each peer group member in turn to lean forward and to light their own candle from the candle in the middle. Each participant – and you too – should then hold their lit candle in their hand. Ask for three minutes' silence to reflect on the lives of people we know around us with HIV, together with their families and friends.

6. Thank all participants for doing this exercise which may have been very difficult for some people.

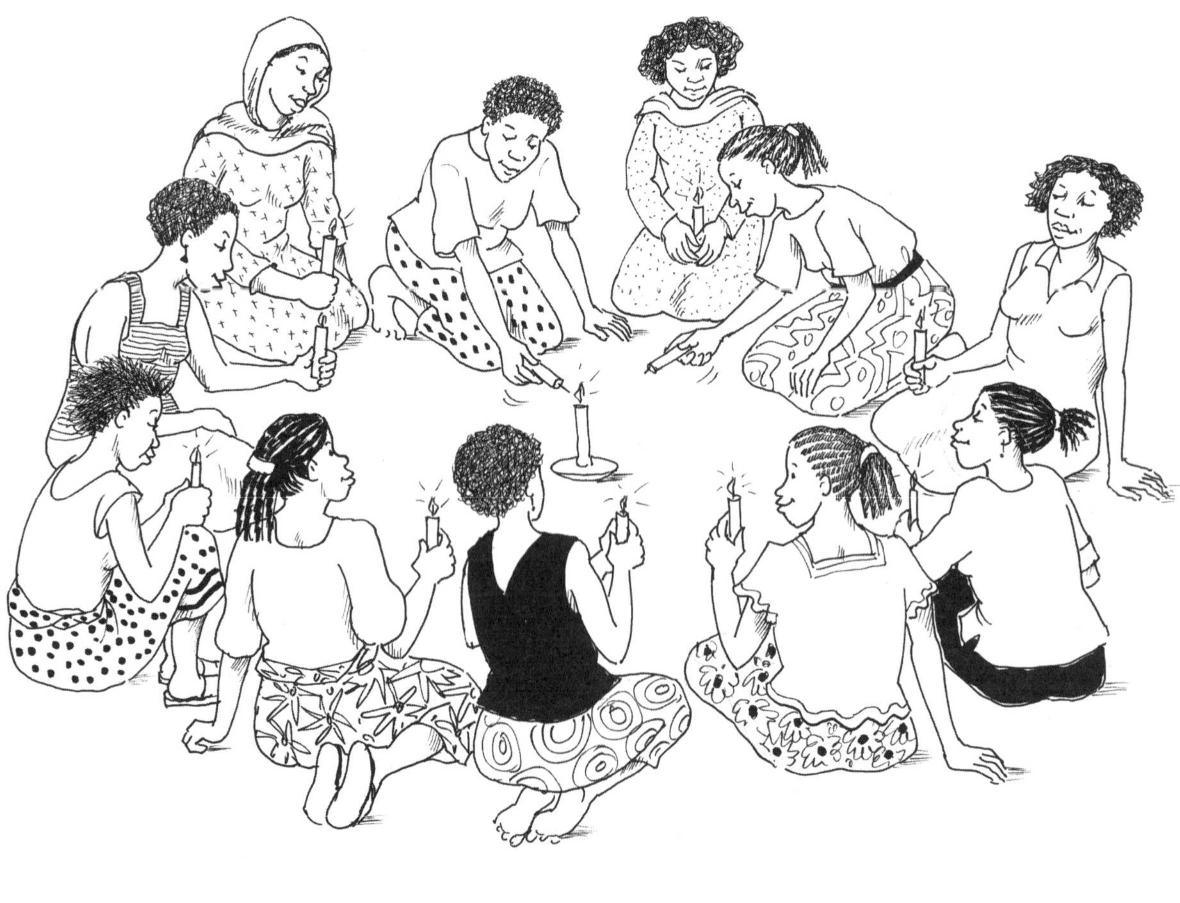

EXERCISE P.6: CLOSING CIRCLE – IF I WERE A BIRD

This is another fun energiser, to bring participants back to the present. Birds have many different characteristics, which can connect us to many of our dreams!

1. Ask each person in turn in the circle to say 'One thing I have learnt from today's session is ...' and 'If I were a bird, I would like to be a ... because it can ...'. Start with yourself.

2. This should be quite a quick game. Encourage participants not to spend too long on their choice.

3. As a going-home exercise, you could ask participants to reflect on their choice of bird, on the basis of what they have learnt at these sessions. Ask them to think at home about whether they would like to be another kind of bird instead of, or as well as, the one each of them has just chosen.

4. Finish off by thanking everyone once more for coming to this session. Remind everyone that the next time you meet there will be some more exercises. Encourage participants to talk in general about the kinds of issues they have been discussing in these sessions with their friends and neighbours, if they like, but not to share any confidential information with others.

5. Remind everyone of their role as guardian angel.

FACILITATORS' TEAM FEEDBACK

After the end of Session P, meet again with your co-facilitators, to compare notes on how your sessions went and the information which you learnt from them. Your co-facilitators could have found useful information that could help you to structure your next session more effectively. Remember, however, not to share individual confidentialities between groups. This is the easiest way to ruin the trust that you have begun to build and to wreck the whole workshop! The next meeting is the third optional session. Remember that this is for members of the four peer groups (meeting separately), and not for the general public.

ENDNOTE

1. Strategies for Hope (2006a)

REFERENCE

Strategies for Hope (2006a) *What can I do? Strategies for Hope*, [website and film], Strategies for Hope, <http://www.stratshope.org/resources/dvds_item/what-can-i-do> [accessed 11 December 2015].

YOUR NOTES...

SESSION Q SUPPORTING MOTHERS AND THEIR CHILDREN: OUR COMMUNITY'S FUTURE IN THEIR HANDS

PURPOSE

To promote understanding, respect and support for mothers and children in our communities.

CONTENTS	**TIME NEEDED**
Introduction	
Q.1	Spider's Web Revisited
Q.2	Our Memories from Childhood
Q.3	Supporting Our Mothers to Nourish their Children Safely
Q.4	The Voices of Orphans
Q.5	Closing Circle – One Thing I Remember

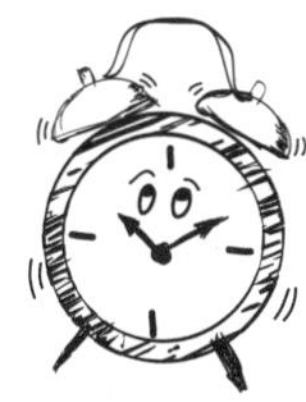

3–4 hours

MATERIALS NEEDED: A ball of string, flip-chart paper and marker pens, chalk (optional), '*Children First*!' DVD, laptop with DVD player, projector.

PARTICIPANTS: Four separate peer groups.

SPECIAL INFORMATION

Don't forget to read 'Before you Begin ...!' before using this section of the manual.

INTRODUCTION

1. Sit in a circle with the group, preferably on the ground. Everyone should be at the same level, including yourself.

2. Welcome everyone to the new session. Thank everyone for coming. Enquire about late-comers or non-attenders.

3. Ask each participant to recount quickly something good which has happened to them since the last session.

4. Review the last session. Ask participants to remind us what we learnt – thoughts about respect, care, and support for people with HIV. Remind them if they have forgotten.

5. Explain that we are going on to discuss other things in this session, but will start with a reflection.

EXERCISE Q.1: SPIDER'S WEB REVISITED

AIMS: Energiser. To remind everyone that they are each an important part of the group and of the wider community.

DESCRIPTION: A ball of string is unravelled and held taut by everyone, like a spider's web.

MATERIALS NEEDED: Ball of string.

DIRECTIONS

1. Make sure everyone is sitting in a circle. Produce a big ball of string. Ask participants if they can remember what this exercise was about last time you did it with them (Exercise G.1). Remind them that last time it was about how important each individual is to this group. Explain that this time we are going to do this exercise again, thinking about a wider network.

2. Hold on to the end of the string, then roll the ball across the ground to someone sitting opposite you, saying his/her name as you roll it to him/her. Keep holding on to your end, tightly.

3. Ask the recipient to hold on to the string so that it makes a taut line on the ground between you both. Then ask him/her to roll the ball back across the circle, along the ground, to someone else, saying that person's name as it rolls to him/her.

4. Everyone keeps on with this, until the circle is full of taut criss-crossing lines. Each person should be holding on tightly to a bit of string. The ball of string should finally be rolled back to you, so that you hold the beginning and the end of the string.

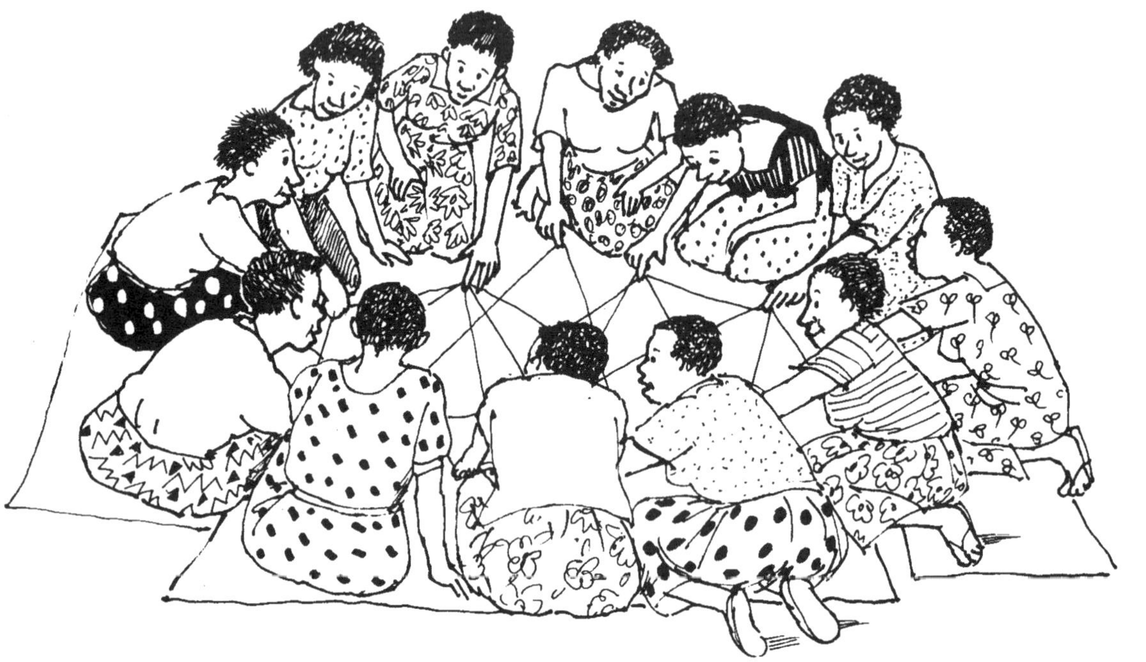

5. Next ask everyone to look at how the string connects you all, like a spider's web. Remind them what you learnt together last time – that you are all dependent on one another to keep this web firm and supported. If anyone were to take their hand away from the web, that part of it would collapse.

6. Ask people to suggest how this spider's web exercise relates to the lives and futures of our communities. Then ask who is the future in our communities. The answer to this that you are looking for is 'the children'. Encourage participants to go on answering until someone says this. Then ask who has most direct contact with our children in their earliest years? Who makes sure they are well and happy? The answer you are looking for here is 'their mothers'.

7. After a few comments, ask everyone to let go of the string. Gather it up in a loose pile so that it can be rewound later. Explain that in this session we are going to explore how we can best work together to support children and their mothers in this community, to ensure and secure the future of our community for all of us. Ask everyone to think about our dependence on one another – and our need to support one another – during the course of today's session.

EXERCISE Q.2: OUR MEMORIES FROM CHILDHOOD

AIM: To remind participants of memories from their childhoods.

DESCRIPTION: The facilitator asks each participant to remember one sad and one happy time in their childhood and share them, if they like, with the rest of the group.

MATERIALS NEEDED: Flip-chart paper and marker pens, chalk (optional).

NB: This exercise may look simple but it can raise deep emotions in participants, particularly if they had a difficult childhood — or if they had a happy childhood but now have a difficult adulthood.

DIRECTIONS

1. Ask each participant to reflect quietly by him – or herself for five minutes about two events which they remember from their childhood — one event that made them feel sad, and one event that made them feel happy. Explain that you would then like to ask them to share these two events with the rest of the group, but that they don't have to share if they don't want to.

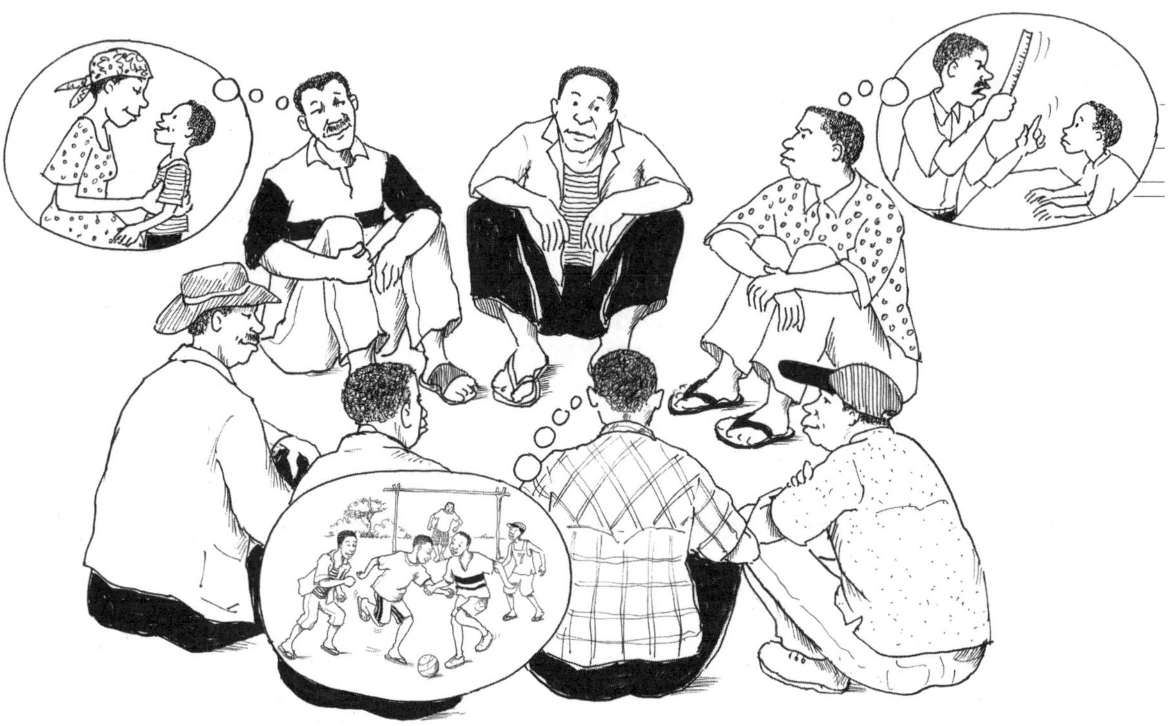

2. After five minutes are up, ask who would like to tell their two memories to the rest of the group. Ask each participant to start with their sad memory and then to tell their happy memory.

3. When all participants who have felt ready to share their memories have done so, thank them for doing so.

NB: The next two questions encourage participants to think about the roles of other people – such as parents, grandparents, aunts, uncles, and older siblings – in their lives which may have affected how they felt as children.

4. Ask everyone whether they have noticed any common themes about the sad memories which have been shared – for instance, children not feeling respected, feeling excluded, feeling lonely, feeling bullied, feeling hungry, being hit or abused in other ways, feeling frightened and confused. Also, ask them how these sad events made them behave afterwards?

5. Then ask everyone whether they have noticed any common themes about the good memories which have been shared – for instance, children feeling valued, respected, wanted, welcomed, included, loved, cared for, having a loving mother who is happy with her own life and well, having a loving father who is happy with his life and well? How did these happy events make them behave afterwards?

6. Ask participants what they think this exercise may help them to appreciate about the children in the community now, and how they might like to change the way in which children are treated in this community.

7. Suggest that **participants might like to draw some action points** (Drawing 5), showing how the way children are treated in the community might be changed, in the light of their discussions.

EXERCISE Q.3: SUPPORTING OUR MOTHERS TO NOURISH THEIR CHILDREN SAFELY

Now that ARV medication is available, if a woman with HIV is stable on medication with an undetectable viral load after her baby is born, she can breastfeed her baby with almost no danger of passing HIV to the baby through the breast milk. This is providing she **continues with the ARVs** while breastfeeding. For the latest information on this in your country, please contact your Ministry of Health. Alternatively, please check the WHO website.[1,2] If a woman is in any doubt, she should follow earlier WHO recommendations, from before ARVs were available, to ***only*** breastfeed for the **first six months** and then immediately change to other foods. Alternatively, a woman can use a bottle with formula milk to feed her baby and not breastfeed at all. However, it is important to ensure that all the equipment is kept clean at all times and that she only uses boiled water to prepare the formula milk. Sometimes this can be very difficult for a woman, especially if she has limited access to firewood or clean drinking water.

HOW CAN COMMUNITY MEMBERS HELP WOMEN IN THIS SITUATION?

During this exercise, please do make it clear that both breastfed and formula-fed babies can grow really well. If participants are worried about lack of bonding with a baby who is bottle-fed, explain that a baby can still be held closely and cuddled a lot, with good eye contact, whilst being bottle-fed. If bottle-feeding is done correctly, babies fed on formula milk can still make good developmental progress, just like a breastfed baby. This information may be especially helpful if women would prefer to formula-feed their babies.

AIMS: For participants to raise questions and learn facts about infant feeding among women living with HIV who are mothers.

DESCRIPTION: Group discussion and feedback.

DIRECTIONS

1. Start off by saying that we are now going to look at the care of children from when they are first born. Ask participants what the best way to support infants is. The answer you are looking for is to **keep their parents alive**, physically well, and psychologically supported. This is what the previous exercises in this session have been about. Go on prompting participants with 'how' or 'why' questions until someone suggests this. If people are focusing more on details of infant care here, you may need to prompt them by saying 'yes, but what comes before that?' each time, until they get to this.

2. Then explain that this exercise is now going to look at the particular issues facing mothers as they try to keep their newborn infants well-nourished and well cared-for.

3. Remind the group that in Session O, we discussed concerns that we have about perinatal care services. We now want to discuss infant feeding in the context of HIV.

4. Ask the group members:

- What are some of the issues that women who are pregnant face in this community today?
- What are some of the beliefs and practices about breastfeeding in our community?
- What concerns do couples living with HIV have about feeding the newborn baby?
- What are the views of family and community members about a woman who does not breastfeed her baby?
- What problems is a child whose mother has HIV and who is not being breastfed likely to face?
- What problems is a child whose mother has HIV and who is being breastfed likely to face?

5. Explain the facts about breastfeeding, both the advantages and disadvantages, in relation to HIV. (Refer to the table in Exercise O.2.) Give additional information from the QQR Fact Sheet.

6. Ask participants what practical steps they think this community might take to support women to feed their infants as safely as possible. If you have time, it would also be good to talk about the types of food that are available in your community and are good for weaning children.[3]

7. **Action point:** (Drawing 6) Suggest that participants draw these steps on a piece of flip-chart paper.

EXERCISE Q.4: THE VOICES OF ORPHANS

AIMS: To consider and take action to improve the situation of children who are vulnerable to HIV and/or orphaned by AIDS.

DESCRIPTION: Watching DVD, followed by discussion.

MATERIALS NEEDED: ***'Children First!'*** **DVD, laptop with DVD player, projector. Flip-chart paper, marker pens.**

DIRECTIONS

1. Watch the *Children First!* DVD with participants. Then ask them what they thought about it and what struck them most about what orphaned and vulnerable children need. (Expected responses: food, care, medicine, love, shelter, protection, education, information.) What do you think such children now have which they didn't have previously? (Their parents? Love? Respect? Trust? Openness?) If participants find it hard to answer these questions, watch the DVD again with them, so that they can listen carefully for the answers.

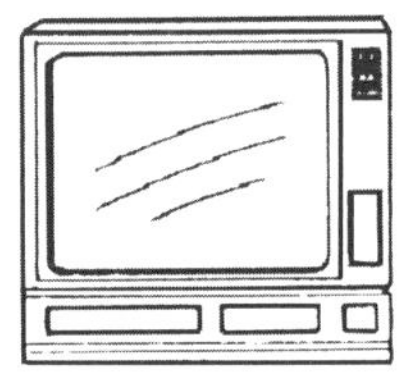

2. Next sit with the participants in a circle. Ask: 'Are there orphans in this community?'

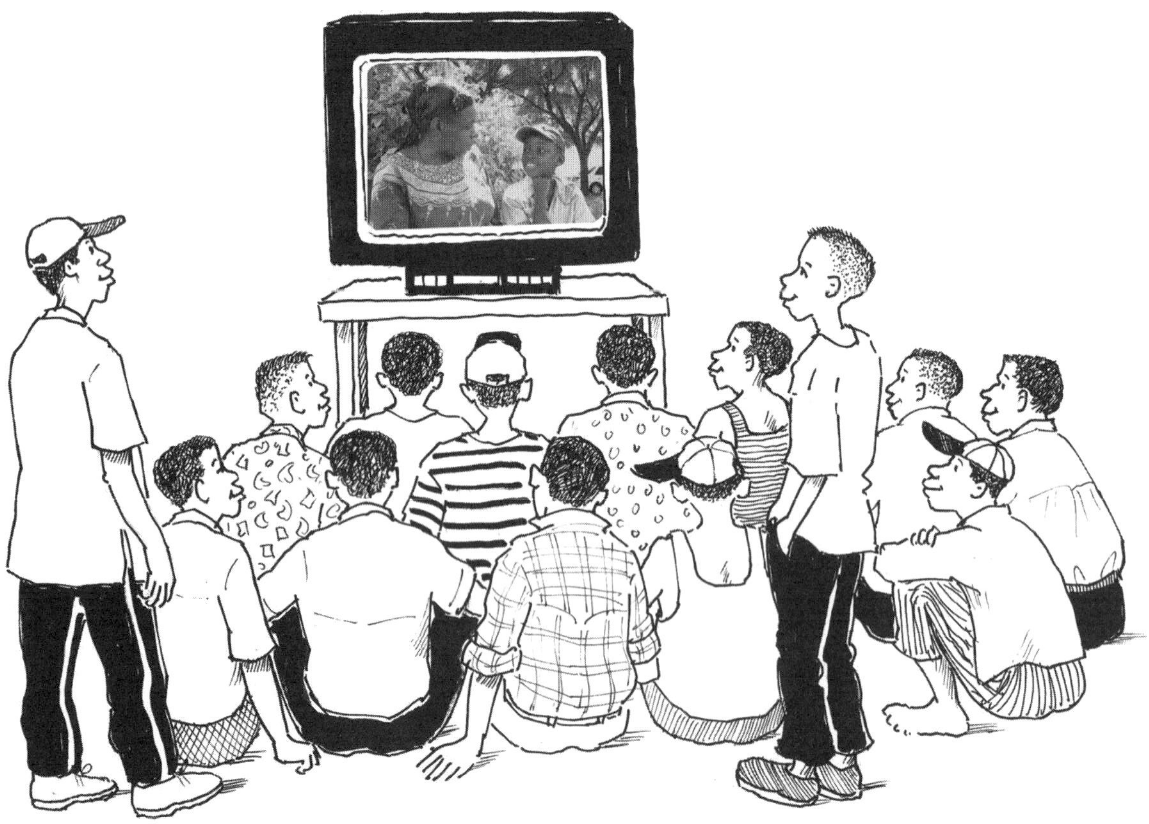

- How is an orphan defined by this community? (A child without a father? A child without a mother? A child without both parents? Different communities may define an orphan in different ways.)
- What is the estimated number of orphans in this community?
- What are some of the causes of orphanhood in this community?

3. Explain that, because children are especially vulnerable to negative attitudes from others, we are going to look into their situation.

In small groups, discuss the following:

- What are the critical problems that children face in our community today?
- How are children whose parents are bedridden, and children from poor families, treated in our community today?
- Do boys or girls face particular or different issues that we also need to think about?
- When children are orphaned, what extra issues do they face? (Again, are there different issues facing boy orphans and girl orphans?)
- Why are they treated like this?
- Should the orphans and vulnerable children be treated this way?

4. Back in the big circle, ask the groups to present the outcome of their discussions. Identify and try to resolve areas where opinions may differ by asking the following questions about points mentioned by each group:

- Do we all see it that way?
- Does it happen that way?
- Do we all agree with that?

Point out that:

- Children are the future ambassadors of our community and they need proper care, preparation, and up-bringing.
- Children have a right to life, to social care and healthcare, to education, and to parental, family, and community love.
- Children may often be blamed for their parents' illnesses and death. Is this fair on them – or on their parents?
- If there is HIV in their family, the children may be excluded from school and family life because of fear of the virus. Is this reasonable, given our knowledge about how HIV is – and isn't – transferred?
- Orphans are often treated differently from other children in families and are often accused of carrying on their parents' 'bad behaviour'. Is this fair?
- Street children are seen as dirty and out of control although many are on the streets because their parents have separated, or have died from AIDS-related illnesses, which means they must survive on their own.
- Explain that children who have little support when they are growing up often have few skills or resources to become good parents, and so cycles of neglect and deprivation continue. How could communities break these cycles?
- Emphasise that all children, especially orphans and those affected by HIV and AIDS, need love, care, and support from those around them.

5. Ask the participants to find out what the law says about the rights of children. Children are the responsibility of adults, families, and communities, so ask the participants to come up with a concrete plan for improving the situation of children in their community.

6. **Action point:** (Drawing 7) Help the participants to draw the issue analysis and planning chart below, to fill in with pictures. The diagram can be drawn first on the ground or on flip chart paper – it doesn't need writing. But it is good to transfer the completed drawing to flip-chart paper, so that your participants can keep a record of what they have suggested and can share these ideas with the other peer groups later.

IMPROVING THE SITUATION OF VULNERABLE CHILDREN				
What is the issue? e.g. picture of an issue	**Issue 1:** e.g. child bullied at school	**Issue 2:** e.g. girl having to leave school to look after sick family members	**Issue 3:** e.g. orphan treated badly by aunt	**Issue 4:** e.g.orphan having to sell sex to feed younger siblings
What's the cause in the community?	A picture of the cause: e.g. other children don't understand enough about how HIV can affect everyone			
What are the **effects?**	Another picture: e.g. child crying, refusing school, bad marks from teachers			
Possible solutions?				
What we want to do **ourselves?**	Another picture to request e.g. more education for all children about HIV from their parents, older siblings			
What do we need?				
Available resources	Another picture: e.g. our own faces and voices; support from our husbands, from young men …			
Resources **needed** from outside our group or our community (there may be several)	Another picture: e.g. support from teachers to notice and ban bullying; support from faith leaders, health staff, elders etc.			
How to obtain the resources we lack				
When to implement				
What changes expected and by **when**				

7. Explain that the next exercise is to bring the session to a close but that if participants would like to discuss more about caring for vulnerable children in this community, there is another training programme like this one, called *Stepping Stones with Children* that they might like to consider.[4]

EXERCISE Q.5: CLOSING CIRCLE – ONE THING I REMEMBER

This is another fun energiser, to bring participants back to the present.

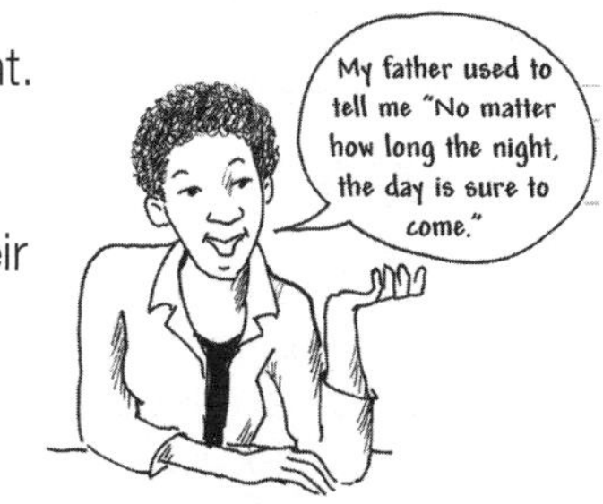
My father used to tell me "No matter how long the night, the day is sure to come."

1. Ask participants to divide into pairs and think of a particular song, rhyme, story, game or proverb which they like and associate with their childhood in this community, remember hearing, saying, singing or playing, or one good thing that their mother or father used to say to them when they were young.

2. After five minutes, ask each person in turn in the circle to say 'I remember from my childhood that we used to ...', followed by 'and one thing I have learnt from today's session is ...'. Start with yourself.

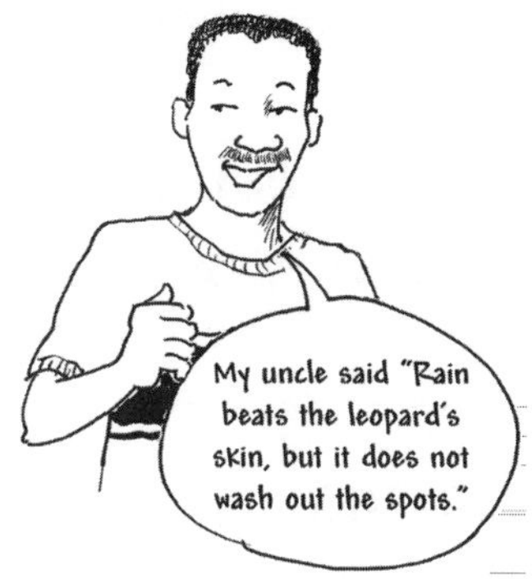
My uncle said "Rain beats the leopard's skin, but it does not wash out the spots."

This should be quite a quick game. Encourage participants not to spend too long on their choice.

3. As a going-home exercise, you could ask participants to reflect on their memories on the basis of what they have learnt at these sessions. Ask them to think at home about whether they would like these old songs, stories, games or proverbs to be heard again in this community, and what they could do to help bring them back for the young people in their community today. For instance, are there some young children in their household with whom they could play an old game or to whom they could tell an old story?

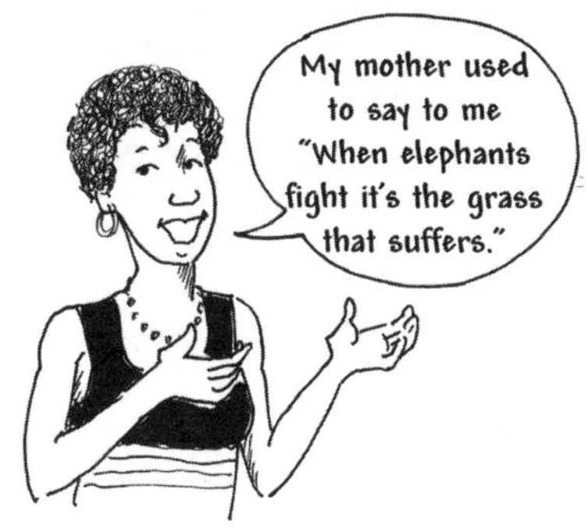
My mother used to say to me "When elephants fight it's the grass that suffers."

4. Finish off by thanking everyone once more for coming to this session. Remind everyone that the next time you meet there will be some more exercises.

Encourage participants to talk in general about the kinds of issues they have been discussing in the session with their friends and neighbours, if they like, but not to share any confidential information with others.

5. Remind everyone of their role as guardian angel.

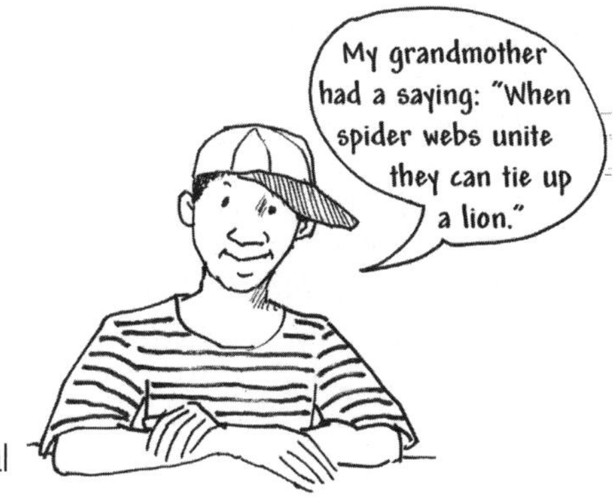
My grandmother had a saying: "When spider webs unite they can tie up a lion."

6. Explain to participants that in the next session, Session R, there will be an election. Three representatives of each peer group will work together for a year on an action planning committee in the community, to take forward all the suggestions from these workshops. Ask everyone to think about whether they would like to be considered or not. Also encourage members to encourage others in their group to put themselves forward for election.

7. Ask all the peer group members who acted in the special request role play at the end of the original *Stepping Stones* workshop (second open community meeting), to meet together in their own time, and re-rehearse their special request for the next session. Explain that there will soon be a further open community meeting, where community members can once more learn what these

sessions have been about. The idea is that all community members will also have another chance to see the special request role play of each peer group, and that it will enable the action planning committee to be set up.

8. Finally, remember to ask for three volunteers to stay behind for ten minutes for a quick review of this session. (See Annex 4 for details.) Make sure that everyone has agreed a mutually convenient time and place for your next session, before saying goodbye.

FACILITATORS' TEAM FEEDBACK

After the end of Session Q, meet again with your co-facilitators, to compare notes on how your sessions went and the information which you learnt from them. Your co-facilitators could have found useful information that could help you to structure your next session more effectively. Remember, however, not to share individual confidentialities between groups. This is the easiest way to ruin the trust that you have begun to build and to wreck the whole workshop! The next meeting is the fourth optional session. Remember that this is for members of the four peer groups, meeting separately, and not for the general public.

SPECIAL INSTRUCTIONS

Please follow the instructions in the box on page 276 before you run Session R.

ENDNOTES

1. In July 2015, WHO stated: 'Antiretroviral drugs now allow these children [of women with HIV] to exclusively breastfeed until they are 6 months old and continue breastfeeding until at least 12 months of age with a significantly reduced risk of HIV transmission.' (2015b). For more information on breastfeeding studies and recommendations see Doherty et al. (2010).
2. See also WHO (2010)
3. See WHO guidelines on infant feeding in the context of HIV for more details.
4. For more information on caring for vulnerable children in the community, see our accompanying new training programme, *Stepping Stones with Children*

REFERENCES

Doherty, T., Sanders, D., Goga, A. and Jackson, D. (2010). Implications of the new WHO guidelines on HIV and infant feeding for child survival in South Africa. Bulletin of the World Health Organization, 89(1), pp.62-67.

Gordon G., with Chiziza N., Holden S, Kilonzo F, Manyama W, McAdam E, Kiwia P, and Welbourn A. (2016) *Stepping Stones with Children* Practical Action, Rugby

WHO (2015b) Infant and young child feeding Fact sheet No. 342. July. WHO. Geneva. http://www.who.int/mediacentre/factsheets/fs342/en/ [accessed 7 November 2015].

WHO 2010 Guidelines on HIV and infant feeding Principles and recommendations for infant feeding in the context of HIV and a summary of evidence http://apps.who.int/iris/bitstream/10665/44345/1/9789241599535_eng.pdf [accessed 24 January 2016].

WHO (2010) *Breast is always best* [webpage] WHO, Geneva, <http://www.who.int/bulletin/volumes/88/1/10-030110/en/> [accessed 16 November 2015].

YOUR NOTES ...

SESSION R ACCEPTING HIV WITHIN THE FAMILY: SUPPORTING FAMILY MEMBERS WHO ARE LIVING WITH HIV

PURPOSE

To address and overcome negative and challenging issues around HIV facing people in their own families and relationships.

CONTENTS	TIME NEEDED
Introduction	
R.1	Sharing Information with Sexual Partners: Challenges and Possibilities
R.2	Sharing Information with Wider Family Members: Challenges and Possibilities
R.3	Looking After Yourself if You are HIV Positive: Challenges and Possibilities
R.4	Review of all Drawings from Sessions O–R and Preparation for the Further Open Community Meeting.
R.5	Closing Circle

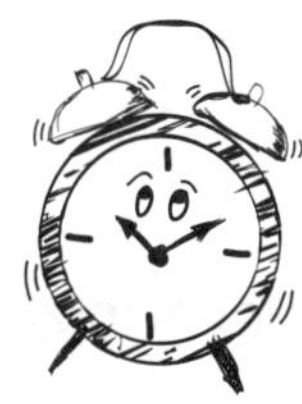

3-4 hours

MATERIALS NEEDED: Flip-chart paper and marker pens, chalk (optional).

PARTICIPANTS: Four separate peer groups.

SPECIAL INFORMATION

Don't forget to read 'Before you Begin …!' before using this section of the manual.

> It would be great if you were able to enlist the help of four older and younger men and women who are living with HIV (one for each of your four peer groups) from a local HIV-support group, or from the community itself, for Exercise R.3 so that they could talk to the peer groups about their experiences of living positively.

INTRODUCTION

1. Sit in a circle with the group, preferably on the ground. Everyone should be at the same level, including yourself.

2. Welcome everyone to the new session. Thank everyone for coming. Enquire about latecomers or non-attenders.

3. Ask each participant to recount quickly something good which has happened to them since the last session.

4. Review the last session. Ask participants to remind us what we learnt then – thoughts about childhood and what it means to us. Remind them if they have forgotten.

5. Explain that we are going on to discuss other things in this session.

EXERCISE R.1: SHARING INFORMATION WITH SEXUAL PARTNERS: CHALLENGES AND POSITIVE POSSIBILITIES

AIMS: To help participants consider and take action to improve communication with their own sexual partners and relatives.

DESCRIPTION: Group discussion.

MATERIALS NEEDED: Flip-chart and marker pens, or chalk.

DIRECTIONS

1. Explain to participants that we have been addressing ways of improving attitudes towards people with HIV and their families amongst health workers, within faith communities, and in the community in general. But often the hardest places for a person living with HIV to be open about their status are in their relationships with their own intimate sexual partner[1] or partners and family members. Ask participants to brainstorm a few ideas about why they might think that this is so, thinking first of all about sexual partners. They should start by thinking about why it is difficult for people of their own gender, and then for men if they are women or women if they are men.

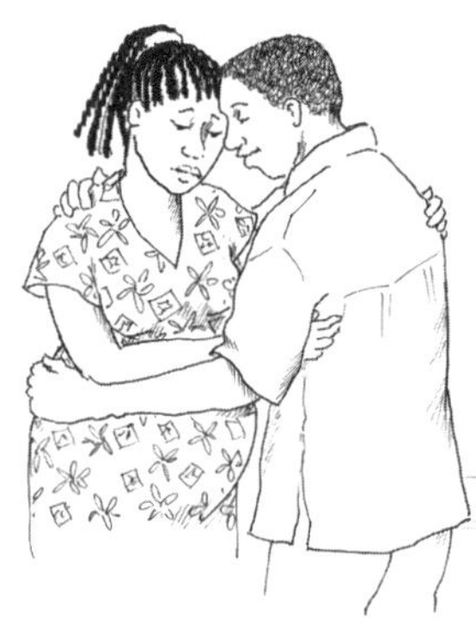

Below are some of the suggestions which participants might make – if they don't, it would be good if you could raise them yourself. They may also make other suggestions, which can be added to this list. If they would like to, participants can draw these suggestions on flip-chart paper with marker pens, or with chalk on a concrete floor, or with a stick on the mud or sandy ground.

For women and girls living with HIV

Some women are given love, care, and support by their partners, who realise that they need all these things and more on the news of their diagnosis. However:

- If you are a woman you might be blamed, beaten up, thrown out of the house, or/and divorced by your partner and you may also lose your older children.
- If you are pregnant, a positive diagnosis can be a disaster for you, for your older children, and for your unborn baby.
- Your in-laws may also blame you and reject you.
- If you are thrown out of your partner's house, your own parents may also refuse to let you go back to their house.
- You may want to have a child so that you can both be a mother and be respected as one.
- You may have had a sugar daddy when you were younger and you may have acquired HIV from him without realising.
- If you are a girl living with HIV, you may have acquired HIV at birth or through child rape. But your partner might accuse you of having loose morals just because you are living with HIV. Also, your partner may reject you as a girlfriend or wife if he knows you are living with HIV.

For men and boys who are living with HIV

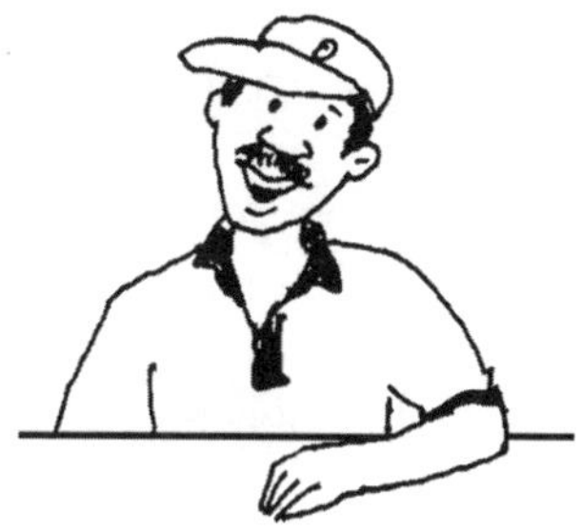

Some men are given love, care, and support by their partners, who realise that they need all these things and more on the news of their diagnosis. However:

- If you are a man, your partner may accuse you of having had sex with other women.
- You may fear that your wife will tell everyone else about your having HIV.
- You may fear losing respect from your wife and others whom she tells.
- You may fear that your wife will now want to use condoms when you have sex with her.
- You may want to have a child and both be a father and be respected as one.
- If you are a boy or man living with HIV, you may have acquired HIV at birth or through child rape. But your partner might accuse you of having loose morals just because you are living with HIV. Also, your partner may reject you as a boyfriend or husband if she knows you are living with HIV.

2. Ask participants, bearing in mind everything they have learnt during this workshop, how fair or unfair, real or unreal, each fear listed above might actually be in this community. Go through each fear that they have listed in turn, and ask participants what they have learnt about this issue in this workshop. It might also help to ask participants: 'What difference do blame, anger and violence make? Are they going to help or cure anyone?'

3. Next ask participants to describe the kind of person who gets HIV in their community.

 By now, the participants should really be very clear that people with HIV are people just like themselves — and indeed could well be any of us. If for any reason, participants go back to the same old stories of people with HIV being sex workers, drug users, homosexuals, truck drivers, foreigners, etc., remind them of all the different exercises that they have done about this throughout the workshop, such as 'Miming the Lie', 'Fixed Positions', 'Who's Labelling Whom', Exploring Why', and 'What Happened Next'. If anyone goes on questioning this, it may be necessary to ask participants gently why they still feel they need to resist the possibility that all these exercises may have no relevance to our own lives, and those of our relatives. Don't get cross with anyone, but it would probably help to encourage those in the group who feel more open to accepting the reality that HIV can affect us all to support you – and to support the group members who are still finding this idea difficult. This should mean that you are doing as little of the talking as possible, and just guiding the discussion.

4. Next, ask participants whether they think someone with HIV goes out of their way to catch HIV and to spread it to others or not.

☞ Again, by now, it would be good if participants feel confident that the great majority of people do NOT intend to get HIV – OR to pass HIV on to others. It would be great if participants were able to say clearly that the reality is that we all tend to live our lives in denial: imagining, hoping, and trusting that such a thing could not happen to us. Point out also that the way in which many of the public health messages have been created only serves to reassure us that HIV could not possibly happen to us or to our families. For instance, many public health messages have focused on people who, they suggest, are in some way to blame for getting HIV through their supposedly 'immoral' lifestyles, rather than focusing on the reality that HIV can and does affect many people from all walks of life, no matter who they are.

Indeed, in societies around the world, it is the culture of silence and taboos related to talking about sex, gender inequalities, violence, and death, along with the ability of those in power to ensure these silences are maintained, which have been the prime causes of HIV spreading across the globe.

What is more, it would be great if participants realised by now that anyone who feels and looks healthy may also have HIV without realising it. When I (Alice, the author of *Stepping Stones*) was diagnosed in 1992, I had no idea at all that I have HIV. I was fit and healthy. Even when, eight years later, in 2000, my CD4 count had fallen to 170, and I needed to start taking antiretroviral therapy, I was easily able to swim 1.5 kilometres for charity. Just because you feel well, it doesn't mean that you don't have HIV.

5. Explain to participants that in the next part of this exercise you would like them to make suggestions about the possible benefits of sharing their HIV status with their sexual partner(s).

☞ Participants may still find this very difficult but encourage them to draw again on what they have been learning together. If they are living with HIV, they could work with their sexual partner(s) to plan for the future of themselves and their children (if they have or want them), to provide emotional support to one another when they feel depressed or overwhelmed, to seek treatment, and so on. Keeping a secret can be a huge burden, both emotionally and physically. It may mean, for instance, feeling guilty about exposing one's partner to HIV or other STIs, having to hide medicines, spending money going off to the city to see a doctor and be treated … Not having to keep any of that secret can be a huge relief. Furthermore, working together to support one another can help everyone to learn from what has happened.

But all this involves a willingness on the part of a sexual partner to appreciate the courage of the person who is telling him or her about their status. If one partner is not prepared to thank the other and to be supportive about being told this news, then people living with HIV are going to go on being afraid to tell their partners. What do your participants feel about this?

6. Finally, ask participants how they think they might be able to support their friends or family members who are living with HIV, or who they think might have HIV, to share this information with their sexual partners in ways which produce responses which are caring, supportive, and respectful – *not* blaming or critical.

You or one of your group may think that one of your friends has HIV, but you fear that she or he may be 'in denial' and afraid to tell their partner. How do you think you could sensitively support them to accept their own HIV status, and to be more open about it, without worsening their fears, their sense of isolation, or their treatment by others?

7. Ask participants **to draw some of the benefits of sharing information about having HIV** on the ground with chalk first, if they like. Eventually they will need to draw them on flip-chart paper with marker pens (Drawing 8).

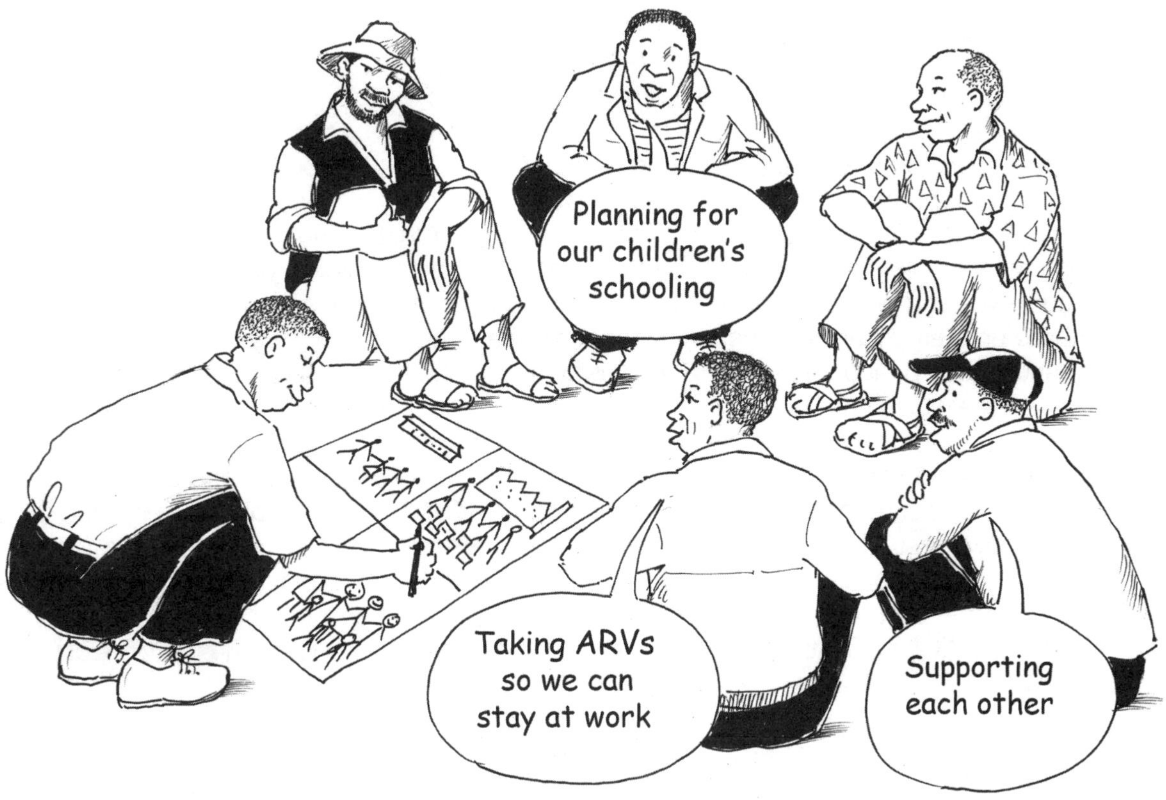
Planning for our children's schooling
Taking ARVs so we can stay at work
Supporting each other

EXERCISE R.2: SHARING INFORMATION WITH WIDER FAMILY MEMBERS: CHALLENGES AND POSITIVE POSSIBILITIES

AIMS: For participants to consider and take action to improve communications with their family members.

DESCRIPTION: Group discussion.

MATERIALS NEEDED: Flip-chart and marker pens, chalk (optional).

If a woman tests positive for HIV there is a strong possibility that any children she already has could also have contracted HIV. Testing of these children is ideally recommended to ensure that they are kept well, especially the under-fives. However, this raises huge issues for their mother — grief, self-blame, and guilt, as well as unjust condemnation from other family members. Similarly, if a woman tests positive for HIV, and her partner hasn't yet had a test, this result can raise feelings like these in him, even though outwardly he may blame and punish her. The shock of discovering that there is HIV in the family can be immense and can create violent responses. Often it is impossible to find out who first contracted the virus and who passed it to whom (although there is widespread documentation of the high risk of young women contracting HIV when they have sex with older, sexually experienced men). But in the end, is it worth arguing about it? Remember the story of the scorpion or snake? The important question surely is how best to look after and support everyone who has the virus — the children, their mother, their father. Access to care, treatment, and support for everyone should surely be the top priority of everyone in a community.

In my (Alice's) 24 years of meeting people with HIV all around the world, there have been extremely few who willingly set out to pass on their virus to others. I could have spent the past 24 years blaming the person who passed HIV on to me. But what use would that have been? It would not have stopped me having it. Do we spend our energies on looking after ourselves and ensuring, as best we can, that others don't contract it or do we waste all our energy blaming others? I feel certain that the person who gave me HIV did not intend to do so, and I believe that the vast majority of people in the world who pass HIV on to others also had no specific intention of doing so. HIV is just a virus. Nothing else. Those very few that do want to pass it on to others intentionally have somehow or other been rejected and therefore have developed a sense of vengeance. The best we can all do is to ensure that everyone who has HIV, or who thinks they may have HIV, and who may have passed it to others, still feels that they are and will be loved and cared for, despite what has happened. In that way, they can dare to be tested, can dare to disclose their status to — and use a condom with — those they love and/or have sex with, and, through protective medication, condoms or other means, can avoid passing the virus on to others.

It would be great if you are able to share these issues in discussions with participants during this session and it would be best if you could talk through these issues with your co-facilitators before you run this session.

DIRECTIONS

1. Explain to participants that in this exercise we will explore how hard it often is for a person living with HIV to be open about their status with their parents or siblings or children. Ask participants to brainstorm a few ideas about why this is so: firstly for people of the participants' own gender, and then for men if they are women or women if they are men.

In Exercise R.1 we listed some of the suggestions which participants might make. Once again, if they don't, it would be good if you could raise them yourself. They may also make other suggestions to add to the list. Participants could draw these suggestions on flip-chart paper with marker pens, or with chalk on a concrete floor.

An additional possibility with a family member is that they might completely reject you and blame you for having let them down – after all, they invested in you when you were growing up. Are such accusations fair or helpful? Do they support the person living with HIV? Do they help him or her to stay well and look after himself or herself? Explain to participants that such remarks can be more hurtful and harmful to the person with HIV than anything else in their lives. Nobody asks to get HIV. Extremely few intend to pass it on. Ask participants what they think of this.

2. Ask participants what they think might be an alternative, more positive response from family members and the wider community. If they need prompting, suggest that family members also need support — from their peers, their faith leader, their health care provider, their village leader, their employer, etc. — to understand what HIV and AIDS are about, to accept that anyone can be affected, and to give all the care and support they can to the family members who are living with HIV.

3. Finally, ask participants what they think might be the benefits of people living with HIV telling their family members about their status, in terms of their own health and well-being. Again, if they need prompting, suggest that, if a family understands about HIV and AIDS, they can provide assistance and emotional support to the person living with HIV in taking care of the household, the children, planning for the future care of the family, and so on.

4. Participants could **draw some of these benefits** on the ground with chalk on concrete and then copy it onto flip-chart paper with marker pens. (Drawing 9).

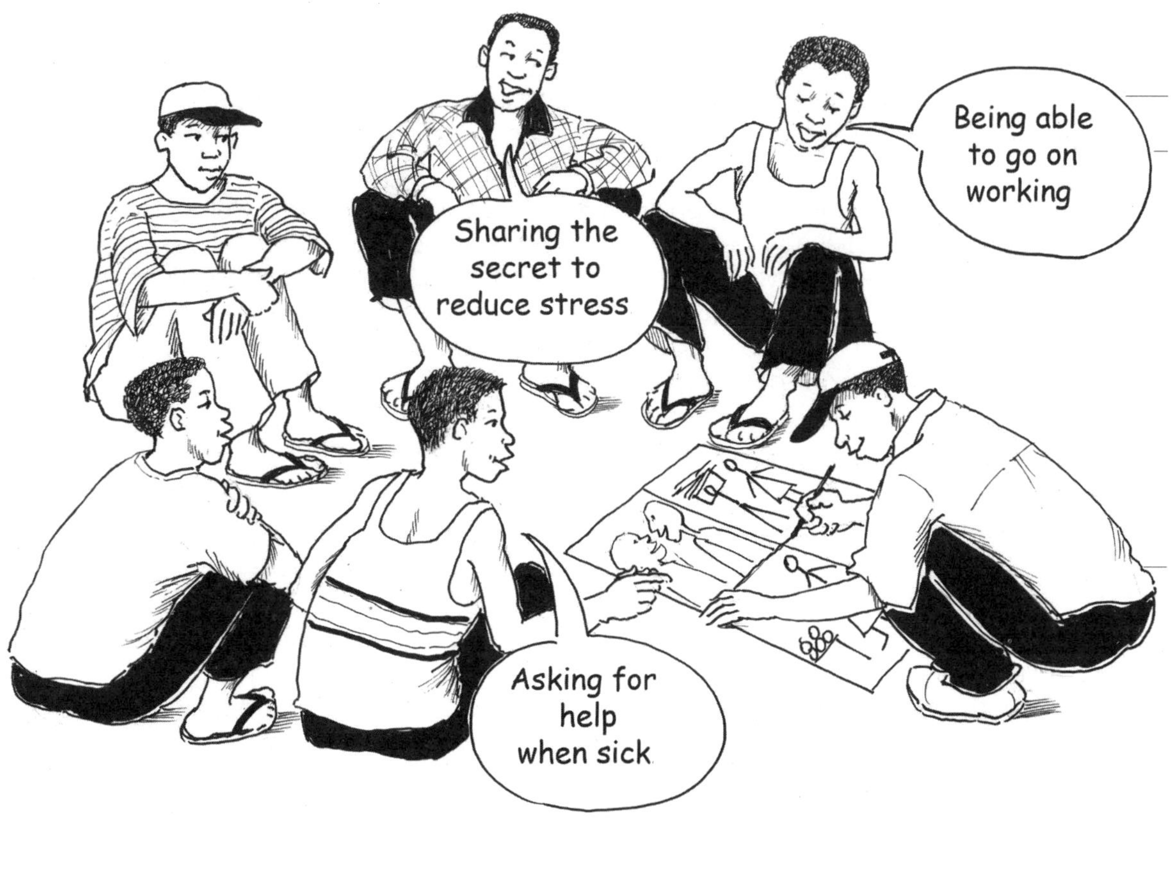
Sharing the secret to reduce stress
Being able to go on working
Asking for help when sick

EXERCISE R3: LOOKING AFTER YOURSELF IF YOU ARE LIVING WITH HIV: CHALLENGES AND POSITIVE POSSIBILITIES

AIMS: To help participants to consider and take action to improve communications with their family members.

DESCRIPTION: Group discussion.

MATERIALS AND PEOPLE NEEDED: Flip-chart paper and marker pens, chalk, (optional). Ideally, a local person living openly with HIV, of the same gender as and similar age to the peer group (one person for each peer group), to talk about his or her own experiences of living positively.

DIRECTIONS

1. Explain to participants that in this exercise we will explore how hard it often is for a person to feel good about herself or himself, and to look after their own health and well-being, once they think they might be, or have had it confirmed that, they are living with HIV. Ask participants to brainstorm why they think that this is so: firstly for people of the participants' own gender, and then for men if they are women or women if they are men.

Here are some of the suggestions which participants might make: if they don't, it would be good if you could raise them yourself. They may also make other suggestions to add to this list. Participants could draw these suggestions on flip-chart paper with marker pens, or with chalk on a concrete floor, or with a stick on the ground.

- Refer to the lists of reasons mentioned in the previous two exercises. As well as these reasons, you might (irrationally) feel that you are somehow to blame for what has happened to you: for instance, because you didn't insist on condom use with your sexual partner, perhaps because you might have faced a violent reaction; because you were in the wrong place at the wrong time and were raped; because you did what all your friends were doing and had many casual sexual partners; and so on.... But ...
- ... are such accusations of self-blame fair to yourself or helpful? Do they help you to accept your condition? Do they help you to stay well and look after yourself – and those around you? Explain to participants that such feelings of self-blame can often be harmful to the individual and not help him or her to deal with their HIV status at all.

2. Ask participants what they think might be an alternative, more positive response from family members and the wider community. Encourage them to repeat the positive suggestions just mentioned in the previous exercise. In addition, ask if there are others living with HIV in your community or in a nearby town with whom they can meet, to form a support group? Can others help people with HIV to attend such a group or clinic, by providing practical or financial support with child care, with transport or with household tasks?

3. Finally, ask participants how they think people with HIV might be supported by everyone in the community to feel good about themselves and accept their status without self-blame or depression.

Participants could draw or write some of their thoughts about the importance of positive living, the possible disadvantages of positive living, and possible solutions to overcome those disadvantages, in a chart as follows (Drawing 10). Some examples are included in the table below, but it is best for participants to come up with their own ideas.

<table>
<tr><th colspan="3">Looking after yourself if you are living with HIV</th></tr>
<tr><th>Advantages Of Positive Living</th><th>Disadvantages Of Positive Living</th><th>Possible Solutions</th></tr>
<tr><td>• A person living with HIV can lead a productive, valuable and long life, just like anyone else.
• You can make the most of your life in many ways, for instance by being an active and caring parent to your existing children, if you have any, and to new children you may wish to have.
• If you know that you have HIV, you can better plan for your future and the future of your family.
• If you want, you can form or join a self-help support group, to help yourself and others understand more about what HIV is and what it isn't, to offer support to others who are newly diagnosed, and to campaign for better services for people living with HIV in your community.
• You could also, with training and support, become a facilitator of workshops like this one – and get paid for your work.
• You become a great inspiration to others as you break down the barriers of silence, ignorance and fear.</td><td>The only disadvantages are connected with how the positive person is treated by everyone around them. If they are treated badly, it can cause deep depression, sickness, and, ultimately, death.</td><td>Receiving:
• psychological support
• physical support
• emotional support
• material support
from:
• family members
• friends
• the whole community
for:
• the individual who has HIV and
• his or her family and friends
to:
• live well and with dignity and respect.

NB: This has to be a whole-community effort — and when that happens the results are great — for everyone</td></tr>
</table>

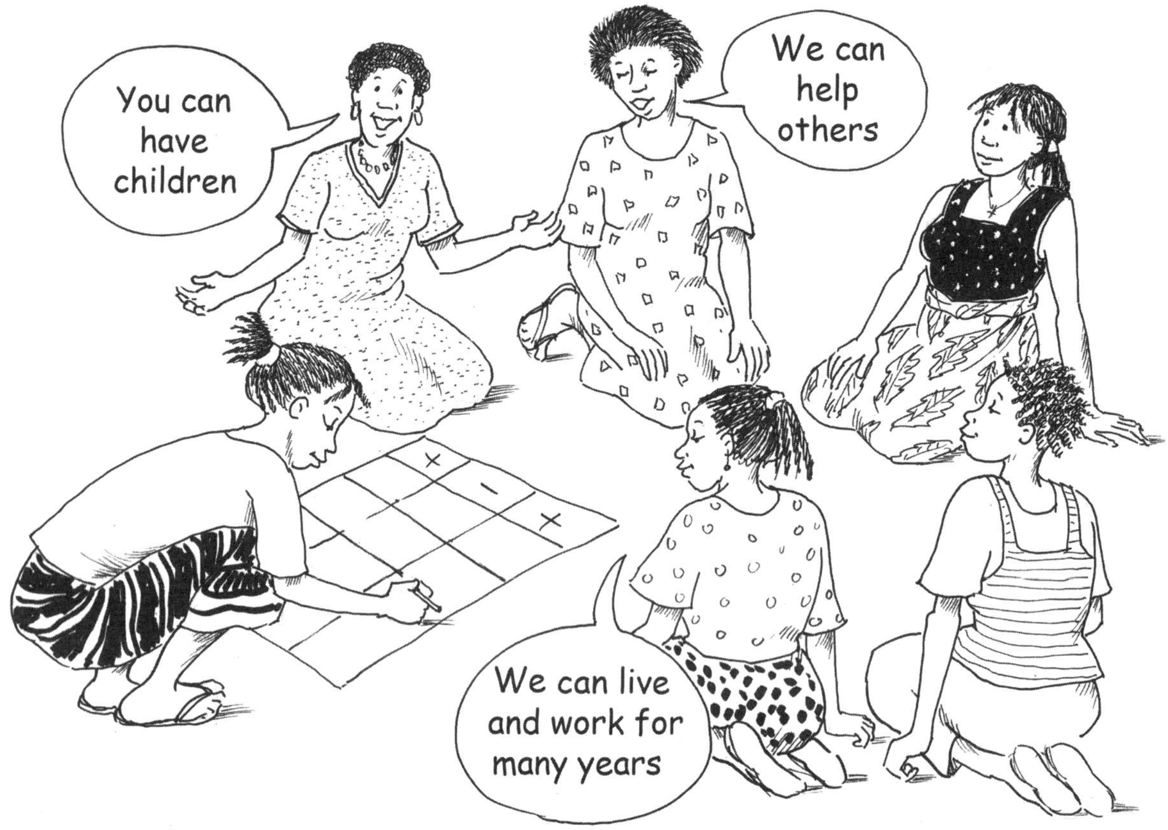
You can have children
We can help others
We can live and work for many years

EXERCISE R.4: REVIEW OF ALL DRAWINGS FROM SESSIONS O–R AND PREPARATION FOR THE FURTHER OPEN COMMUNITY MEETING

AIMS: For participants to review their drawings and charts and prepare for their presentation at the further open community meeting.

DESCRIPTION: Group discussion.

MATERIALS NEEDED: Flip-charts from all the sessions O–R.

DIRECTIONS

1. Explain to participants that you now have up to 12 drawings from the exercises which you have done in this session and the three before it. We now need to look at all these drawings together in order to remind everyone what each drawing shows, and to think about how best to present them in the further open community meeting. (Refer to the table of drawings just before Session O to remind you which flip-charts or drawings were produced.)

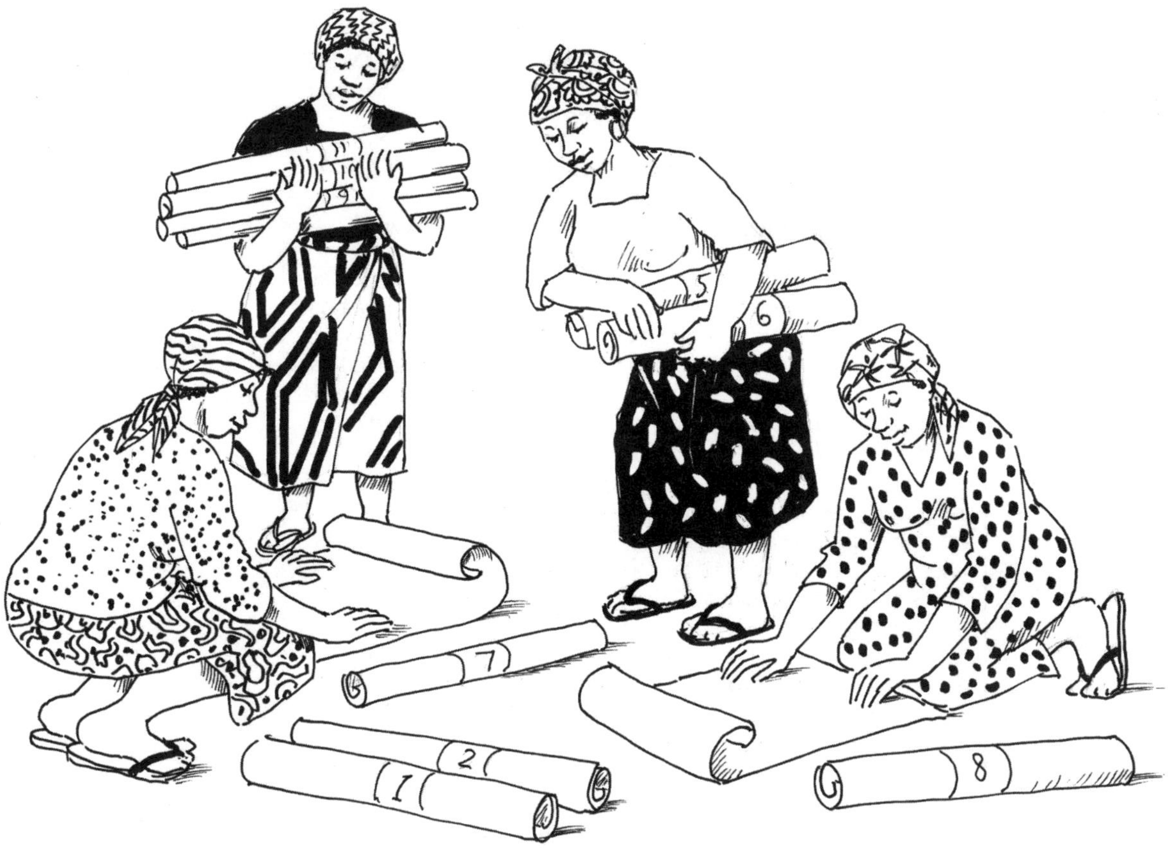

2. Explain that it would be good to hold the further open community meeting in a square or rectangular village hall or large school room that has a lot of wall space so that each peer group can stick their flip charts on one of the four walls. It will then be possible for members of other peer groups and the wider community to walk round and view the drawings for themselves. The idea is that members of each peer group will stand by their own drawings, explaining the contents to the visitors.

3. Here is an example of the possible layout of a village hall, seen from above:

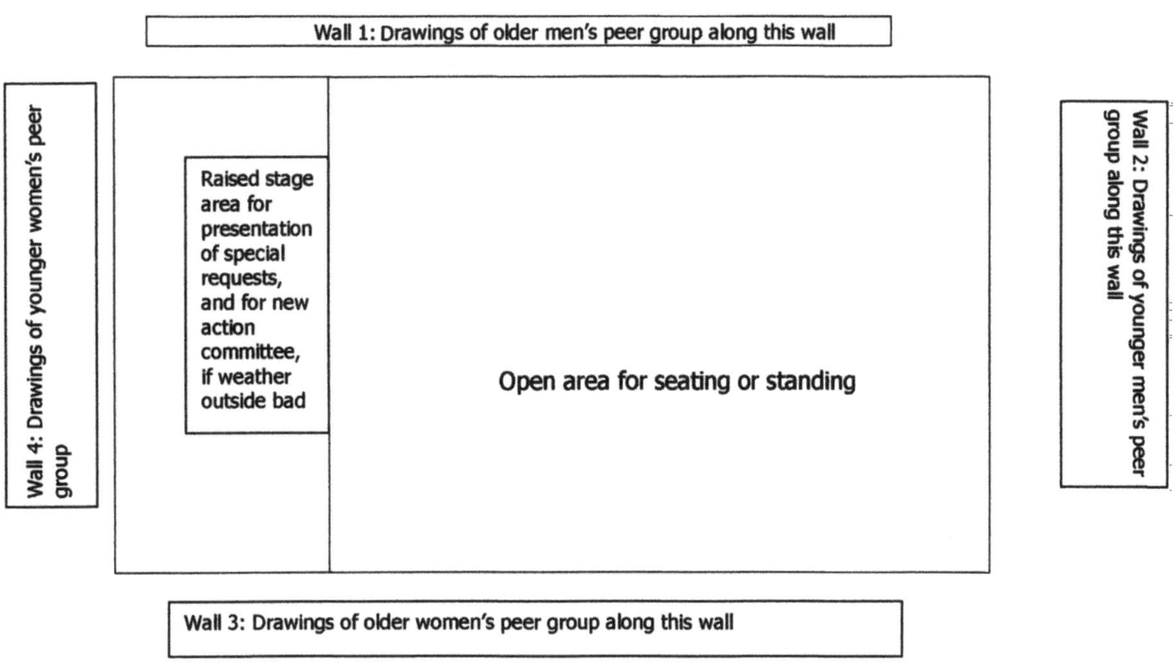

SUGGESTED AGENDA AND TIMETABLE FOR FURTHER OPEN COMMUNITY MEETING (PLEASE SEE THE NEXT SESSION FOR FURTHER DETAILS ON SOME OF THESE STEPS)			
Introduction and song/dance (see next session for details)			
Tugs of war and peace (see next session for details)			
Timing	**What**	**How**	**Materials needed**
Introductory 80 minutes: Viewing exhibition	Visitors from the community who have not been part of the workshop, together with members of other peer groups, have the opportunity to walk round the exhibition of drawings. They spend 20 minutes by each set of drawings, learning about what the drawings contain from the peer group members who are standing beside their own drawings, and asking questions for clarification, where necessary. (You can divide visitors up into groups of 20 or so, so that each group can spend the suggested time with the drawings of one group before being asked to move on to the next set of drawings. In this way, you have four separate sets of visitors moving from wall to wall at the same time, without any group getting too big to see the drawings.)	Peer group members stand by the drawings produced by their own group and explain their contents to the viewers, answering questions of clarification where necessary.	Up to 12 drawings from each peer group, fixed on the wall with tape, pins, or Blu Tack.
Next 80 minutes	All visitors stand – or sit – in the open area of room, while each peer group in turn presents its special request drama on stage. Ideally you could start outside, then show the drawings inside, then move outside for the remaining activities. Or you can hold everything outside if you don't have a suitable hall and if the weather and ground is dry. You could then place the drawings on the ground, but make sure they don't get damaged.	Peer group members represent their special requests to the audience. Up to 10 minutes drama and 10 minutes of questions and answers for each peer group.	Props, clothes etc. for acting, as in previous open community meeting.
Final 30 minutes	All visitors agree to set up an action committee to support special requests with regular 3-monthly whole-community review meetings.	Lead facilitators invite three peer group representatives from each group to come up on stage, to present themselves and seek acceptance from the community of their role as members of the new *Stepping Stones* action steering committee. (See more detail in Exercise 4.3 in the next session.)	Someone from each peer group to record what is agreed.
Five to ten minutes	Candles distribution, silent reflection, announcements (see details in next session). Then all peer group members go round to visitors from the rest of the community, thanking them for coming to this presentation and for agreeing to take part in the action plan for change.		

4. Describe the agenda and timetable for this meeting suggested above to participants.

If, for any reason, any peer group is unhappy with this plan, ask them for an alternative plan and explain that you will need to check it out with the other peer groups, through their facilitators. Explain that the idea, as before, is to give each peer group equal time in the open meeting.

5. If participants are ready to accept this plan, explain that we need now to allocate roles.

a) Ask peer group members who were in the special request role play for the second open community meeting to step forward to remind everyone who they were.

b) Ask for four volunteers from the group, ideally people who are *not* involved in the role play, to volunteer to stand by the group's drawings to present them to the public in the further open community meeting.

6. Now ask the actors to present the special request role play to the rest of the peer group, so that other members have a chance to make any final suggestions for altering any of it if they want. Make sure that the whole role play doesn't run over 10 minutes – or else it will be too long and take time away from the other peer groups' presentations.

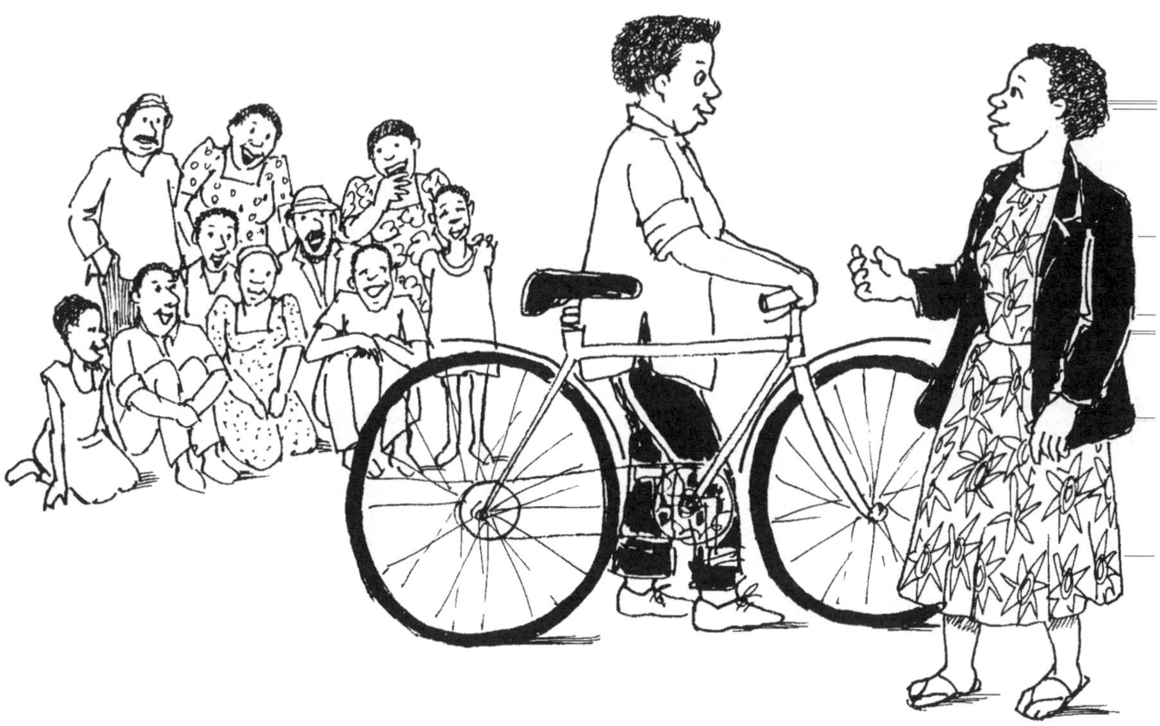

7. Now it's time to ask the four volunteers who will present the drawings to step forward. Each of them needs to choose drawings from one of the four sessions to present. Emphasise to the volunteers that they need to give a summary of the highlights or key points of each drawing rather than a complete description. This is very important, because otherwise your peer group will completely run out of time. Bear in mind that your peer group has 12 drawings altogether.

This means that in 20 minutes the volunteers must present all 12 drawings and leave time for questions from the onlookers. Therefore each drawing should be summed up in a maximum of one minute, so that 12 minutes are spent pointing out key things about the drawings and 8 minutes are left for three or four questions from the audience. This is a tight schedule and needs practice!

Once you have explained all this, ask the four volunteers to decide which of them wants to speak about the drawings from which of the four sessions. Then ask the peer group to divide into four separate sub-groups, with one volunteer presenter in each sub-group. Then the sub-group with the volunteer presenter for session O should study all the drawings from that session and decide which are the highlights of each drawing. The other three sub-groups should do the same with their volunteer presenter.

After about 10 minutes of discussion in these sub-groups, ask all the participants to form a big group again.

8. Then invite the volunteer presenter for Session O to come forward to the front of the group and present the highlights of the drawings from that session to the rest of the group. Get one of the other participants to be timekeeper, giving the presenter one minute maximum to present the highlights of each drawing.

Explain also the importance of the volunteer standing so the drawings are not hidden from the audience behind the presenter, and the need for the volunteer to speak up clearly, face the audience, and make eye contact with everyone – remind them of the body language and assertiveness exercises you have done together. It's no good if the audience just sees the presenter's back and can't hear what they are saying!

After all the drawings from that session have been presented, invite the audience first to clap the presenter and then to comment – kindly – on what they thought was good about the presentation, and then what they thought could be improved.

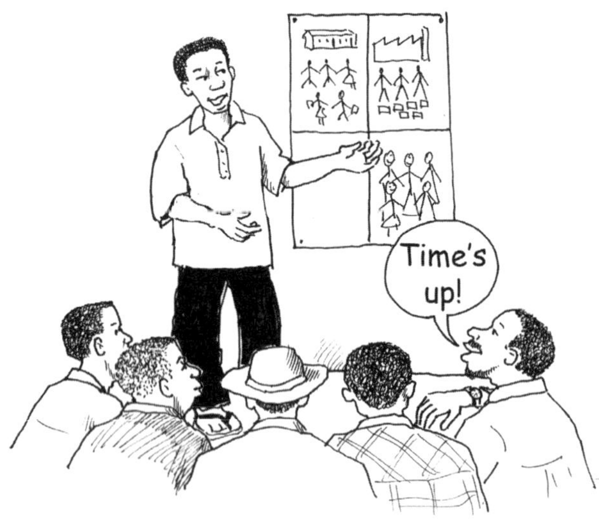

Then ask the volunteer presenter how she or he felt about their own effort and whether she or he feels good about the presentation and the comments made, or whether they want to have another go or ask for some clarification from the rest of the group.

9. Once everyone feels good about the presentation of the Session O drawings, move on to Session P and go through the process described in point 8 above. Then repeat the process for Session Q and Session R. You may need to go on emphasising the need for sticking just to highlights and not going into too much detail.

10. Next, ask the peer group members which of them have decided to nominate themselves for election as one of the three representatives of the group on the action steering committee which will follow up on all the ideas from these workshops over the next year. These three representatives could be anyone in the peer group.

11. The idea of an action steering committee, with three representatives from each peer group, has come out of *Stepping Stones* workshops around the world. Communities and organisations have felt that there is a need for such a group to plan ahead for change in the community once the main workshop sessions are over. There is not room in this publication to explore how communities could plan ahead and monitor change in their community. But it would be good for representatives of peer groups to be chosen by members of each group at this stage. All the people who have nominated themselves should leave the area, while everyone else decides who would be their best representatives. Then call the candidates back, thank them all for standing, and announce which three of them have been chosen for now. Remind them that they will need to step down after one year of service and three new representatives will then need to be chosen from the group.

EXERCISE R.5: CLOSING CIRCLE

1. Thank participants for all the effort they have put into this final optional session. Ask them if they are happy with the preparations they have made for the open community meeting and whether they feel they are ready for it or would like to meet once more to prepare further.

2. Then ask each participant in turn to mention one thing that they have liked about this last session together. Encourage participants not to spend too long on their choice.

3. As a going-home exercise, you could ask participants to reflect on their discussions in this session, and how they think they can work to support their own friends or family members who may be struggling with the issues that were discussed.

4. Finish off by thanking everyone once more for coming to this session. Ask them for convenient dates for the open community meeting, so that you and the other facilitators can finalise a date which suits all the peer groups and community leaders.

Encourage participants to talk in general about the kinds of issues they have been discussing in these sessions with their friends and neighbours, if they like, but not to share any confidential information from the peer group with others.

5. Remind everyone of their role as guardian angel.

6. Remember to ask for three volunteers to stay behind for ten minutes for a quick review of this session before saying goodbye. (See Annex 4 for details.)

FACILITATORS' TEAM FEEDBACK

After the end of Session R, meet again with your co-facilitators to compare notes on how your sessions went and the information which you learnt from them. Your co-facilitators could have found useful information that could help you to structure the further open community meeting more effectively. Remember, however, not to share individual confidentialities between groups. This is the easiest way to ruin the trust that you have begun to build and to wreck the whole workshop! The next meeting is the further open community meeting. This is for the general public.

ENDNOTE

1. Violence is a particular risk for women in heterosexual relationships who tell their partner about their positive HIV status after antenatal testing. However this exercise could equally be of use to people with HIV in same-sex relations who want support to disclose their status to their partners and families.

YOUR NOTES ...

FURTHER OPEN COMMUNITY MEETING

PURPOSE

To enable all four peer groups to share their special requests with the rest of their community.

TIME NEEDED: Maximum 4 hours.

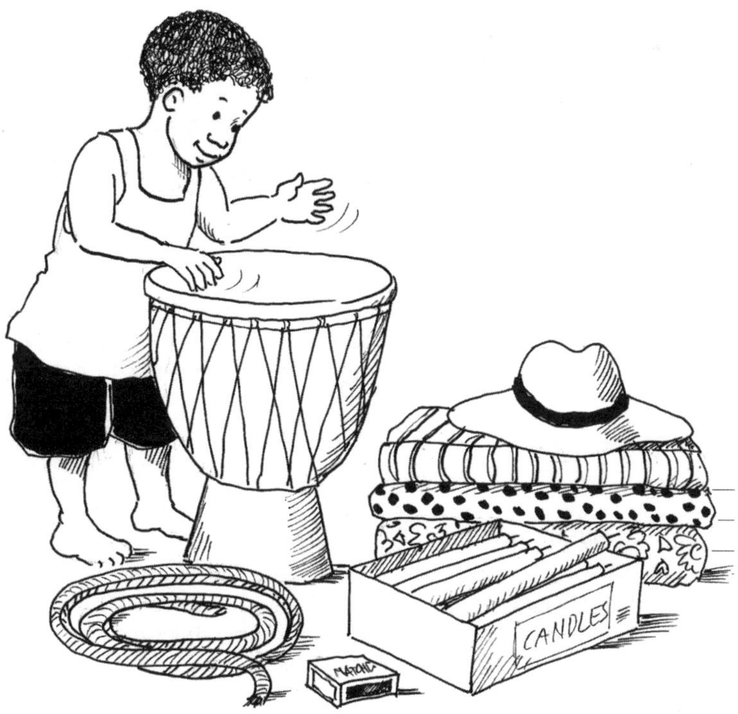

MATERIALS NEEDED: A long, **strong** rope. The drawings from each of the last four sessions, on flip charts. Something to stick them up with. One candle for each person attending and several boxes of matches. Musical instruments? Special clothes and/or props (eg a bicycle or head scarf) for the acting and dancing? Refreshments? Food? (The materials with question marks are not essential, but would be good to have if participants would like a general public celebration of the end of the workshop. Providing food means that no-one needs to worry about cooking food for their families afterwards. See more details below.) You may also need to plan ahead for extra candles for additional community members who may wish to join the candlelit procession in a few days' time.

PARTICIPANTS: All workshop participants and any other community members who want to attend.

SPECIAL INFORMATION

Don't forget to read 'Before you Begin ...!' before using this section of the manual.

Your participants may like to turn this further open community meeting into a bit of a celebration. Would it be possible for them or for you to find money to pay for some light refreshments for everybody? Could a meal be provided for all the workshop participants to share, before or after the meeting? Can some of the participants do some singing or dancing to entertain everyone at the start and the finish of the meeting? Is it possible to welcome children of all ages to join in the audience?

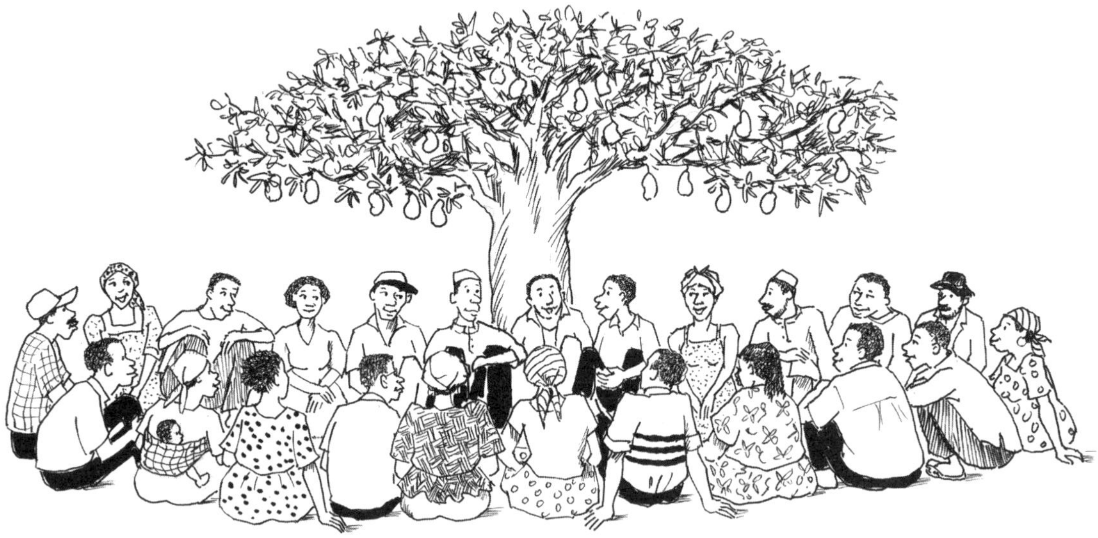

You will also need to think through how the special requests which are to be presented can be taken up seriously by the community leaders and others. Read through the notes for this meeting carefully and talk with your colleagues and others about how best you could begin this process during the meeting.

LOCATION

It would be good to hold at least some of this meeting in a village hall, or a large school room, where there is a lot of space on four separate walls for the peer groups to display all their drawings (see the proposed plan of the meeting hall, shown in the notes for Session R). If the weather is good, perhaps you can hold the tugs of war and peace and the presentations of the special requests outside, but go inside for the exhibition, then return outside for the other activities.

INTRODUCTION

DIRECTIONS

As in the previous public meetings, one or two lead facilitators should do any talking required. The following points need to be made to the audience:

1. Thank everyone for sparing the time to come to the meeting. Give a special welcome to any community leaders, faith leaders, health staff, or other officials who may have turned up.

2. Reintroduce yourself and let each of your co-facilitators reintroduce themselves to the audience.

3. Explain that, as everyone is probably aware, there has been a workshop running in the community in recent weeks. The participants have recently completed four extra optional sessions and now they would like to share their new discussions with the community. This meeting today will provide everyone with an opportunity to see and hear a bit more about what the participants have done in these additional sessions. The participants will also re-present the special requests they have made of one another and the whole of the community.

4. At this stage, perhaps, some of the participants could sing or dance for everybody.

5. Next, say that you have often used games during the workshop, to lighten the proceedings and to illustrate some of the issues which you have been discussing. Say that you would now like to ask the participants to come forward to play one of the games again, for everyone to see.

EXERCISE 1: TUGS OF WAR AND PEACE

AIMS: Warm-up exercise to illustrate to everyone some benefits of working together.

DESCRIPTION: All workshop participants pull together on a rope, whilst others watch.

MATERIALS NEEDED: A long, strong rope.

DIRECTIONS

1. Divide all the workshop participants into two teams, one of all the women and the other of all the men. Ask these two teams to stand up and hold opposite ends of a long strong rope. Mark a line across the middle of your training area, over which each team must try to pull the other.

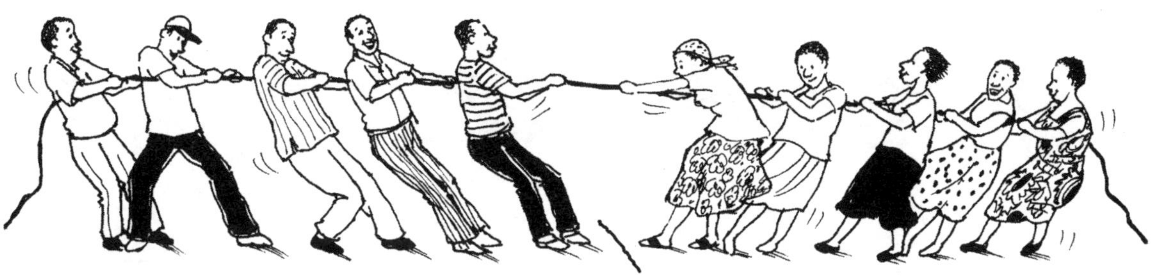

2. When you have said 'One, two, three, go!', the teams should start pulling against each other. Let them go on until one team has ended up falling over the dividing line.

3. Next, ask everyone to divide into two different teams to repeat the contest: this time the older men and women can pull together against the younger men and women. If they would like to try it again, what other two teams can they think of to divide into?

4. Next, ask all the participants – or as many as possible, depending on the length of the rope - to sit in a circle with the members of the different groups mixed up around it. Now tie the same strong rope in a large circle and hand it to all the participants so that they are sitting round the edge of it (see illustration in Session K).

5. Ask all the participants to pull together on the rope so that they can all stand up.

6. Now ask the onlookers, i.e. the people who were not involved in the workshop, what this game illustrates to them.

> The idea is to give the onlookers an idea of what the workshop was all about: i.e. how, instead of pulling on opposite ends – a tug of war, where only one team wins – we can respond to situations in a way that benefits everyone. True, the tug of war might be much more fun for the victors in the short term – but how do the losers feel? How does all this relate to our lives in general?

EXERCISE 2: WALK-ROUND EXHIBITION OF DRAWINGS

Now organise the walk-round exhibition of drawings, as described in the previous session. Divide all the attendees into separate groups of no more than 20 or so, so that they can move round the hall or schoolroom in a clockwise direction. One group can start off at wall 1, another group at wall 2, a third group at wall 3, and a fourth group at wall 4. After 20 minutes, you need to call 'time' and encourage the group viewing wall 1 to move to wall 2, the group viewing wall 2 to move to wall 3, and so on, so that everyone is moving at the same time to hear the presentations of a new peer group. You may want to give the participants time earlier in the day to look at the drawings from each of the other peer groups so that all have seen them all and so that you don't have too much of a crowd now.

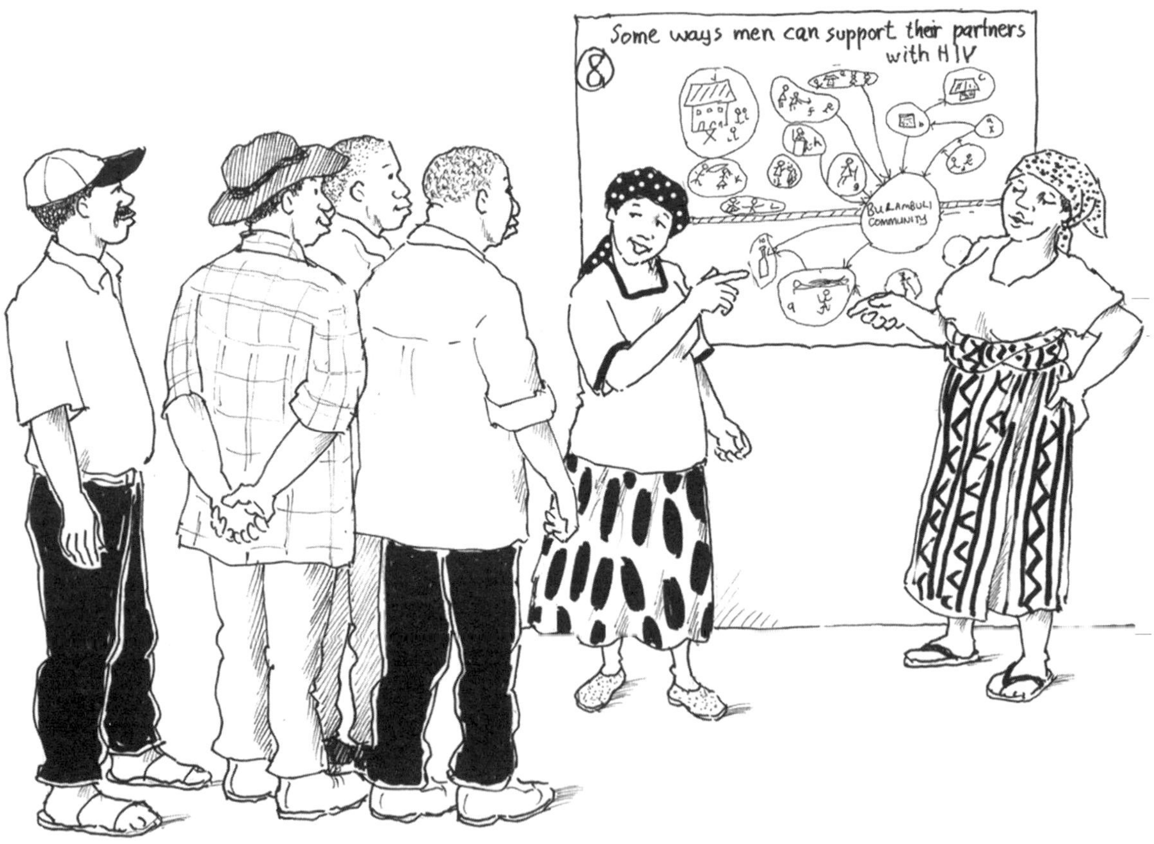

EXERCISE 3: PRESENTATION OF SPECIAL REQUESTS

1. Each peer group has about 20 minutes to present its piece and respond to questions from the onlookers. Make sure each peer group has the same time. Participants should decide for themselves the order in which they make their presentations.

2. One of you should act as timekeeper, to ensure that every peer group has equal time. Another of you should chair the discussion, to ensure that a number of different people in the audience have a chance to ask questions of the participants.

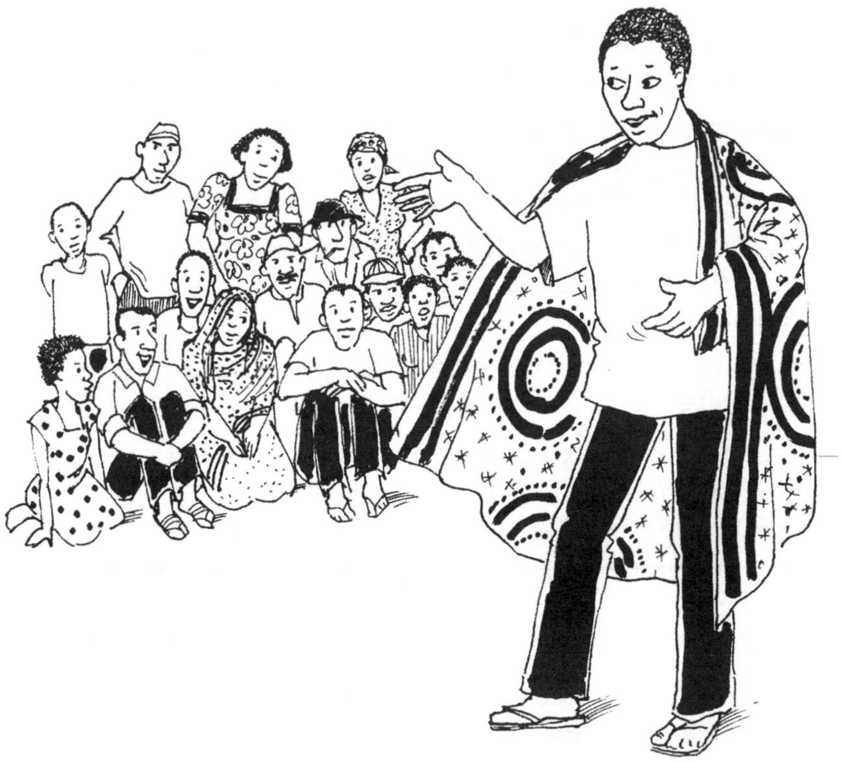

EXERCISE 4: FINAL COMMENTS AND COMMUNITY PROCESSION

1. You could ask any of the community leaders who have come to the meeting whether they would like to make any comments about the drawings or the special requests, or both. If there are community leaders amongst the workshop participants, they should, of course, also be asked to say something.

2. Try to encourage community leaders to adopt the special requests, have them considered by the community, or at least to discuss them further at the next community council meeting or other appropriate time.

3. Explain that the peer groups would now like to set up an action committee, made up of three representatives from each peer group chosen by their own peers. Ask the permission of the elders and other leaders in the community for this action committee to be supported in its efforts to develop all the ideas generated by the workshop.

> ☞ You may well need to do some background work on this in advance. It might be too easy for everyone to agree to adopt a special request or to set up an action committee in public, but for nothing to happen about it afterwards. With your co-facilitators and any community leaders who are attending your workshop, think about what the best way might be to set up the action committee and develop related activities in the community.
>
> The first thing the action committee will need to do will be to plan the candlelit community procession, which is explained in point 8 below.
>
> Later, one related activity might be to set up a meeting with the local health service director to present to him or her the improvements in health services that the different peer groups have requested, and to discuss the possibility of setting up a Community Advisory Board.

Another may be a meeting with faith leaders in the community to discuss how the church, mosque, or other faith community might improve their support for people living with HIV.

A third may be a meeting with the local school authorities to discuss support for students who are living with HIV, or have family members who are, in order to ensure they can go on attending school and don't get bullied by other students or by teachers.

A fourth might be a meeting with community elders to see how widows can be supported in the community without being forced out of their houses, or into new marriages, or to sell their possessions.

If there are local employers, perhaps they could be approached too, so that people with HIV are assured that they can keep working and earning.

No doubt your committee can think of many other activities also. Perhaps you could hold another public event with all the health, faith and education officers, to present to them the role plays and drawings which you are presenting to the community today.

4. If any of the peer groups intend to go on meeting, you could announce this publicly now.

5. You could encourage all participants to continue in their role as guardian angels for one other, whether their group continues to meet or not.

6. If there seems to be enough interest in starting up a repeat workshop for new participants, you could also make an announcement about this now.

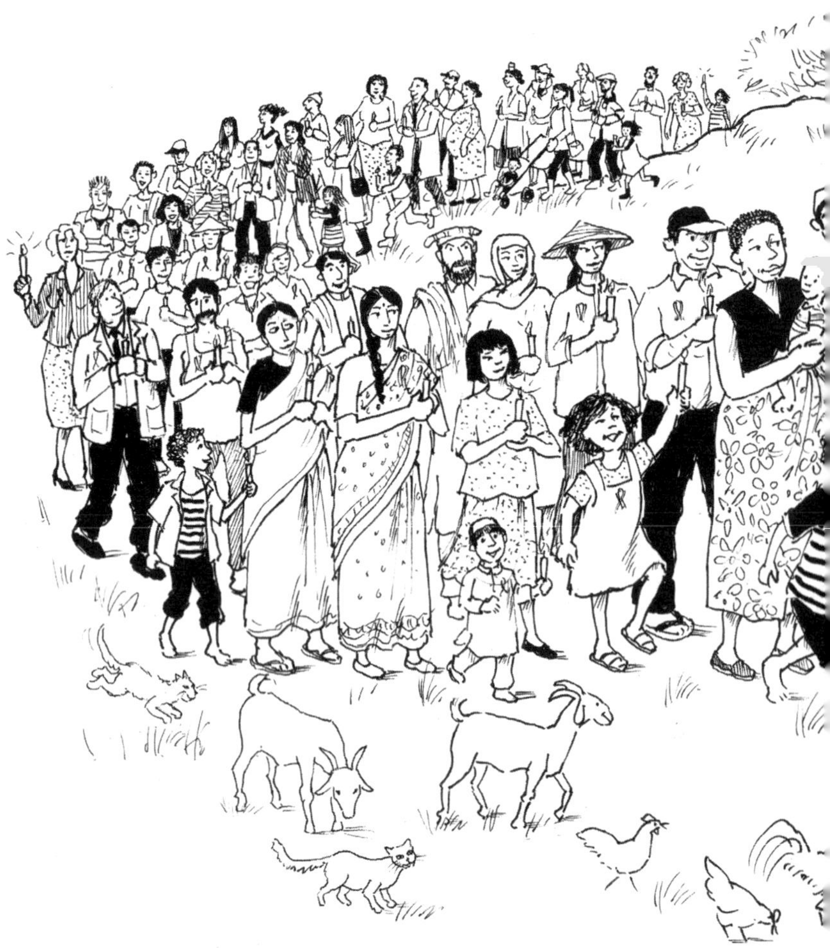

7. Now for passing lit candles around the gathering for three minutes' silence here. Distribute candles to all the peer group members present and get their candles lit. Then ask each of them to move around the meeting area with four or five extra unlit candles. Ask each of them to distribute these candles to the other community members present lighting these candles from their own as they hand them out. Make sure that there are enough candles to go round, and that each attendee has received a candle from a participant. Explain that you would now like to ask everyone to stand together in a big circle for three minutes, reflecting silently upon all the people with HIV and their families and friends, in this community, and around the world.

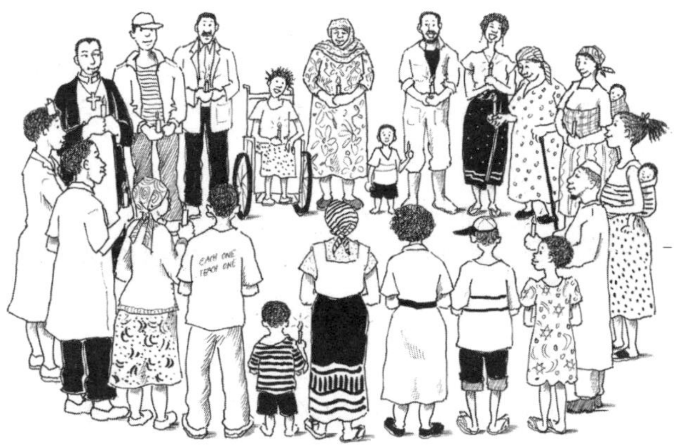

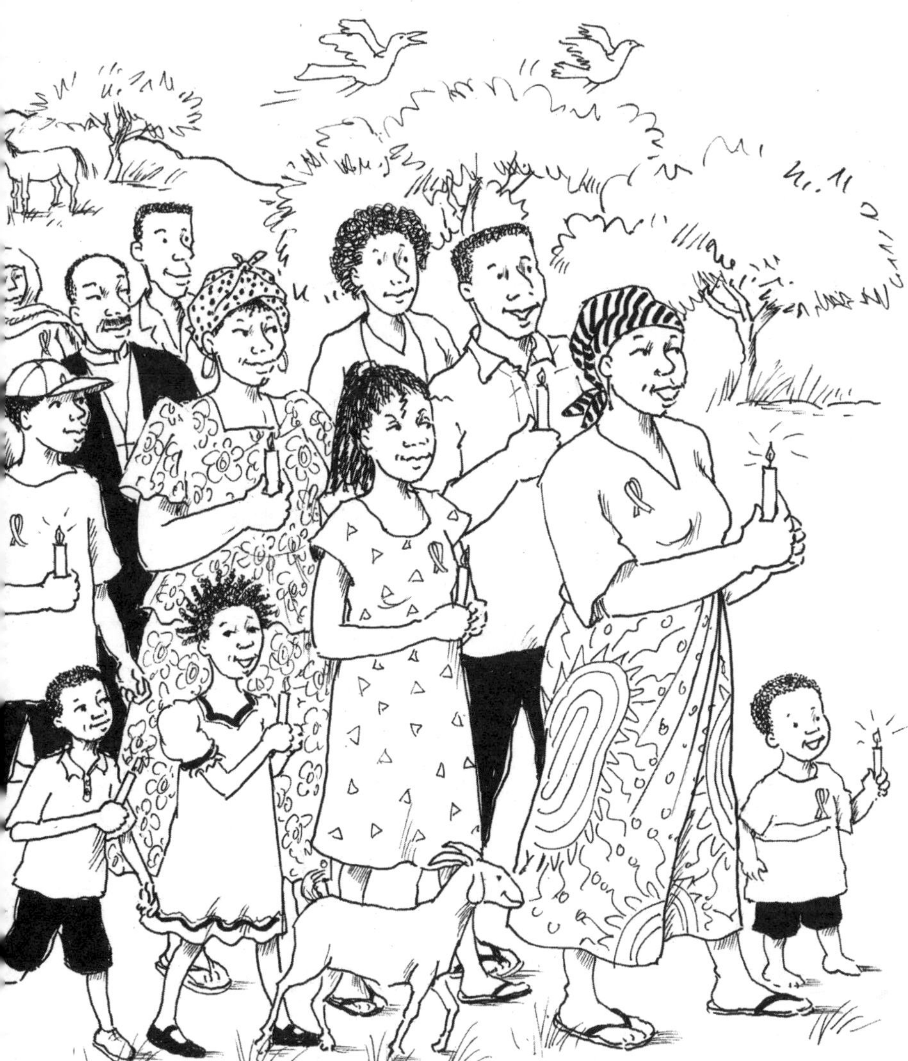

8. Once these three minutes of silence are over, explain that you would also like to request everyone there to take part in a candlelit procession around the local area in a few days' time as a symbol of the commitment of the whole community to supporting one another in relation to HIV and AIDS, and also as a symbol of the fact that HIV can affect everyone in a community. Explain that anyone who wants to can join the procession, carrying a lit candle as they walk. It would be great if the procession could pass by every home in the community, and for someone from every home to receive a lit candle from someone in the procession. Remind people also that, if there are people who are homeless, or people with disabilities, or others who are often marginalised in the community, it would be good to ensure that they take part in the procession, if they would like, or receive a lit candle if they don't join in themselves.

Ask the permission of all those present for this procession to take place. Then, if they agree, ask them to give the community action committee members permission to make plans for it to take place soon.

9. Ask once more for three participants from each peer group to meet for a few minutes with their own facilitator, after you have finished, in order to conduct a quick review of this final meeting (see Annex 4).

10. Finish the proceedings by thanking all the participants for their great support and hard work throughout the workshop and thanking the community leaders for their support. You could then ask everyone to join in more singing and dancing.

FACILITATORS' TEAM FEEDBACK

Don't forget to share your views of this last meeting. Annex 4 gives you ideas about how you can conduct a full evaluation of the whole workshop. You could make plans now about when and how you can do this. You can also make plans about how you will organise the follow-up sessions. Guidelines for these are in Annex 5.

FINALLY, CONGRATULATIONS TO YOU!

YOU HAVE NOW COMPLETED THE WORKSHOP.

But remember, this is only a beginning. Participants may continue to need your continued support and hard work. No-one can be expected to change the habits of a lifetime in a few weeks. In Annex 5, you will find some ideas about how you can continue to support those with whom you have worked, if they would like you to.

We hope you have enjoyed using this manual and have found it easy enough to follow. We would very much like to hear from you. Please look at Annex 8, which asks you some questions about how you have found the work.

We look forward to hearing from you soon!

There are also a lot of reports available about how *Stepping Stones* workshops have been adapted and developed for many different countries and contexts.

If you would like to hear more, please contact: enquiries@steppingstonesfeedback.org so that we can send you the relevant information.

Or ask a local faith leader, health worker, school teacher, community leader or an NGO staff member to contact us for you.

THANK YOU for all your efforts! We wish you the best of luck and success with all your work.

ANNEX 1 NOTES ON ROLE PLAYS AND TABLEAUX

Throughout this workshop, we frequently suggest that you use role plays to help participants address different issues. Tableaux are also occasionally suggested. Participants are always asked to draw on their **own** experiences for these.

For exercises where role play is suggested, participants should be encouraged to think of a situation of their choice, relevant to the particular exercise. Each participant should adopt a different character, so that together they can act out the situation they have chosen. What they say to each other should be agreed only roughly beforehand — it needs no written script. What is important is the spontaneity of the performance and the clarity for everyone of what is being communicated between the actors. Body language can often be as important as words in these scenes.

A role play really only needs to last a **maximum** of 4 minutes. In truth, the **shorter** and more simple the role play, the more effective it is in presenting a situation clearly. Longer role plays start to ramble and the audience quickly gets lost.

Tableaux are similar to role plays in that they present a situation. But they are different in that no one says anything and no one moves: everyone is **frozen** in their position. So people's relationships to one another are shown only through their frozen body language and facial expressions — no words are used at all.

With both tableaux and role plays, participants who are looking on ask questions after the presentation. Those acting can stay in their positions to answer — which often works very well. They can answer either as the person they are playing, or as themselves. Alternatively, you can just bring everyone back to a group circle for discussion.

The **discussions** which follow a role play or a tableau are **the most important part** of the learning process. This is when the **analysis** of what has been heard and/or seen takes place. Onlookers should be encouraged to ask 'why', 'who', 'what', 'when', 'how', and 'where' as much as possible, so as to explore the reasons behind what happened in the situation.

Therefore you should make sure that your participants don't concentrate too much on their performances. This would take valuable time away from their discussions, and repeated rehearsals would also quickly make their performances rather stale and less realistic.

Next, you will often realise that exercises suggest that your actors do another role play or tableau after the discussion. In the second presentation, you will be asking them to show how the situation could have turned out **differently**. This second presentation must also be followed by a discussion, so that everyone has a chance to think about and talk through what has changed.

Acting and role play need **no literacy skills** at all. People who can't read can be just as good — or even better — at acting as those who have had a formal education. However, they often lack confidence. So make sure that non-literate participants are given a lot of encouragement to involve themselves throughout and do not just watch quietly from the sidelines. Examples of both role plays and tableaux are on the DVD.

Finally, remember to remind peer groups that when they present their role plays or tableaux at larger meetings, they should **not** think that they are having a competition! Some groups may feel nervous about performing in front of others. So each peer group should receive as much encouragement and praise as possible from the other peer groups. Everyone will be surprised by what they find they can achieve.

ANNEX 2 TECHNICAL NOTES ON USING DVD

By Jamie Hartzell, revised by Nell Osborne

THE EQUIPMENT YOU NEED

To show a DVD you will need, at the very least, a laptop computer which is well enough charged to play the DVD clips needed for each session, maybe up to eight times (twice for each peer group). Ideally the laptop should have an inbuilt working DVD player. Otherwise, you need a separate DVD player and relevant lead(s). If you have a noisy environment or more than about 10 people, you will also need a loudspeaker that plugs into the laptop or DVD player, to make sure everyone can hear the DVD. In addition, if you have a large audience, you would be best to use a projector and either a mobile projector screen or a clear wall on which the DVD can be viewed by each peer group in turn. Make sure you have the leads to connect the laptop to the projector, to the DVD player and to the loudspeaker. You may also need an extension lead with multiple sockets. We find it helps to keep these all together in one box and clearly labelled, so as not to misplace anything.

BEFORE YOU GO

Before you take the equipment anywhere, check that it works. Plug the DVD player and the laptop in to your mains power or generator, join them to the loudspeaker and projector, play the DVD, and see if the picture and sound work properly. Play the DVD in the same kind of size of room or open space that you plan to use it, to see if you can see and hear it properly. A big mobile screen, with a good quality loudspeaker, is best.

Before you take the laptop, DVD player, projector, and loudspeaker anywhere, make sure that there is mains power, or a generator and enough fuel, or solar power in the place where you are going. If there isn't, you cannot show the DVD.

If there is no electricity where you are going, you will need a generator and fuel to run it. The equipment can also be run off car or motorbike batteries, or solar power. You will need a device called an inverter to enable you to do this.

Before you start showing the DVD, set up everything and check again that it works. If not, go through the steps below. Once the equipment is working, insert the DVD and choose the film clip you want to watch.

VIEWING CONDITIONS

If you use a mobile screen or a community wall, avoid bright light or people won't be able to see the film. You may need to drape fabric over windows, especially if there is bright sunlight outside. Make sure that everyone can see the screen from where they are sitting. You may have to put the projector higher up.

Make sure that you can easily stop and start the DVD player. If it has a remote control, use it. Remember also that a DVD player has a PAUSE button. This button freezes the picture on the DVD and stops the sound, until you press the PLAY button again. This can be useful if you want to go over the clip again with participants and wish to stop it at a particular point.

Make sure that everyone can hear the sound.

If the faces on the screen still look too dark or too light, you may need to adjust the BRIGHTNESS of the laptop.

Make sure that you have everybody's attention before you start playing the DVD.

NOW YOU ARE READY TO START.

GOOD LUCK!

WHAT TO DO IF IT DOESN'T WORK

If the DVD does not work, the most likely reason is that there is no power to it, so the first thing to do is check that the DVD player and the laptop and projector are plugged in and turned on. If you are sure that the laptop and DVD player and projector and loudspeaker are in working order, test whether there is power in the mains socket by plugging in something that you know works. Then also check that the sockets of the extension lead work, by plugging something which you know works into each of these sockets in turn. If the equipment still doesn't work, try changing the fuse in the mains plug on the extension lead first. Then try changing the fuse in each of the laptop and projector and DVD player plugs in turn.

It may also be that the laptop is broken or the DVD is scratched. We find it helpful to have back-ups available in case they are.

ANNEX 3 SYNOPSIS OF DVD CLIPS

There are brief summaries of each DVD clip below. They are for your guidance only. Do not read them out to the participants! However, do remember to read out or translate the written title, shown at the start of each clip, for your participants. They may not all be able to read.

Remember also that each time one of these DVD clips is shown, participants may want to view the clip again. If so, it is usually best for them to have some discussion about it first, then to have further discussions after the second viewing.

1. 'STEPPING STONES'

An introduction to the workshop, to the village of Buwenda in Uganda, and to some of the members of the community who took part in the workshop held there. Some comments on the value of the workshop to them.

2. 'WHAT IS LOVE?'

A presentation of two couples, the Senyondos and the Kaumas. The Senyondos each have their own views of life and earn their incomes separately. The Kaumas work together in the house and field and are mutually faithful.

3. 'THE CONDOM'

Two peer groups — older women and younger men — are shown separately familiarising themselves with condoms.

4. 'HOPES AND FEARS: THE YOUNG WOMEN'

A presentation about two young women of Buwenda. Saitun has left secondary school before completing it, but would like to go to university. Her father has enough money, but does not believe in education for women. She doesn't want to have children until she has graduated and married. Mega left school at Primary 7. She has three children and lives with her mother. She works as a hairdresser at home. She wants no more children. These young women also discuss options for other young women in their community.

5. 'HOPES AND FEARS: THE YOUNG MEN'

The younger men's group of Buwenda perform a role play of a disco At this pretend disco, the 'father' of a young man warns him off the young women. But after his father has gone, he goes off with a young 'woman'. Upon returning to the disco, his friend rebukes his foolishness. The young 'woman', however, protests that 'she' does not have HIV and the young man regrets his actions. Next, Julius (who acted as the young man above) describes his own situation and strategy for living. Whenever he has sex with a woman, he uses a condom, if he has one. John then presents his situation and strategy. For the last few years, he has abstained from sex. One day, he would like to get married but he is afraid of acquiring HIV from his future wife.

6. 'ALCOHOL'

The older women of Buwenda begin with a song about drinking. This is followed by a role play by the older men's group of a drunkard dragging a 'woman' off into the bushes. There follows a discussion about the pros and cons of alcohol amongst drinkers of banana beer.

7. 'TRADITIONS'

The older women's group perform a role play where a man is killed by a car. His 'father' decides to marry off his younger son to the new widow, according to traditional practice. The widow feels worried about this decision.

8. 'MONEY'

The older women's group perform a tableau where a wife prepares to leave home because of money disputes. This is followed by a discussion among some members of a women's income-generating group in Buwenda. Then the older men's group perform a role play where a husband and 'wife' have a problem over the use of money in their household. Finally, the role play of the older men's group is acted out again, this time with a happier outcome.

9. 'SAYING 'YES'?'

The younger women's group perform a role play where a young woman is picked up and seduced by a 'sugar daddy'. When she is pregnant, she goes to 'his' office, asking him for help, but he throws her out.

10. 'SAYING 'NO'?'

The younger women's group practise saying 'No!' and re-enact the role play. However, this time the young woman refuses to be picked up by the 'sugar daddy' and rejects 'his' advances very clearly.

11. 'COMING HOME'

The older women's group perform a role play, where a 'man' comes home from a journey to his wife and children. He is anxious to have sex with his wife and quickly gets the children out of the house in order to do so. In asides to the audience, both the wife and the 'husband' voice their fears about HIV and whether this should affect their actions. The wife then decides to propose to her 'husband' that they use a condom ...

12. '"I" STATEMENTS'

Different groups practise and discuss 'I' statements. The younger women's group role play a scene between a 'husband' and wife where he goes out to drink and leaves her, feeling upset, at home. They then re-enact the scene. This time, the wife manages to express her needs by being assertive. Her husband then agrees to bring beer back home, to share with her. Some members of the older women's group then recount some of their own experiences in learning to be more assertive.

13. 'TRUST'

A younger couple from Buwenda talk about their lives together and the decisions they have made. Their relationship is based upon mutual trust, cooperation, and shared responsibility. The husband explains that his friends question his approach, but he believes that it is right for them.

14. 'THE LONG JOURNEY'

Mr and Mrs Mulumba are shown. Mr Mulumba is preparing for his death. His aunt is writing out his will for him. Together they explain the other preparations that they have made. The older men's group is also shown. They reflect on what they have learnt from the exercise 'The Long Journey'. They say that they have recognised the value of ensuring the future security of their dependents.

15. 'THE COMMUNITY CHALLENGE'

The purpose of this clip is to show participants how the Buwenda community arranged their final open community meeting. The older women's group and the younger men's group perform their role plays and present their special requests. These are followed by audience discussion. Several participants comment on their views of the workshop. Now it is up to your participants to design their own finale!

ANNEX 4 EVALUATION OF THE WORKSHOP YOU RUN

1. MONITORING

It is really important to keep a running check on how your participants feel about the workshop. If they do not like it, you may find that participants drop out and it is too late for you to change anything.

We suggest that you adopt the following approach.

First of all, we strongly recommend that you contact us for the Word version of the *Stepping Stones Facilitators' Journal* created by users of the programme in the Pacific, which is an excellent handbook that facilitators can use to record information from each session.[1] If you have a modified version of this, you may not need a notebook too.

The best way to monitor your progress is to have a quick review **after each session**. Each time, you can ask for three people from your peer group to stay behind for a few minutes to tell you how they think things are going. This means that, if you have about 20 participants in your peer group, each will be asked to stay behind and comment after two or three of the sessions you have together, after the first open community meeting.

In this way, all your participants can feel involved in the review process and will thereby feel some ownership of it.

It is just as important for you to have feedback from non-literate people as it is from literate people. Therefore we suggest that you perform the review in a way which uses drawings so that everyone is equally capable of understanding it.

Please ask participants to be as honest and open as possible with you about their views. In this way you will be able to improve subsequent sessions.

MATERIALS NEEDED

For every session: one new large piece of flip-chart paper, two marker pens, 15 small stones, one note-book and pen for you.
After each session, draw a chart on a piece of flip-chart paper, putting the following headings across the top:

CONTENT **PRESENTATION** **TIMING**

Explain that:

- The **content** of an exercise means what it taught us, whether it felt enjoyable, relevant, or worthwhile.
- The **presentation** of an exercise means how well or badly you, the facilitator, introduced and ran the exercise with the participants.
- The **timing** of the exercise means whether it was too long, too rushed, or just right.

Ask your participants to draw a symbol under each word on the flip chart, so that they remember what each word means. (For instance, they could draw a book under 'content', a face under 'presentation', and a clock under 'timing'.) Check that they all understand the meaning of the three symbols.

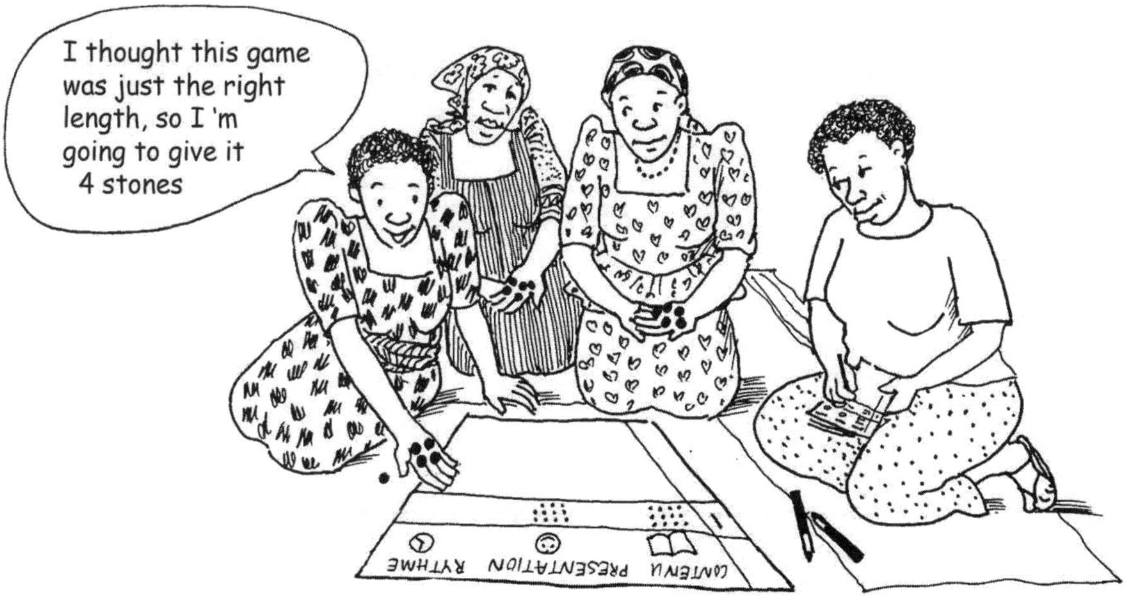
I thought this game was just the right length, so I 'm going to give it 4 stones

Then give your three participants five stones each. Explain to each participant that you are going to ask them to give scores out of five with the stones for each different exercise.

A score of five stones by a participant would mean that they thought something was very good. A score of one or no stones would mean that they thought something was very poor.

Next, go through each exercise in the session which you have just run, asking all three participants to give a score with their stones. For instance, in Session A, you would start off with the 'Adjectival Names' game.

- Ask each participant to use the stones to give a score out of five for content. They should all place their stones at the same time. If all three participants were to give a score of four stones, there would be 12 stones lying below the content symbol.
- Remove the stones and write a note in your notebook, for example, 'Adjectival Names: Content: 12/15' You could also keep a record on the flip chart, by asking your participants to draw a symbol in the left-hand column which reminds them of each exercise, and then marking with dots the number of stones they have scored under content, presentation and timing. (See the diagram above, which illustrates this.)
- Then ask each participant to give a score out of five for presentation. If two participants gave a score of 4 stones and the third gave a score of 3 stones, the total score for presentation would be 11/15.
- Remove the stones and write this score in your notebook and on the chart if you have decided to do this.
- Repeat the process for timing for this exercise and record the result as before.
- Then move on to the next exercise in the session and repeat the scoring process, until you have covered all the exercises in the session. So, in Session A, for instance, your next exercise would be 'Expectations'.
- After each individual exercise has been judged, ask your scorers to give scores on content, presentation and timing for the session **as a whole**.
- If at any stage, your scorers give a score of **3 or less** for something, it is helpful to ask them to explain why they felt the score should be low. You can make a note of their comments in your notebook.

- After this, ask your volunteers whether they thought the **location** of the session was alright: whether there was enough privacy and lack of disturbance, whether there was enough shade or light, and so on. If there are problems with any of this, it is best to find a better location as soon as possible!
- Finally, thank your scorers very much for their help.

The whole scoring process should not take more than ten minutes at the end of a session.

You should share the results of this instant review with your co-facilitators, so that you can discuss together any problems which you may have come across.

Then please share them with us! In particular, we would be glad to know what you think and participants think of the optional materials, (Sessions O-R), since they are newer and we have had less feedback on them so far.

> ☞ Don't feel put off or defensive if the participants criticise the sessions in any way. Nobody ever scores full marks for everything! It shows that they feel they can trust you enough to be honest with you. Allow yourself to listen and learn from their comments and make use of them in your plans for future sessions.

2. POST-WORKSHOP REVIEW

MATERIALS NEEDED

The flip-chart paper from Exercise N.6, all the drawings from the optional sessions (O–R), new flip-chart paper, marker pens.

In Session N, Exercise 6, you and your co-facilitators asked participants in each peer group to think of several changes which they would like to see over the next six months in their community. They should have drawn symbols representing between five and ten hoped-for changes on a piece of flip-chart paper, as a record of this.

There were several drawings and charts produced in Sessions O–R, if your participants decided to have these sessions, and these were shared in the further open community meeting.

Six months after the whole workshop has finished, it is a good idea for you and your co-facilitators each to run a review session with your peer groups.

DIRECTIONS

1. Let each peer group meet separately with its facilitator. Ask them to bring the flip chart from Session N on which they drew the hoped-for changes, together with all the drawings and charts from Sessions O–R (if relevant). You could then ask participants to discuss the changes they hoped to see. For each change they mentioned in Session N, ask if they have seen it happen or not. If it has, to what extent has it happened? If it has not happened, why do they think it has not? In what ways do they think they could help the change to happen in future? You can also do the same review with each of the other drawings and charts.

2. Ask participants (again, if relevant), also to consider the special requests which their peer group made to the community in the second and further open meetings. To what extent have

these been accepted? If they have not been accepted, why do they think they have not? What could be done to help the special requests be accepted in future?

3. Next, ask participants what **unexpected** changes they have seen in individuals or in their community over the last six months. Don't ask them to name names but to talk in general about changes they have noticed. Ask them to mention both negative changes and positive changes. For each one, ask them to what extent do they think it was connected with the workshop. What could be done to stop the negative changes from happening in future? What could be done to help the positive changes happen more?
It would also be a good idea to encourage each peer group to draw up a new set of indicators on a new flip chart. These would show what changes they hope to see over the *following* six-month period. Some changes may be the same, others may be new ones. By repeating this exercise every six months, participants will be able to see and judge for themselves their own community's progress over time.

In Buwenda, six months after their workshop, participants said that the programme had helped not only the participants but also other members of the community who had benefited by learning from their neighbours about knowledge and skills they had acquired in the workshop. So the effect of the programme was more widespread than had originally been hoped.

Finally, ask participants what they thought of the workshop programme as a whole. To what extent did they feel it was a positive or a negative experience? Looking back, what do they think could have been done differently to enable it to have a more positive effect on their lives?

Once each facilitator has conducted this discussion with his/her peer group, you might like to have another full workshop meeting, where the findings of each peer group could be presented to participants from other groups. This may be a good way of highlighting whose hopes have been met and whose hopes have not been met. We often find that the hopes of most men are met more than those of most women. The hopes of women – and of younger people – are often forgotten about. So this would be a good way of encouraging all the workshop participants to take joint responsibility for addressing the needs and hopes of *all* the peer groups.

It is very important for you to write up all these discussions in full. You can then make use of what you have heard in planning future workshops, either with this community or with others. The community itself should find the discussions very useful in re-assessing the needs of its own members, and in deciding on future plans for its own development.

We also really want to hear about your experiences, so we can learn from them and share them with other members of the international *Stepping Stones* Community of Practice. So do please send us a copy of such write-ups.

3. FULL WORKSHOP FORMAL EVALUATION

Over the past two decades a great deal has been learnt about the importance – and also the challenges – of formal evaluation processes. We recommend that you seek to conduct, at least, a formal qualitative evaluation of your workshop, alongside the *participatory* evaluation described above.

If the evaluation is positive, it will help you to find further funding for your work. In any case, it will help the international community of *Stepping Stones* users, who will be able to benefit from your experiences and will also help us all to expand the global evidence base of what works in relation to reducing gender-based violence and HIV around the world.

If you also have resources to conduct a quantitative evaluation also, then all the better. However, we recommend strongly that the questions you formulate in the quantitative workshop are based on quantitative evaluations that have been carried out elsewhere, so that you are sure that the questions being asked make sense to participants.

For more information about how to conduct formal qualitative and quantitative, and participatory evaluations of *Stepping Stones* you can:

a) contact us
b) read our newsletter on monitoring and evaluation[2]
c) look at the many evaluation reports from around the world on the website
d) ask us for the ALIGHT Framework, which will be published in 2016 by UNAIDS.

Please send any requests and evaluations to us at: enquiries@steppingstonesfeedback.org

Alternatively you can send them by post to:
Stepping Stones Coordinator
Salamander Trust
Positively UK
345 City Road
London EC1V 1LR, UK

ENDNOTES

1. *SPC/FSPI (2009)*
2. *Salamander Trust (2012)*

REFERENCES

Salamander Trust (2012) Stepping Stones Newsletter about Monitoring and Evaluation, <http://us2.campaign-archive1.com/?u=24d198c33ed45c3d1513bf5ff&id=f624da86a1>, [accessed 18 November 2015]

Secretariat of the Pacific Community/ Foundation of the Peoples of the South Pacific International (2009) Stepping Stones Community Facilitators' Journal

ANNEX 5 DISCUSSION TOPICS FOR FOLLOW-UP WORKSHOPS AND NOTES FOR STRUCTURING SESSIONS

In this annex you will find the following:

1. Why follow up?
2. Who to follow up with.
3. What to follow up with.
4. How to structure sessions you plan.
5. Extra tips on session styles.

1. WHY FOLLOW UP?

In this kind of peer-group work, when behaviour change is discussed and planned, it is extremely valuable for participants to continue to meet regularly. This gives them a lot of mutual support, encouraging them to share news about how they are getting on and to cheer one another up, if they feel discouraged.

In Buwenda, six months after the workshop was finished, the peer groups were all still meeting regularly. Sometimes they met with a facilitator from Redd Barna, sometimes on their own.

Having an outside facilitator can often help participants to address issues which they would find hard to tackle on their own. At other times, peer groups may prefer to meet without outside help. You should encourage peer groups to decide for themselves what is best for each of them.

2. WHO TO FOLLOW UP WITH

The follow-up work can be carried out with:

- Peer groups continuing to meet on their own.
- Older men and women meeting and working together, and younger men and women meeting and working together.
- All men meeting and working together and all women meeting and working together.
- All participants meeting and working together.

Any or all of these combinations may work, occasionally, sometimes, frequently, or always. Encourage peer groups to try out different combinations. Perhaps the one golden rule is that all participants should always listen to and respect the views of others. This rarely happens without having someone chosen as facilitator or moderator. But you can help to make it begin to work by reminding everyone of the ground rules and by ensuring, for instance, that each group has equal time to present its ideas to the others. You need to beware especially of men dominating women in mixed meetings, or of older community members ignoring the needs of younger ones. Otherwise, there is a danger of such meetings turning into shouting matches, creating or developing more arguments and resentment, rather than resolving differences.

3. WHAT TO FOLLOW UP WITH

In this list of possible topics for discussion, we suggest three different types of work:

- Conducting optional sessions O–R and the further open community meeting.
- Repetition of exercises which participants have already done.

- New topics which participants could explore, especially further work on assertiveness and on conflict resolution.

Conducting optional sessions O–R and the further open community meeting

These are all in this volume. They explore key issues such as supportive health care, support from partners, families, faith leaders and neighbours, support for women living with HIV during pregnancy, and support for other family members. These are all topics highlighted by previous *Stepping Stones* facilitators and trainers as needing more attention. Also, new research has shown[1] that these are the areas where women, once diagnosed with HIV, experience gender-based violence (GBV), often for the first time. So we highly recommend these additional sessions.

Repetition of exercises already done

Hold regular discussions about **condoms** and condom practices. Use a banana to putting a condom on properly and taking it off again properly with your eyes closed. It's dark at night, so people normally have to do this without looking. Can they?

Have further practices on skills to **overcome manipulation**.

Practise further standing your ground and **saying 'no!'**

Practise more **assertiveness**. Try other contexts for role play, such as in a shop, at the market, at the health centre, on buses, at a job interview, with extension workers, with the police, with more educated people, with government officials, and so on.

Discuss the issues of **wills and inheritance rights** further. Is anything changing? If so, how? If not, why not? What else can be done to help people with these?

Repeat any other exercises the participants may want to repeat.

New topics for participants to explore

Encourage participants to use **assertiveness** techniques to discuss the good and bad things about sex with their partners. Encourage them to role play, for instance, discussions about contraception, family planning, fears of impotence, pain on intercourse, what feels good about sex, and so on. Role play using 'I' statements in these discussions.

Explore participants' views on who it is **acceptable** to have sex with and who it is **unacceptable** to have sex with. Ask participants to draw diagrams on flip-chart paper, or on the ground, to explore their views on this. Peer groups can share their opinions with one another in a bigger meeting. (For instance, this may help in discussions about the rights and wrongs of girls being forced into sex by their uncles, or cousins, or older men.)

- Who pays for, or should pay for, **condoms**?
- Who pays for, or should pay for, **family planning?**
- Who should take **responsibility** for using condoms?
- Who should take responsibility for using family planning?

Hold discussions about how some people can find condoms difficult to use, to encourage them to keep going with them (which is better – discomfort or disease?).

- Discuss women's **access** to condoms and family planning.
- Also discuss men's access to condoms and family planning.

Help participants to develop further their own **self-esteem**. This can be particularly valuable for the young women's peer group but is important for everyone. For instance, ask each participant in turn to share answers to questions such as: "What is one thing that makes me feel really good? Do I give myself time to feel good each day? If so, how? If not, what could I start to do for myself for five minutes each day? What is one thing which I really like about myself?"

Questions like these can be extremely difficult for some people to answer and so they can be very helpful in encouraging people to develop some self-respect for themselves and a sense of self-worth. Refer to the manuals mentioned below for more exercises on this. Often, when people have developed their own sense of self-worth, they find themselves able to become more assertive and, in turn, more respected by other people. Even loud young men may actually be hiding a lack of self-confidence behind a brash exterior!

Explore exercises in **conflict resolution and mediation together**. There is no room to go into details here, but one conflict resolution technique is seven point problem-solving. Individuals or groups in dispute can attempt, either by themselves or with the help of a mediator whom both sides respect (you or a neutral third person in the community, whom both sides respect) to reach agreement by use of the following formula:

1. Each person states the problem as s/he sees it.
2. Each person tells the other what s/he heard him/her say.
3. Participants brainstorm possible solutions.
4. Select from these solutions ones which are acceptable to all.
5. Draw the solutions agreed upon, with symbols understood by everyone. Get each person to sign or put their thumbprint on the agreement.
6. Agree upon a time to review the agreement (e.g. one or two months' time).
7. Affirm the other person. This means that the two people involved in the conflict should shake hands, or acknowledge each other in some other way.

See *Stepping Stones for Peace and Prosperity* for more exercises on conflict resolution.

(See Annex 7 for more details about this and other publications.)

4. HOW TO STRUCTURE SESSIONS

Here are some brief ideas to help you structure the follow-up workshops, or to help you divide sessions in this manual into two meetings.

A good format for any session is shown below. It is the format which we have followed most often in this manual. Steps 2 to 4 are needed when a group has not met for a while, otherwise you can go straight from step 1 to step 5.

1. Warm-up exercises – ice-breakers, energisers to help participants feel at ease.
2. Trust games.
3. Ground rules – no smoking? no interruptions? listen to others? respect for others' views? etc.
4. Expectations (very important in the first session).
5. What do participants already know about the issue which is going to be discussed?
6. Main exercises – these can be longer and more detailed and should build on participants' existing knowledge, helping them to develop their ideas.
7. Wind-down exercises, to help participants come back to the reality of life.
8. Quick session review, with at least some volunteers. (See Annex 4 for details of this.)

5. EXTRA TIPS ON SESSION STYLES

It is always a good idea to vary the pace of a session quite a lot – to have pair work or small-group work followed by plenary feedback. Otherwise, people can get bored and fall asleep.

You can have energising games, like 'Fruit Salad' (which is a marvellous game to make people feel relaxed and refreshed) followed by more serious games, made up of groups named with the fruit salad fruit (e.g. mangoes over here, bananas in that corner, oranges over there ...). Techniques you could use include:

- Brainstorms (for instance 'Think of as many words as you can that mean "happiness" to you': One of the peer group could draw them all on a flip-chart and you would soon run out of paper!).
- Pair work, where individuals take it in turns to talk and to listen.
- Role plays and tableaux, as described in Annex 1.

If someone asks questions or raises issues which you don't want to answer or discuss at that particular stage of the session, you could just say that you will make space for further discussion at the end of the session. Or you could arrange to have an extra meeting to cover the issue(s) before the next session as scheduled in the manual. As a reminder, ask someone to draw a quick picture representing the issue(s) on a 'further issues' flip chart.

Last but not least, in training work, it always seems to be a good idea to use openness and humour. If you don't know something, be ready to say 'I don't know' and ask if anyone else knows. Or say you'll try to find out, if people would like you to.

ENDNOTE

1. Orza, L. Bewley, S., Chung, C., Crone, E.T., Nagadya, H., Vazquez, M., Welbourn, A., (2015) '"Violence, Enough Already": findings from a global participatory survey among women living with HIV'. *Journal of the International AIDS Society 2015*, 18 (Suppl 5): 20285, <http://dx.doi.org/10.7448/IAS.18.6.20285>.

ANNEX 6 WHO NEEDS WORKSHOPS?

In 'Before you Begin ...!' we emphasised the importance of recognising the needs of people of different genders and ages in the community where you plan to run the workshop. This annex also draws your attention to people with different positions or roles in the community. Before you run the progamme, it is also important to think about how these people could be involved.

LEADERS OR OFFICIALS

We have already recommended that permission should be sought from community leaders, before you start a workshop in a location. You may feel that some of these people should also be trained before the community workshops take place, or at the same time in a different setting.

For instance, you could run **separate**, smaller group workshops at people's places of work. Participants could be community leaders, local officials (e.g. government administration and extension staff and workers), other community development workers, religious leaders, voluntary agency workers, school teachers, and so on. Draw up with local community members a list of all such people they can think of in the area. Don't forget to ask each community group separately whom they think should be on the list!

Alternatively, the community with whom you plan to work may feel that it would be better for some officials to be involved **as ordinary participants** in the community workshops.

There are no hard and fast rules on the best time to involve leaders and officials. But beware: the presence of these people may influence what others say – or don't say – in the workshop. And often officials dominate or want to demonstrate their knowledge – which may not always be relevant or even correct. Alternatively, if they are not included, they may feel reluctant to support the workshop.

MARGINALISED PEOPLE

In all communities there are people who have lower social or economic status than others. These people rarely attend meetings. Often they are not told about them. Or, if they are told, they may not be able to attend because they have to work or are sick. Or they see no point in attending because they have never benefited from such meetings in the past. Or they are made to feel uncomfortable or unwelcome by other participants. **It is particularly important to ensure that these people are told about, and are enabled to be involved, in the workshop programme, if they want to be.** This is because poor and marginalised people are often very vulnerable to acquiring HIV and exploitation by others. They have the least say, the most ill-health, and the most work to do. They often work for other members of the community and have no land or savings to call their own. They tend to have very low level of self-esteem and are looked down on by others in the community.

In different communities, different people fall into the lowest socio-economic categories. They may be widows with many dependants, they may be young single mothers, they may be disabled people, they may be refugees who have settled in the community, they may be sex workers, or people who use drugs, or lesbian, bisexual or gay, or they may be transgender people. Who they are varies from one community to another. If you find it hard to know who the most vulnerable people in the community are (and even community members are often surprised by the vulnerability of their own neighbours), you could read RRA Notes No. 15. This describes how you can conduct a well-being ranking exercise with the community members. (See Annex 7 for full details of this resource and also of other resources related to different groups of vulnerable people.)

Once you have identified who the most vulnerable people in the community are, it would be best if they could attend the workshop sessions from the beginning. On the other hand, you may discover that their workloads are much heavier than those of others and that they are just not able to turn up to sessions as regularly as better-off community members. Or they may feel safer meeting separately.

Therefore you could think about running separate workshop sessions just for these most vulnerable people, at times of the year and day, and in locations, which fit in best with their limited availability and mobility.

OTHER KEY PEOPLE

Every community has a number of skilled practitioners who are respected by their neighbours. These include traditional birth attendants, traditional healers, traditional leaders, herbalists, circumcision practitioners, and so on. It is important to bear in mind what quality of contact you have with these key people. If you have developed a good relationship with them and they respect what you have to offer, their support in the community will be invaluable. It is of course also important to determine in a sensitive way the extent to which their practices may influence HIV transmission. If they are traditional healers, birth attendants, or circumcision practitioners, for instance, do they ever draw blood or use syringes? If so, is this done in a hygienic way? Your questions and any necessary follow-up need to be handled very delicately, in order to help the practitioners to feel included in, and not alienated by, your work.

In one part of Uganda where circumcision is practised, health officials recognised that shared use of the circumcision knife and the cloths used to clean and nurse circumcised people could promote HIV transmission. Therefore, circumcision practitioners were involved in sessions which explained about HIV transmission. The circumcisers explained, however, that it was relatives of the candidates for circumcision who insisted that they all be circumcised together, so that a blood bond be forged between them through the act of sharing. Therefore, the health officials realised that circumcision candidates themselves and their relatives also needed to understand the dangers of sharing. Once they too understood this, then a safer way of performing the operation could be worked out between the circumcisers and their clients

OTHER COMMUNITY MEMBERS

You may find that other community members come forward to join the peer groups when they see how much the participants are enjoying the sessions.

In Buwenda, the participants themselves discouraged late joiners. They said: 'It would be like having primary school students joining secondary school students, since we have already learnt so much.' It was agreed instead that a new course would start for new participants once the first course was finished. This decision met with everyone's agreement.

CONCLUSION

You and your co-facilitators will need to consult with one another, and with community members themselves, to decide on the best strategy to adopt for each of these groups of people in your community.

ANNEX 7 FURTHER RESOURCE MATERIALS

Revised by Nell Osborne and Sophie Dilmitis

A wide range of manuals, books, newsletters, and videos has influenced the material in this manual. This section includes additional resource materials to support your work. The list is not comprehensive and several organisations could be listed under several categories. but the resources listed will help you find websites and other references from which you can get additional information.

If you find other resources or websites helpful and they are not listed, do please let us know by writing to enquiries@steppingstonesfeedback.org

A. STEPPING STONES MATERIAL AND RELATED SUPPORT

B. RECOMMENDED FURTHER RESOURCES

1. Useful NGO websites for general information about HIV
2. Support networks for people living with HIV
3. Support networks and resources for other key populations
4. Training and manuals
5. Guidelines and checklists
6. Faith-based resources
7. Communication skills and conflict management
8. Sexual and reproductive health and rights
9. Participatory, inclusive approaches
10. Monitoring and evaluation (M&E)
11. Caring for health workers living with HIV
12. Legislation regarding HIV transmission
13. Education
14. Food security, livelihoods, and HIV
15. Gender equality
16. Health-related issues
17. Home-based care
18. Male circumcision
19. Men
20. Violence against women - safety and security: physical, sexual, psychological and financial dimensions
21. Supporting safe parenthood
22. Voluntary counselling and testing
23. Workplace
24. Young people

A. STEPPING STONES MATERIAL AND RELATED SUPPORT

(See www.steppingstonesfeedback.org)

- **Implementing Stepping Stones.** This manual, published by ACORD and based on its research in Ugandan, Angola and Tanzania, provides an excellent resource for anyone wishing to adapt and use the *Stepping Stones* manual or other community training manuals. Please contact us if you want to adapt the material and we could then send you this resource.

- **Stepping Stones Facilitators' Journal.** This reporting book, published by the Secretariat of the Pacific Community and the Foundation of the Peoples of the South Pacific International in 2009, is an invaluable additional resource for all using the manual. It enables facilitators to write down what emerges from each session. Contact us for a Word version if you would like to adapt it. http://www.steppingstonesfeedback.org/resources/33/SS_FSPI_FacilitatorJournal_Fiji_2009.pdf
- **The Stepping Stones International Community of Practice.** This is a 1,200-strong global network of people who have used, or are using, *Stepping Stones* material. It is free and open to join. Members receive a free email newsletter three to four times a year and, through this, learn across countries and continents about others' innovations in relation to the programme. www.steppingstonesfeedback.org
- **Stepping Stones For Peace and Prosperity.** This manual is specifically designed to support facilitators to run community workshops to improve communication and relationship skills and to promote peace and prosperity through reducing conflict and violence. It is recommended for *any* community affected by small arms proliferation, sexual violence and conflict. To order please email: ststk@steppingstonesfeedback.org
- **Stepping Stones with Children.** This manual is designed to work with children aged 5–14 affected by AIDS and their caregivers. It is designed to build resilience, mutual trust, and shared coping strategies and incorporates sessions on physical, psychological, sexual, and material well-being, including how our brains work. This is published by Practical Action Publishing. Please contact enquiries@steppingstonesfeedback.org
- **Stepping Stones Revisited: Stories from the village of Buwenda.** This short film takes us on a journey back to the village of Buwenda in southwest Uganda, to see what had happened 12 years after the original *Stepping Stones* workshop was conducted in 1994. Watch online at: https://vimeo.com/salamandertrust/steppingstonesrevisted
- **Seeking Safety: Stepping Stones in Malawi.** In this short documentary, members of the Coalition of Women Living with HIV and AIDS in Malawi (COWLHA) and their partners meet to discuss their use of the *Stepping Stones* programme to overcome gender-based violence, improve communication and relationship skills, and restore peace and prosperity in their families and communities. Order a DVD and accompanying interactive training handbook from: http://www.steppingstonesfeedback.org/index.php/page/Resources/gb?resourceid=74 or watch online at: https://vimeo.com/salamandertrust/seekingsafety
- **Stepping Stones Community of Practice Newsletter on Monitoring and Evaluation.** This newsletter edition highlights several ongoing challenges regarding effective monitoring and evaluation. http://us2.campaign-archive2.com/?u=24d198c33ed45c3d1513bf5ff&id=f624da86a1

RECOMMENDED FURTHER RESOURCES

1. USEFUL NGO WEBSITES FOR GENERAL INFORMATION ABOUT HIV

All the following organisations focus a lot of their work on HIV in the context of their particular experiences and expertise. Do contact them through their websites for further information.

- **What Works For Women and Girls.** What Works for Women and Girls provides the evidence to inform country-level programming. This website contains a comprehensive review, containing 2,500 articles and reports with data from close to 100 countries, that has uncovered a number of interventions for which there is substantial evidence of success:

from prevention, treatment, care, and support to strengthening the enabling environment for policies and programming. http://www.whatworksforwomen.org

- **International HIV/AIDS Alliance.** The Alliance exists to end AIDS through community action. The Alliance was founded in 1993 to support community groups in countries that were most affected by the global AIDS crisis and are building knowledge, mobilising people, inspiring leadership, and allowing all voices to play significant roles in the response to HIV. The Alliance work with communities in over 40 countries to take local, national, and global action on HIV, health and human rights. http://www.aidsalliance.org/resources
- **NAM Aidsmap.** NAM works to change lives by sharing information about HIV and AIDS. They believe independent, clear and accurate information is vital in the fight against HIV and AIDS. http://www.aidsmap.com/
- **i-Base HIV.** i-Base is a treatment activist group committed to providing timely and up-to-date information about HIV treatment to people living with HIV and to health-care professionals. This includes technical and non-technical publications that are available online and in different languages. i-Base also has a Q&A service (by phone, email and online). All resources are produced by and with the involvement of people living with HIV and are reviewed by a medical advisory group. www.i-base.info
- **The Body.** An online source of information on HIV and AIDS including news, research and resources on HIV prevention, testing, care, and treatment. http://www.thebody.com
- **AIDSPortal.** An online resource supporting the community response to HIV. http://www.aidsportal.org
- **AVERT.** AVERT is an international HIV and AIDS charity, based in the UK. Founded in 1986, AVERT provides people with knowledge about HIV to protect themselves and others from HIV, reduce stigma, and break down barriers to treatment and support. www.avert.org
- **HIV InSite.** University of California, San Francisco. http://hivinsite.ucsf.edu/
- **AVAC.** AVAC advocates for HIV prevention to end AIDS. http://www.avac.org/
- **Women4GF.** Women4GF brings together women's rights advocates – especially women living with HIV, and directly affected by TB and malaria — to advance gender equality through the Global Fund. Women4GF mobilises women in all their diversity to ensure that the world's most important finance mechanism for HIV, TB, and malaria supports programmes that meet the rights and needs of women and girls. http://women4gf.org

2. SUPPORT NETWORKS FOR PEOPLE LIVING WITH HIV

- **International Community of Women living with HIV.** ICW is the only global network run by and for women living with HIV. It was established in 1992 by women living with HIV as a response to the consistent silencing and marginalising of their concerns. http://www.iamicw.org
- **East Africa (ICW EA).** The International Community of Women living with HIV East Africa. http://www.icwea.org
- **The Well Project.** Online information for women living with HIV. http://www.thewellproject.org
- **The Global Network of People living with HIV (GNP+).** GNP+ exists to improve the quality of life of people living with HIV by facilitating equitable access to treatment, care, and support services for people living with HIV around the world. www.gnpplus.net
- **Unzip The Lips.** Unzip the Lips is a platform of individuals and organizations working for the rights and meaningful participation of key affected women and girls in the context of HIV and its intersections with other gender issues in the Asia-Pacific region. http://unzipthelips.org/
- **Salamander Trust.** Salamander aims to protect, promote, and enhance the health and rights of people particularly, but not exclusively, marginalised by societies worldwide as a result of their gender, HIV status or sexual and reproductive health. www.salamandertrust.net/
- **SHE Programme.** The SHE Programme is a safe, friendly information resource for HIV positive women and the issues surrounding HIV in women. http://www.shetoshe.org/

- **Positively UK.** Talk to and meet other people living with HIV and receive support around all aspects of your HIV. http://positivelyuk.org/

3. SUPPORT NETWORKS AND RESOURCES FOR OTHER KEY POPULATIONS

Here are some resources for sex workers, people who use drugs, gay and lesbian and transgender communities

Sex work

- **Global Network of Sex Work Projects (NSWP).** NSWP influences policy and builds leadership among sex workers and it facilitates the development of regional and national networks of sex workers and sex work projects. http://www.nswp.org
- **WHO.** *Implementing Comprehensive HIV/STI Programmes with Sex Workers: Practical approaches from collaborative interventions.* For overview and access to this document, see http://www.who.int/hiv/pub/sti/sex_worker_implementation/en/ [Accessed 30 January 2016]

People/women who use drugs

- **International Network of People who Use Drugs (INPUD).** INPUD is a movement of people who support the Vancouver Declaration. The Vancouver Declaration sets out our demand that the human rights of people who use drugs should be respected and for harm reduction measures to be put in place to protect individual and public health. http://www.inpud.net
- *Women who use drugs, harm reduction and HIV.* http://www.inpud.net/en/women-who-use-drugs-and-hiv
- **The Reference Group to the United Nations on HIV and Injecting Drug Use**. *Women who inject drugs: A review of their risks, experiences and needs.* http://www.unodc.org/documents/hiv-aids/Women_who_inject_drugs.pdf
- **Open Society Foundations**. *By Women, For Women: New approaches to harm reduction in Russia.* http://www.soros.org/publications/women-women-new-approaches-harm-reduction-russia

Gay and lesbian

- **OUTRIGHT Action International.** (Formerly known as the International Gay and Lesbian Commission.) Works to document and expose human rights violations against LGBTIQ people across the world. http://www.outrightinternational.org
- **Naz Foundation International.** Naz Foundation is a charity working in England, America, India, and Bangladesh, providing sexual health and HIV prevention, education, and counselling and support services. http://www.nfi.net
- **The Global Forum on MSM & HIV.** MSMGF is working worldwide against HIV for the health and human rights of men who have sex with men. http://www.msmgf.org/
- **Violence Against Women & Girls (VAWG).** *Brief on violence against sexual and gender minority women*. (Phil Crehan and Jennifer McCleary-Sills, 2015). Published in conjunction with the World Bank, Global Women's Institute, Inter-American Development Bank, International Center for Research on Women. http://www.vawgresourceguide.org/sites/default/files/briefs/vawg_resource_guide_sexual_and_gender_minority_women_final.pdf

Transgender

- **Transgender Law Center.** Transgender Law Center works to change law, policy, and attitudes so that all people can live safely, authentically, and free from discrimination regardless of their gender identity or expression. http://transgenderlawcenter.org

4. TRAINING AND MANUALS

- **ACORD (Agency for Cooperation and Research in Development).** An Africa-led international alliance working to promote social justice. Their HIV and AIDS Support and Advocacy Program – HASAP – provides training, technical support, and information-sharing. http://www.acordinternational.org/index.php/base/hiv
- **Strategies for Hope.** Strategies for Hope, the original publisher of this manual, promotes care, support and prevention in the field of HIV/AIDS in sub-Saharan Africa. They produce a wide range of materials available in English, French, and other languages, including practical handbooks such as the *Called to Care* toolkit and videos such as *What Can I Do?* featuring the HIV ministry of Canon Gideon Byamugisha of Uganda. All materials are available as free electronic downloads on the SFH website. www.stratshope.org
- **Raising Voices.** Raising Voices is a nonprofit organization based in Kampala, Uganda that is working toward the prevention of violence against women and children. They strive to influence the power dynamics shaping relationships between women and men, girls and boys by catalyzing social change in communities, rigorously studying and learning from the work they do, and sharing experiences to shape the field. http://raisingvoices.org/resources/
- **IPAS**, **The AIDS Society of the Philippines, and Health and Development Networks**. *Gender or sex: who cares?* Adaptable and practical educational and training materials on gender and reproductive health for healthcare and other service providers who work with youth. http://www.genderandaids.org/index.php?option=com_content&view=article&id=403:gender-or-sex-who-cares-notes-for-training-of-trainers&catid=45:training-materials-andor-tool-kits&Itemid=92
- **GNP+, ICW, Young Positives, EngenderHealth, IPPF, UNAIDS.** *Advancing the Sexual and Reproductive Health and Human Rights of People Living With HIV: A Guidance Package*. A training manual for healthworkers on SRHR (Sexual Reproductive Health and Rights) for people living with HIV. This provides information and structure for the care and support of women and adolescent girls living with HIV in the local context. The Resource is designed for programme managers and healthworkers for a four-day training and a two-day planning workshop for integrated SRH counselling and programme planning that links SRH and HIV/AIDS services. http://www.gnpplus.net/images/stories/SRHR/090811_srhr_of_plhiv_guidance_package_en.pdf
- **ACORD.** *Trainers' Handbook on HIV & AIDS Mainstreaming.* http://www.acordinternational.org/silo/files/trainers-handbook-on-hiv--aids-mainstreaming.pdf
- **ACORD.** *Condom Commandos*. A film showing how ACORD adapted *Stepping Stones* for use with soldiers in a barracks in Angola. http://www.acordinternational.org/silo/files/condom-commandos.mp4
- **FHI 360/C-Change**. *Compendium of Gender Scales*, by Geeta Nanda. https://www.c-changeprogram.org/content/gender-scales-compendium/pdfs/4.%20GEM%20Scale,%20Gender%20Scales%20Compendium.pdf

5. GUIDELINES AND CHECKLISTS

- **GNP+.** *Policy framework to implement Positive Health, Dignity and Prevention*. This policy framework highlights the importance of placing the person living with HIV at the centre of managing their health and wellbeing. http://www.gnpplus.net/resources/policy-framework-to-implement-positive-health-dignity-and-prevention/
- **UNAIDS.** *UNAIDS Gender Assessment Tool* (2014). The gender assessment tool for national HIV responses is intended to assist countries assess their HIV epidemic, context, and response from a gender perspective, helping them to make their HIV responses gender transformative and (as such) more effective. http://www.unaids.org/sites/default/files/media_asset/JC2543_gender-assessment_en.pdf

- **WHO.** *Consolidated guidelines on the use of antiretroviral drugs for treating and preventing HIV infection* (2013). http://www.who.int/hiv/pub/guidelines/arv2013/en/
- **WHO.** *Maximizing The Treatment and Prevention Potential of Antiretroviral Drugs: Early Country Experiences Towards Implementing a Treat-All Policy: Programmatic Update* (2015). http://apps.who.int/iris/bitstream/10665/183599/1/WHO_HIV_2015.35_eng.pdf
- **AIDS Accountability.** The AIDS Accountability Scorecard on Women. http://aidsaccountability.org/?page_id=920
- **Salamander Trust.** *The Participation Tree*. Recommendations for approaches to supporting, enabling, accompanying, and promoting the meaningful participation of HIV-positive women's networks, organisations and community support groups. http://salamandertrust.net/resources/13ICWWECARE_Policy%20briefing_ENGDakarSep2013.pdf
- **FIGO.** *Integrating human rights and health: A checklist for quality care*. http://www.figo.org/sites/default/files/uploads/wg-publications/wsrr/Introduction%20to%20HRWH%20Framework.pdf
- **WHO.** *Countdown to Zero: Global plan towards the elimination of new HIV infections among children by 2015 and keeping their mothers alive.* http://www.unaids.org/en/media/unaids/contentassets/documents/unaidspublication/2011/20110609_JC2137_Global-Plan-Elimination-HIV-Children_en.pdf
- **WHO.** *Tool to set and monitor targets for HIV prevention, diagnosis, treatment and care for key populations* (July 2015). http://www.who.int/hiv/pub/toolkits/kpp-monitoring-tools/en/

6. FAITH-BASED RESOURCES

- **INERELA+.** INERELA+ is an international network of religious leaders – lay and ordained, women and men – living with, or personally affected, by HIV. http://inerela.org/
- **World YWCA.** The World YWCA works to promote social, economic, cultural, religious, and political rights of women and girls through advocacy and services in priority areas including young women's leadership, sexual and reproductive health and rights, HIV and AIDS and violence against women. http://www.worldywca.org/
- **Christian Aid.** Christian Aid works on HIV awareness raising to supporting human rights and tackling the route causes of poverty. See, in particular, the SAVE Approach. http://christianaid.org.uk/images/HIVSAVELeaflet2010.pdf
- **CAFOD.** CAFOD is the official aid agency of the Catholic Church in England and Wales and part of Caritas International. Selected resources responding to HIV are available on its website. http://www.cafod.org.uk/search?basicsearch%5Bterm%5D=HIV
- **Ecumenical Advocacy Alliance.** The Ecumenical Advocacy Alliance is a diverse global network of churches and related organisations committed to campaigning together on common concerns for justice and human dignity. www.e-alliance.ch
- **Strategies for Hope.** Strategies for Hope promotes care, support and prevention in HIV/AIDS in sub-Saharan Africa. The *Called to Care toolkit* is a set of practical, action-oriented booklets and mini-manuals on issues related to HIV/AIDS that are designed for use by church leaders, especially in sub-Saharan Africa. http://www.stratshope.org/resources/called_to_care
- **Islamic Relief.** *Positive Living*, the Islamic Relief awareness programme, is aimed at prevention, care, and support for people living with HIV and gender-based violence. http://www.islamic-relief.org/feature-hiv-aids-prevention-and-care/
- **American Jewish World Service (AJWS).** AJWS supports women, girls, and LGBT people, as they organise to end discrimination, stop violence, and live with dignity, safety, and health. https://ajws.org/what-we-do/sexual-health-and-rights/
- **UNICEF and Sangha Metta Project.** *A Buddhist Approach to HIV Prevention and AIDS Care: A training manual for monks, nuns and other Buddhist leaders*. (Lawrence Maund, 2006) http://www.unicef.org/eapro/A_buddhish_approach_to_HIV.pdf

7. COMMUNICATION SKILLS AND CONFLICT MANAGEMENT

- **GNP+.** *Language, identity and HIV: The responsible use of language.* http://www.gnpplus.net/resources/language-identity-and-hiv-the-responsible-use-of-language/
- **Understanding Violence.** To read about violence and its causes, especially in young men, we recommend *Preventing Violence* by James Gilligan (Thames and Hudson, 2001).
- **Infectious Diseases Institute.** *Using a clinic based creativity initiative to reduce HIV related stigma, at the Infectious Diseases Unit, Mulago National Referral Hospital, Uganda.* http://www.ncbi.nlm.nih.gov/pubmed/23056033
- *Drugs, hopes and dreams: appreciative inquiry with marginalized young people using drugs and alcohol.* Elspeth McAdam and K. A. H. Mirzab. http://www.thinklocalactpersonal.org.uk/_library/News/Jan15/JOFT_2009_Appreciative_Inquiry__Elspeth_and_Mirza.pdf
- **Mainstreaming HIV in German Development Cooperation.** *Crisis, Conflict and Peace Building.* https://sites.google.com/a/ms-hiv-gdc.org/mainstreaming-hiv-in-german-development-cooperation/Home/sectors-priority-areas/development-oriented-emergency-aid

8. SEXUAL AND REPRODUCTIVE HEALTH AND RIGHTS

- **Salamander Trust.** *Building a Safe House on Firm Ground: Key Findings from a global values and preferences survey regarding the sexual and reproductive health and human rights of women living with HIV.* http://salamandertrust.net/resources/BuildingASafeHouseOnFirmGroundFINALreport190115.pdf
- **Salamander Trust.** *There is life after HIV: The Mama's Club Psychosocial Care and Support Programme, Uganda.* A short documentary that can be watched online at https://vimeo.com/salamandertrust/lifeafterhiv or order the hard copy DVD and interactive training handbook. http://salamandertrust.net/index.php/Projects/UNAIDS_Participatory_Film_Project/
- **The Pregnancy Journey when you are living with HIV.** A short documentary about the 'From Pregnancy to Baby and Beyond' project. The film highlights the key importance of peer network support, led by and for women living with HIV, through the pregnancy journey. Order a DVD and accompanying interactive training handbook from: http://salamandertrust.net/index.php/Projects/Rights_Camera_Action. Watch online at: https://vimeo.com/salamandertrust/pregnancyjourney
- **Protection The Film.** A training programme for condom use as a crucial strategy to help men and boys avoid HIV. The film shows men and youth in South Africa, Kenya and Sierra Leone addressing the condom challenge in different ways. Created by Jill Lewis. http://protectionthefilm.org/
- **ATHENA Network.** *In Women's Words.* Action agenda translating the 2011 political declaration of the High Level Meeting on AIDS into action for women, girls, and gender equality. http://www.athenanetwork.org/assets/files/Action%20agenda/womenswords_0531-%20FINAL.pdf
- **UNAIDS.** *Achieving sexual and reproductive health and rights for women and girls through the HIV response.* http://www.unwomen-eseasia.org/docs/2009_Diamonds.pdf
- **APN+ and UN Women.** *Diamonds: Stories of women from the Asia-Pacific network of people living with HIV* by Susan Paxton. http://www.unifem.org/materials/item_detail.php?ProductID=163
- **UNFPA.** *Preventing HIV and unintended pregnancies: strategic framework 2011–2015.* http://www.unfpa.org/public/home/publications/pid/10575
- Chitembo A, Dilmitis S, Edwards O, Foote C, Griffiths L, Moroz S, et al. Towards an HIV-free generation: getting to zero or getting to rights? Reprod Health Matters J. 2012;20(39):513.
- **ATHENA Network.** *Bridging the Gap: Addressing contentious and neglected issues at the intersection of SRHR and HIV.* http://www.athenanetwork.org/assets/files/Bridging%20the%20Gap/Bridging_the_Gap_Report.pdf

- **Reproductive Health Matters Journal.** *Towards an HIV-free generation: getting to zero or getting to rights?* Amina Chitembo, Sophie Dilmitis, Olive Edwards et al. This offers a commentary by women living with HIV. on the Global Plan Towards the Elimination of New HIV Infections Among Children by 2015 and Keeping Their Mothers Alive http://http://www.rhm-elsevier.com/article/S0968-8080(12)39638-9/fulltext
- **Center for Health and Gender Equality.** *What Does Family Planning Have to do with HIV? Everything.* http://www.genderandaids.org/index.php?option=com_content&view=article&id=1085:what-does-family-planning-have-to-do-with-hiv-everything&catid=81:prevention&Itemid=111
- **Engender Health.** For decades, EngenderHealth has improved the lives of men, women, and families through its work in family planning, maternal health, HIV and AIDS, gender equity, and many other programme. https://www.engenderhealth.org/our-work/
- **Female Health Company.** Manufactures female condoms designed for safer sex under female control and dual protection against unintended pregnancy and sexually transmitted diseases. Their website provides information and resources on the use of the female condom including diagrams illustrating how the female condom should be inserted into the vagina. http://www.femalehealth.com
- **International Planned Parenthood Federation (IPPF).** IPPF is made up of national Member Associations that deliver sexual and reproductive health services and advocacy. http://www.ippf.org/

9. PARTICIPATORY, INCLUSIVE APPROACHES

The right of all citizens to participate in decisions about what happens to them in their lives is enshrined in the UN Declaration of Human Rights, created in 1948. People with HIV are still seeking for this right to be meaningfully respected. Below are some references about participation in general and about the greater involvement of people living with or affected by HIV and AIDS (GIPA).

- **IIED.** *RRA Notes 15: Wealth Ranking.* Information about on wealth and wellbeing ranking that you can refer to in order to identify who is most marginalised in the community where you are working. http://pubs.iied.org/6084IIED.html?k=RRA%20Notes%2015
- **IIED.** IIED publishes PLA Notes which covers a large range of participatory tools and approaches. Particularly helpful are *RRA Notes 15: Applications for Health*, and *PLA Notes 23: Section on Participatory Approaches to HIV/AIDS Programmes*. You can access all of these through the search box on the IIED Publications page. http://pubs.iied.org/
- **ATHENA Network.** The ATHENA Network publishes a wide range of information, some of which was highlighted on the previous page. Their *Community Innovations* reports highlight a wide range of powerful community-based interventions from around the world. http://www.athenanetwork.org/our-work/promoting-sexual-and-reproductive-health-and-rights/community-innovation.html
- *Denver Principles 1993.* There is no better way to cite the history of the self-empowerment movement of people living with HIV than to quote the principles articulated in Denver in 1983. They are as relevant and powerful today as they were then. http://data.unaids.org/pub/ExternalDocument/2007/gipa1983denverprinciples_en.pdf
- **UNAIDS.** *The Greater Involvement of People Living with HIV.* Policy brief from March 2007. http://data.unaids.org/pub/BriefingNote/2007/jc1299_policy_brief_gipa.pdf
- **The Institute of Development Studies (IDS).** The IDS is a leading organisation for research, teaching and communications on international development. www.ids.ac.uk
- **ICW.** *The Tree of Participation*, based on UNICEF's ladder of participation, was commissioned over 10 years after the GIPA principle was articulated and highlights the importance of having HIV positive people involved at all levels of decision-making. http://www.icw.org/node/136

- **UN.** *Universal Declaration of Human Rights* (1948). http://www.un.org/Overview/rights.html
- **ICRW.** *Understanding and Challenging HIV stigma: toolkit for action*. http://www.icrw.org/files/publications/Understanding-and-Challenging-HIV-Stigma-Toolkit-for-Action.pdf

10. MONITORING AND EVALUATION (M&E)

These resources are a useful addition to the M&E approaches described in Annex 4, and in our other resources listed in Part A of this annex

- **AWID.** *Strengthening Monitoring and Evaluation: 13 Insights for Women's Organizations* http://www.awid.org/publications/strengthening-monitoring-and-evaluation-13-insights-womens-organizations
- **DM&E for Peace.** Page 10 of this organisation's *Indicator Module* describes SPICED indicators which are used to demonstrate change in a situation, or the progress in, or results of, an activity, project, or program. www.dmeforpeace.org/sites/default/files/3.9%20Indicators.pdf.
- **Global Fund for Women.** A short film about how to measure progress using a change matrix. https://www.youtube.com/watch?v=C92s4k3t2Mg

11. CARING FOR HEALTH WORKERS LIVING WITH HIV

- **Public Health England.** *The Management of HIV infected Healthcare Workers who perform exposure prone procedures: updated guidance, January 2014.* https://www.gov.uk/government/uploads/system/uploads/attachment_data/file/333018/Management_of_HIV_infected_Healthcare_Workers_guidance_January_2014.pdf
- **Kerry, E. U., Nash. J. and Avalos, A. (2007)** 'Caring for the Caregivers: Models of HIV/AIDS Care and Treatment Provision for Health Care Workers in Southern Africa', *Journal of Infectious Diseases*, Dec 07, vol. 196, SUP3. http://jid.oxfordjournals.org/content/196/Supplement_3/S500.long
- **Physicians for Human Rights.** *Epidemic of Inequality: Women's Rights and HIV/AIDS in Botswana & Swaziland* (2007). http://physiciansforhumanrights.org/library/reports/botswana-swaziland-epidemic-of-inequality.html
- **Physicians for Human Rights.** *Bold Solutions to Africa's Health Worker Shortage* (2006), Section 4, on pages 7 and 8, considers healthcare for health workers in Swaziland. http://physiciansforhumanrights.org/library/reports/report-boldsolutions-2006.html
- **World Health Organization (WHO).** WHO is the directing and coordinating authority for health within the United Nations system. Their website provides policy resources and health publications in different languages. See their initiative in relation to care for health workers living with HIV: *Treat, Train, Retain: The AIDS and health workforce plan* (2006). http://www.who.int/hiv/pub/meetingreports/TTRmeetingreport2.pdf

12. LEGISLATION REGARDING HIV TRANSMISSION

Many countries have punitive legislation specific to having HIV on entry and HIV transmission. Some international legal organisations and UNAIDS have raised their concerns about these measures, arguing that punitive legislation does not work.

- **Canadian HIV/AIDS Legal Network.** This network promotes the human rights of people living with and vulnerable to HIV in Canada and internationally, through research, legal and policy analysis, education, and community mobilization. http://www.aidslaw.ca
- **Canadian HIV/AIDS Legal Network.** *HIV Disclosure to Sexual Partners: Questions and answers for newcomers* (2015). http://www.aidslaw.ca/site/hiv-disclosure-to-sexual-partners-qa-for-newcomers/
- **HIV Justice Network.** The HIV Justice Network is a global information and advocacy hub for individuals and organisations working to end the inappropriate use of the criminal law to regulate and punish people living with HIV. http://www.hivjustice.net

- **Edwin Cameron.** Plenary speech at the International AIDS Conference in Mexico 2008. Edwin Cameron is a South African Supreme Court judge who was the first senior official to state publicly that he was living with HIV/AIDS. https://www.afao.org.au/library/topic/government/Cameron_speech_Mexico_International_AIDS_Conference_2008.pdf
- **The United Nations Joint Programme on HIV/AIDS (UNAIDS).** *Background Paper on Criminalisation of HIV Non-Disclosure, Exposure and Transmission: Background and Current Landscape, February 2012, Revised Version.* http://www.unaids.org/sites/default/files/en/media/unaids/contentassets/documents/document/2012/BackgroundCurrentLandscapeCriminalisationHIV_Final.pdf
- **Open Society Foundations.** The Open Society Foundations work to build vibrant and tolerant democracies whose governments are accountable to their citizens. *10 reasons to oppose the criminalization of HIV exposure or transmission* is one useful document. https://www.opensocietyfoundations.org/sites/default/files/10reasons_20081201.pdf
- *Respect, Protect and Fulfill: Legislating for Women's Rights in the Context of HIV and AIDS*. http://www.aidslaw.ca/EN/womensrights/english.htm
- **ATHENA Network.** *10 Reasons Why Criminalisation of HIV Exposure or Transmission Harms Women.* http://www.athenanetwork.org/our-work/promoting-sexual-and-reproductive-health-and-rights/10-reasons-why-criminalization-harms-women.html
- **Commission on HIV and the Law.** *Criminalisation of HIV Exposure and Transmission: A Global Review.* http://hivlawcommission.org/index.php/working-papers?task=document.viewdoc&id=90
- **Commission on HIV and the Law.** *Gender-Based Violence, Criminal Law Enforcement and HIV.* http://hivlawcommission.org/index.php/working-papers?task=document.viewdoc&id=91
- **Commission on HIV and the Law**. *Human Rights, the Law, and HIV among Transgender People.* http://hivlawcommission.org/index.php/working-papers?task=document.viewdoc&id=93
- **UNAIDS.** *Report of the International Task Team on HIV-related Travel Restrictions: Findings and Recommendations.* http://www.unaids.org/en/media/unaids/contentassets/dataimport/pub/report/2009/jc1715_report_inter_task_team_hiv_en.pdf

13. EDUCATION

- **Education as a vaccine.** Education as a Vaccine is a non-profit organization created in 2000 to improve the health and development of children and young people. http://www.evanigeria.org/
- **Eldis.** Eldis is an online database of resources and policy documents on development issues. http://www.eldis.org/education/
- **Kenya Network of Positive Teachers (KENEPOTE).** This network made the film referenced below. It raises the profile of people living with HIV who are continuing to live and work and make a great contribution to society. http://hivhealthclearinghouse.unesco.org/library/documents/kenya-network-positive-teachers-kenepote-hiv-and-aids-planning-workshop-report
- **Imperial College and World Bank.** *Courage and Hope*. Film on teachers living with HIV who are members of KENEPOTE in Kenya. http://www3.imperial.ac.uk/newsandeventspggrp/imperialcollege/newssummary/news_3-12-2008-15-58-23
- **The United Nations Educational, Scientific and Cultural Organisation (UNESCO).** UNESCO encourages international peace and universal respect by promoting collaboration among nations. It conducts studies and facilitates knowledge-sharing. **UNESCO.** The EDUCAIDS initiative is UNESCO's comprehensive education sector response. http://www.unesco.org/new/en/hiv-and-aids/our-priorities-in-hiv/educaids/
- **UNESCO.** *Making the Case for HIV/AIDS/STI Prevention through Schools* provides arguments for communities and schools to benefit from HIV/STI prevention. http://www.ibe.unesco.org/fileadmin/user_upload/HIV_and_AIDS/publications/FRESH_general_all.pdf

- **The World Bank.** The World Bank is an internationally supported bank that provides financial and technical assistance to developing countries for development programmes. http://www.worldbank.org/en/topic/education

14. FOOD SECURITY, LIVELIHOODS AND HIV

- **STOP AIDS NOW!** *Food Security, Livelihoods & HIV/AIDS.* STOP AIDS NOW! aims to expand and enhance the quality of the Dutch contribution to the AIDS response, working with various partners. http://www.stopaidsnow.org/food-security-livelihoods-amp-hivaids
- **Food and Agricultural Organisation of the United Nations (FAO).** *HIV/AIDS, food security and rural livelihoods*. Achieving food security for all is at the heart of FAO's efforts – to make sure people have regular access to enough high-quality food to lead active, healthy lives. http://www.fao.org/worldfoodsummit/english/fsheets/aids.pdf
- **OXFAM.** OXFAM is a non-governmental organization working worldwide to fight poverty and injustice which also has a focus on sustainable food. https://www.oxfam.org/en/explore/issues/sustainable-food
- **UNAIDS.** UNAIDS Policy Brief: *HIV, food security and nutrition* (2008). http://www.unaids.org/sites/default/files/media_asset/jc1515_policy_brief_nutrition_en_1.pdf

15. GENDER EQUALITY

- **ATHENA Network.** This organisation seeks to advance gender equity and human rights in the global HIV response. http://www.athenanetwork.org
- **Association for Women in Development (AWID).** An international, feminist, membership organisation committed to achieving gender equality, sustainable development and women's human rights. http://www.awid.org
- **MENENGAGE.** An alliance of NGOs working together with men and boys to promote gender equality. http://menengage.org
- **BRIDGE.** A specialised gender and development research and information service based at the Institute of Development Studies (IDS) in the UK. BRIDGE supports gender advocacy and mainstreaming efforts of policymakers and practitioners by bridging the gaps between theory, policy, and practice. http://www.bridge.ids.ac.uk
- **Global Coalition on Women and AIDS (GCWA).** A worldwide alliance bringing together civil society groups working on HIV, women, girls, and gender equality, including networks of women living with HIV, women's rights organizations, AIDS service organizations, faith-based organizations, networks of women from key populations, care-giving networks, men and boy's organizations working explicitly for gender equality, the private sector, and the United Nations system, hosted by the UNAIDS secretariat. https://gcwa.unaids.org/
- **UN Women.** Works on human development and human rights issues that have gender dimensions. UN Women focuses on priority areas that are fundamental to women's equality, and that can unlock progress across the board. http://www.unwomen.org/en

16. HEALTH-RELATED ISSUES

- **UNAIDS.** *Women out loud: How women living with HIV will help the world end AIDS.* http://www.unaids.org/en/resources/presscentre/featurestories/2012/december/20121211womenoutloud
- **The Stop TB Partnership.** *Women and Tuberculosis.* http://www.stoptb.org/assets/documents/resources/factsheets/womenandtb.pdf
- **GBCHealth.** *Women and TB: How to Respond*. http://www.gbchealth.org/system/documents/category_1/73/GBCHealth%20Issue%20Brief_Women%20&%20TB.pdf?1314216806

- **Global Coalition on Women and AIDS.** *Tackling TB and HIV in Women: An Urgent Need* Agenda (2010). This is one of a series of briefing papers published by the GCWA to deepen the agenda on women and AIDS, to build consensus among a larger group of AIDS and women's health advocates on key messages and evidence, and to set out clear recommendations and calls for next steps and actions. http://women4gf.org/wp-content/uploads/2013/10/Tackling-TB-and-HIV-in-Women-copy.pdf
- **The Global Fund to Fight HIV, TB and malaria.** The Global Fund was created to finance HIV/AIDS, tuberculosis, and malaria programmes in countries. www.theglobalfund.org/

17. HOME-BASED CARE

Good home-based care of people with HIV and their families forms an essential part of keeping them happy, healthy, safe, and alive. Yet home-based care can also put a huge strain on already overworked women and girls. The following references provide more information about this.

- **Home Based Care Alliance (HCBA)**. HBCA represents over 30,000 caregivers and is organized into multi-district home-based care alliances in 11 African countries. http://homebasedcarealliance.org/
- **VSO International.** *VSO's Position on Community and Home Based Care.* http://www.ivoindia.org/Images/vso-position-on-community-and-home-based-care_tcm78-36846.pdf
- **HelpAge International.** HelpAge aims to improve the lives of disadvantaged older people. http://www.helpage.org/
- **ACORD.** *Caregiving in HIV affected households*. ACORD's vision is that of a society in which all citizens are equally able to achieve their rights and fulfill their responsibilities. http://www.acordinternational.org/our-work/acords-work/hiv/caregiving-in-hiv-affected-households/
- **STOPAIDS.** *Care and Support: The Forgotten Pillar of the HIV Response*. STOPAIDS is the network of UK agencies working since 1986 to secure an effective global response to HIV and AIDS. http://stopaids.org.uk/wp-content/uploads/2013/08/CareSupportAdvocacyDoc2011Compressed.pdf

18. MALE CIRCUMCISION

Male circumcision is now being rolled out in many countries, especially in east and southern Africa, as there is evidence that male circumcision reduces the risk of heterosexually acquired HIV in men by approximately 60%. However there are also challenges with this (see more about these in Session F).

- **WHO.** *Voluntary medical male circumcision for HIV prevention in 14 priority countries in East and Southern Africa.* Progress brief. http://www.who.int/hiv/pub/malecircumcision/brief2015/en/
- **WHO.** *Operational guidance for scaling up male circumcision services for HIV prevention* (2008). http://www.who.int/hiv/pub/malecircumcision/op_guidance/en/
- **AVERT.** *Voluntary Medical Male Circumcision For HIV Prevention.* http://www.avert.org/professionals/hiv-prevention-programming/voluntary-medical-male-circumcision

19. MEN

Other programmes, as well as *Stepping Stones*, seek to work with men as well as women in communities. Here are some references to some of them.

- **Raising Voices**. Raising voices is a small organisation based in Kampala, Uganda, that is recognised internationally for its creative and practical preventative approaches. It provides consultations to international organisations on programme development, technical support and capacity building, particularly in the field of violence against women and children. Its website displays articles and programme tools on violence prevention including ***SASA!***

which (along with *Stepping Stones*) is one of the few community programmes that has been proved in a randomised control trial to be effective in reducing gender-based violence in communities. http://www.raisingvoices.org

- **Sonke Gender Justice.** Sonke's vision is a world in which men, women and children can enjoy equitable, healthy and happy relationships that contribute to the development of just and democratic societies. http://www.genderjustice.org.za/
- **MenEngage.** MenEngage members work collectively and individually toward advancing gender justice, human rights, and social justice to achieve a world in which all can enjoy healthy, fulfilling, and equitable relationships and their full potential. http://www.menengage.org
- **ICRW and Promundo.** *Engaging Men and Boys To Achieve Gender Equality: How Can We Build on What We Have Learned? An evaluation and review of interventions with men and boys.* http://www.icrw.org/files/publications/Engaging-Men-and-Boys-to-Achieve-Gender-Equality-How-Can-We-Build-on-What-We-Have-Learned.pdf
- **EngenderHealth and Planned Parenthood Association of South Africa (PPASA).** *Men As Partners: A Program for Supplementing the Training of Life Skills Educators*. Designed to train community health educators in the facilitation of educational workshops with groups of men on reproductive health issues within a gender framework. http://www.comminit.com/en/node/271316/38#
- **Promundo.** A Brazilian NGO working to promote sexual and reproductive health among adolescent males. It specializes in research, training, policy advocacy, and implementing community-based interventions. They provide a range of materials in Portuguese and in English such as clips that can be used in workshops and trainings dealing with masculinities, gender socialisation and violence against women. See particularly *Once Upon a Boy, Once Upon a Girl* (http://promundoglobal.org/resources/once-upon-a-girl/), *Afraid of What*? (http://promundoglobal.org/resources/afraid-of-what/), and *It's Not Easy* (http://promundoglobal.org/resources/5194/).

20. VIOLENCE AGAINST WOMEN — SAFETY AND SECURITY: PHYSICAL, SEXUAL, PSYCHOLOGICAL AND FINANCIAL DIMENSIONS

Reports by various international organisations document the links between violence and HIV. Violence heightens risk of acquiring HIV and HIV heightens violence.

- **Development Connections & ICW Global.** *Violence against Women living with HIV: A Background Paper* by Fiona Hale and Marijo Vazquez. http://salamandertrust.net/resources/VAPositiveWomenBkgrdPaperMarch2011.pdf
- **UNAIDS.** *Women living with HIV speak out against violence.* http://www.unaids.org/en/resources/documents/2014/womenlivingwithhivspeakout
- **WHO.** *Violence against women. Factsheet number 239.* http://www.who.int/mediacentre/factsheets/fs239/en/
- **UN Women.** *Effective approaches to addressing the intersection of violence against women and HIV/AIDS. http://www.eldis.org/go/home&id=69118&type=Document#.VpvldSqLTcs*
- **WHO.** *Multi-country Study on Women's Health and Domestic Violence against Women: Initial results on prevalence, health outcomes and women's responses* by Claudia Garcia-Moreno, Henrica A.F.M. Jansen, Mary Ellsberg, Lori Heise, and Charlotte Watts (2005). http://www.who.int/gender/violence/who_multicountry_study/summary_report/summary_report_English2.pdf
- **One in Nine Campaign.** *We Were Never Meant to Survive: Violence in the Lives of HIV Positive Women in South Africa.* http://www.phmovement.org/sites/www.phmovement.org/files/We%20Were%20Never%20Meant%20to%20Survive%20-%20Violence%20in%20the%20Lives%20of%20HIV%20Positive%20Women%20.pdf

- **Eldis.** Eldis aims to share the best in development, policy, practice and research. www.eldis.org
- **Raising Voices.** This is a small organisation based in Kampala, Uganda, recognized internationally for its creative and practical preventative approaches. It provides consultations to international organisations on programme development, technical support, and capacity building, particularly in the field of violence against women and children. Its website displays articles and programme tools on violence prevention including the *SASA!* programme. http://www.raisingvoices.org
- **ICW.** *New Research on Women's Experiences of ACTS.* Three reports from Kenya, Tanzania, and Namibia. (2006) http://www.icw.org/node/224
- **Amnesty International.** NGO aiming to protect human rights worldwide by producing reports, press releases, appeals for action, and newsletters. See *'I am at the lowest end of all': Rural women living with HIV face human rights abuses in South Africa.* (2008) http://www.amnesty.org/en/library/info/AFR53/001/2008/en
- **IDS.** *Sexual safety, sexuality & HIV*. http://www.ids.ac.uk/idsresearch/ids-sexuality-and-development-programme
- **Salamander Trust and Namibian Women's Health Network**. *Stop Abusing Widows (2015*). In many parts of the world, women have unequal access to property or inheritance rights. This inequity can make them both more vulnerable to acquiring HIV and more vulnerable to the consequences of HIV. https://vimeo.com/147866910

21. SUPPORTING SAFE PARENTHOOD

Now that more people with HIV are able to access antiretroviral treatment, more people are also able to fulfil their dream of having a family. This topic is a central part of later sessions in this volume.

- **Mama's Club.** A psychosocial support network for young women living with HIV in Uganda. See some films made by members of Mama's Club with support from Salamander Trust here: http://salamandertrust.net/index.php/Projects/UNAIDS_Participatory_Film_Project/ http://www.mamasclubonline.com
- **From Pregnancy to Baby and Beyond.** This project was started by Positively UK in partnership with clinicians to help women living with HIV make informed choices and decisions around pregnancy, birth, and the care of themselves and their babies. *See Rights, Camera, Action* in Section 8 of this annex for more details.
- **i-base.** *Guide to HIV, pregnancy, and women's health.* http://i-base.info/guides/pregnancy/pdf
- **APN.** *Positive and Pregnant: how dare you.* http://www.asiapacificalliance.org/component/content/article/91-resources/413-positive-and-pregnant-how-dare-you-.html
- **GNP+.** *Consultations with people living with HIV on PMTCT.* http://www.gnpplus.net/resources/consultations-with-people-living-with-hiv-on-pmtct/
- *HIV, women and motherhood.* Audio interviews with women living with HIV. http://www.salamandertrust.net/index.php/Projects/The_HIV,_Women_and_Motherhood_Audio_Project/
- **WHO.** *Guidance on Couples HIV testing and counselling including Antiretroviral therapy for treatment and prevention in serodiscordant couples*: *Recommendations for a public health approach* (2012). This document explains how 'serodiscordant' couples, (where one partner has HIV and the other doesn't) can still be supported to conceive safely. http://apps.who.int/iris/bitstream/10665/44646/1/9789241501972_eng.pdf
- **The Body.** A forum on the Body website provides space for discussion of safer sex between 'serodiscordant' couples http://www.thebody.com/Forums/AIDS/SafeSex/
- **Women, Children, and HIV.** Resources on the prevention and treatment of HIV infection in women and children targeted at health workers, programme managers, and policy makers in resource-poor settings. http://www.womenchildrenhiv.org

22. VOLUNTARY COUNSELLING AND TESTING

- **WHO.** *Guidance on Couples HIV testing and counselling including antiretroviral therapy for treatment and prevention in serodiscordant couples: Recommendations for a public health approach* (2012). http://apps.who.int/iris/bitstream/10665/44646/1/9789241501972_eng.pdf
- **WHO.** *Consolidated guidelines on HIV testing services.* The consolidated guidelines on HIV testing services bring together existing guidance relevant to the provision of HIV testing services (HTS) and address issues and elements for effective delivery of HTS that are common in a variety of settings, contexts and diverse populations 2015. http://www.who.int/hiv/pub/guidelines/hiv-testing-services/en/
- **WHO states.** "All HIV testing services must include the 5 C's recommended by WHO: informed Consent, Confidentiality, Counselling, Correct test results and Connection (linkage to care, treatment and other services)." See Fact sheet No. 360 for more on this. http://www.who.int/mediacentre/factsheets/fs360/en/
- **EngenderHealth.** An NGO that aims to improve the health and wellbeing of people in poor communities by sharing expertise in sexual and reproductive health issues. Their website hosts several resources related to counselling and informed choice and consent. http://www.engenderhealth.org/pubs/counseling-informed-choice/index.php

23. WORKPLACE

- **International Labour Office (ILO).** *A workplace policy on HIV/AIDS: what it should cover.* http://www.ilo.org/wcmsp5/groups/public/@ed_protect/@protrav/@ilo_aids/documents/publication/wcms_121313.pdf
- **ACORD.** Workplace policies on HIV. http://www.acordinternational.org/our-work/a/hiv/workplace/
- **NGO Code of Conduct.** The purpose of this code of conduct offers guidance on how international non-governmental organizations (NGOs) can work in host countries in a way that respects and supports the primacy of the government's responsibility for organizing health system delivery. http://ngocodeofconduct.org

24. YOUNG PEOPLE

- **Healthy, Happy and Hot.** A guide for young people on their [sexual] rights. http://ippf.org/resources/publications/healthy-happy-hot
- **Youth Rise.** *Aint I a Woman? Recognising and protecting the rights of young women affected by drug use.* http://youthrise.org/youth-rise-reform-drug-policy-series/aint-i-a-woman
- **IPAS.** An international organization that works around the world to increase women's ability to exercise their sexual and reproductive rights. http://www.ipas.org
- **IPAS.** *Fulfilling reproductive rights for women affected by HIV/AIDS*. This is a tool designed by Maria de Bruyn for monitoring progress toward three of the Millennium Development Goals when working with young people on sexual health.
- **International HIV/AIDS Alliance**. *Orphans and Other Vulnerable Children Support Toolkit*, produced with Family Health International (FHI), contains an electronic library of more than 650 resources about supporting orphans and vulnerable children. These have been gathered from a wide range of organizations, drawing on years of experience. https://www.iywg.org/resources/orphans-and-other-vulnerable-children-support-toolkit
- **Strategies for Hope.** *The Child Within* (Called to Care toolkit number 6). Strategies for Hope promotes care, support and prevention in the field of HIV/AIDS, especially in sub-Saharan Africa. http://www.stratshope.org/resources/called_to_care_item/the-child-within
- **UNICEF.** The United Nations Children's Fund works for children's rights, their survival, development and protection. It is guided by the Convention on the Rights of the Child. http://www.unicef.org/aids

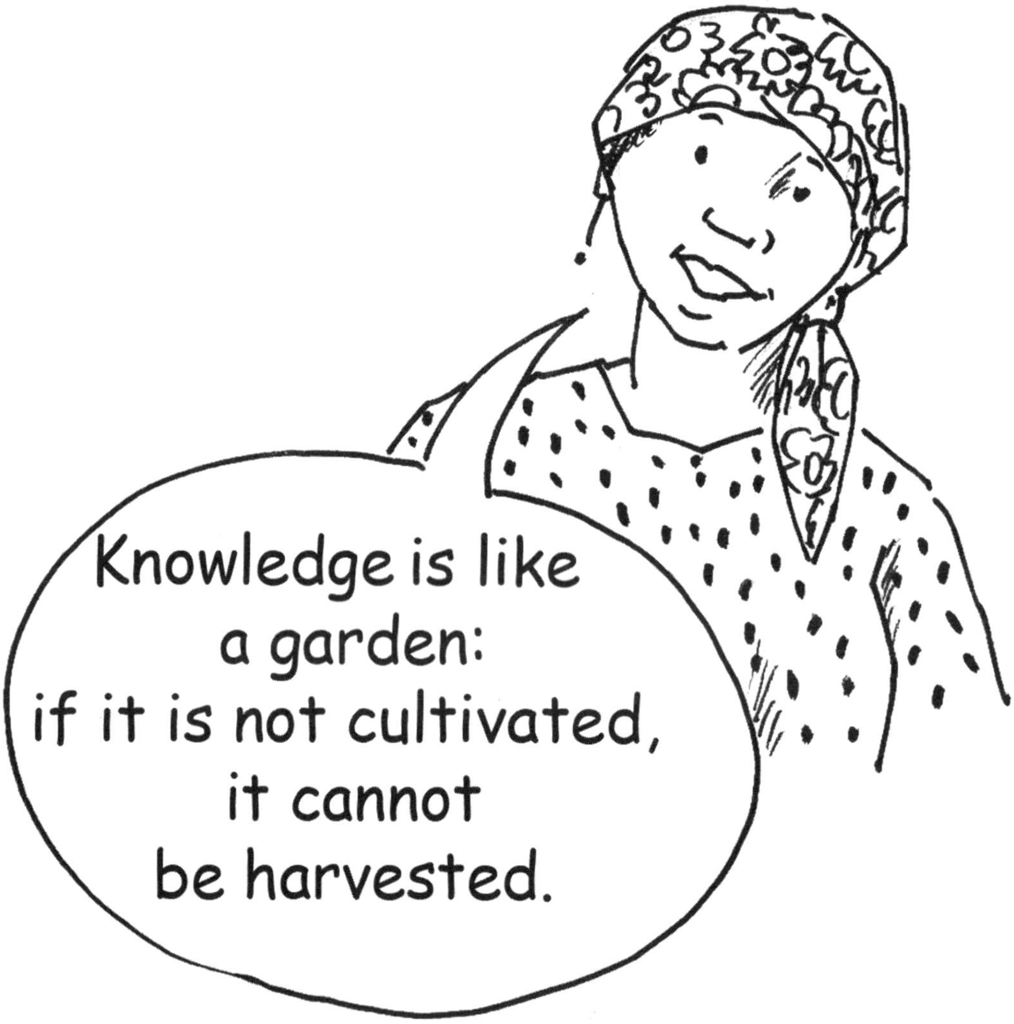
Knowledge is like a garden: if it is not cultivated, it cannot be harvested.

ANNEX 8 QUESTIONNAIRE ON THIS MANUAL AND DVD

Did you find this manual and DVD package useful?
Would you like more material like this?

A lot of time, money, and effort has gone into the production of this manual and DVD. We and our donors would like to know whether this has been worthwhile or not, and whether it might be worth producing more materials of this kind in future. The best judges of this are you, the users. We would be most grateful, therefore, if you could spare the time to fill in this questionnaire, **after you have run the programme with a community for the first time**, and send it to us (address at the end of the questionnaire). If you want to keep your copy of the manual intact, perhaps you could photocopy these pages and fill them in for us. Please note that if, for any reason, you **cannot** run a workshop because of something which you see as a problem with this manual and DVD, we would be very glad to hear from you also. If you would like to, please include your name and address, but you do not have to if you would rather make your comments anonymously. Thank you!

Please note that we would also be very pleased if you could send us your write-up of the six-monthly post-workshop review meetings, which are described in the second half of Annex 4.

QUESTIONNAIRE ON 'STEPPING STONES' MANUAL AND VIDEO

If you would like to give us your contact details, please write them in capital letters below

Your Name:

Organisation:

Address:

Email address: (please write this clearly in lower case if need be!)

Position/Occupation:

Male ☐ Female ☐ Other ☐ (please tick)

Age in years:

Please answer the following statements about yourself and the training material in the most appropriate way.

1. I would consider myself: (please circle)

5	4	3	2	1	0
very experienced trainer					not experienced in training at all

2. I have used this manual and DVD: (please tick)

As part of my work
On a voluntary basis

3. I have trained .... (number of people), who were: (please tick)

Old men	Young men
Old women	Young women
Others (please describe)	

Location of training:

(name of village, nearest town, region, country)

Duration of training:

(number of weeks over which workshop was conducted)

Trainees could best be described as: (please tick the best answer or answers)

Rural people	Employees
Urban people	Armed forces/police
Students	Other (please describe)

4. I have had formal training specifically for use of this manual and DVD: (please tick)

Yes No
If 'Yes', please state where this was, when, who organised it and how long it lasted:
Where:
When:
Organiser:
How long:

5. (If you did have formal training for this manual and DVD) I found this training:

5	4	3	2	1	0
very helpful					not helpful at all

In the following questions, please circle the answer which best fits your experience.

THE MANUAL

6. In relation to my work, the contents of the manual are:

5	4	3	2	1	0
very relevant					not relevant at all

7. The manual corresponds to the needs of the peer group or groups:

5	4	3	2	1	0
very much					not at all

8. The manual helped me to assess my own progress while running the workshop:

5	4	3	2	1	0
very much					not at all

9. The quality of the contents of the manual is:

5 very high	4	3	2	1	0 very low

10. The information is given in an order which makes sense to me:

5 strongly agree	4	3	2	1	0 strongly disagree

11. I can find the information I need in the manual:

5 very easily	4	3	2	1	0 with great difficulty

12. The language used in the text is:

5 very hard to understand	4	3	2	1	0 far too simple

13. The Contents table is arranged in a way which is:

5 clear and easy to use	4	3	2	1	0 very difficult to use

14. The introduction to the manual ('Before you Begin ...!') helps me to understand how to use the manual:

5 very much	4	3	2	1	0 not at all

15. The quiz in the introduction helped me to assess my own capacity as a trainer:

5 very much	4	3	2	1	0 not at all

16. I found the instructions about how to use the DVD in the workshop sessions:

5 very easy to follow	4	3	2	1	0 very hard to follow

17. The way in which each session is presented makes using the manual:

5 very easy	4	3	2	1	0 very difficult

18. The illustrations in the manual are:

5	4	3	2	1	0
very clear and easy to understand					very difficult to understand

19. It does not matter that there is no index:

5	4	3	2	1	0
strongly agree					strongly disagree

20. I find the manual size:

5	4	3	2	1	0
very easy to carry around and use in sessions					much too bulky to carry around and use in sessions

21. I find the manual binding:

5	4	3	2	1	0
good: strong and long-lasting					bad: manual is falling apart

22. The general appearance of the manual is:

5	4	3	2	1	0
very attractive					very unattractive

23. Availability: (please tick)

I have my own copy of this manual or
I have to share my copy of the manual with others.
If shared, please state how many people you share it with.

(If shared) I share a copy because of: (please tick)

High cost of the manual
The few copies available
Other reasons (please explain)

24. I would like more material like this:

5	4	3	2	1	0
very much					not at all

ADDITIONAL INFORMATION

(You can write your comments on a separate piece of paper, if you prefer.)

25. How could we improve the manual to meet your needs better?

26. What additional comments would you like to make about the manual?

THE DVD

27. In relation to the community where I work, I found the contents of the DVD:

5	4	3	2	1	0
very relevant					not relevant at

28. I found the the DVD:

5	4	3	2	1	0
very easy to follow and use					very hard to follow or use

29. I found the length of the various DVD clips:

5	4	3	2	1	0
much too long					much too short

30. I found the themes of the DVD clips:
(please score each clip as follows: A = very clear, B = quite clear, C = OK, D = not very clear, E = not clear at all)

Clip Number:

1	6	11
2	7	12
3	8	13
4	9	14
5	10	15

31. The language version of the DVD which I used was: (please write which language)

32. I would most like the DVD to be translated into: (please write which language)

33. I would like more DVDs like this:

5 very much	4	3	2	1	0 not at all

ADDITIONAL INFORMATION

(You may write your comments on a separate piece of paper, if you prefer.)

34. How could we improve the DVD to meet your needs better?

35. Please write any additional comments you would like to make about the DVD below.

Please send your completed questionnaire either as a scanned document to: enquiries@steppingstonesfeedback.org and mark the subject line 'Stepping Stones questionnaire response'

Alternatively you can send it by post to:
Stepping Stones Coordinator
Questionnaire Response
Salamander Trust
Positively UK
345 City Road
London EC1V 1LR, UK

Thank you!

QUICK REFERENCE PAGE

PRESENTATION OF SESSIONS

There are three open community meetings, two full workshop meetings and eighteen peer group sessions described in this manual. During the first open community meeting and some of the peer group sessions a DVD clip will be shown. In some peer group sessions drawing materials, DVD equipment, rope, or string will be needed. You will also need your own notebook or Facilitators' Journal and pen. In other sessions, nothing is needed except the participants themselves. **At the end of every session (except the first open community meeting), you will need some flip-chart paper, marker pens, and small stones to carry out the instant review. See Annex 4 for details of this.**

In order to help you prepare for each session, a checklist appears of materials required for the exercises on the title page of each session. You will also see special information about each session. Please read this carefully.

Within each session, you will find that each exercise is presented as follows:

AIMS
DESCRIPTION
MATERIALS NEEDED (if any)
DIRECTIONS

Some exercises also have a section called **Feedback and discussion**, where ideas are given for analysis of the exercise.

Some exercises also have other boxes in italics. These are often examples of what happened when the workshop in Buwenda was conducted. They are included to illustrate to you how this exercise worked there. They do NOT mean that your community is expected to come up with the SAME examples!

☞ Many exercises have a box of text, beginning with a pointing finger. In these you will find additional comments which will help you to conduct the exercise more effectively.

Each session concludes with a section entitled **FACILITATORS' TEAM FEEDBACK**. This reminds you to meet, and provides notes relevant to the previous and next sessions.

Your notes ... At the very end of each session, any spare space is left for you to jot down your own notes or comments.

SUPPORTING RESOURCES AND DEDICATED WEBSITE

Our ethos

As users of the *Stepping Stones* materials, we expect you to collaborate with us using the same ethos of shared learning and growth, through regular communication and discussion, that is at the core of this programme. This includes your involvement in the following:

Stepping stones community of practice (COP)

This 1,200 strong community is free to join. It links individuals and organisations, large and small around the world who have used or are using *Stepping Stones* in diverse contexts and cultures. Through our regular COP newsletter, we are especially keen for you to share with us any evaluations you have undertaken of your work with *Stepping Stones*. We can also keep you up to date with new ideas and advice about how others have adapted *Stepping Stones* to their context whilst keeping true to the original 'foundation stones', to maximize chances of its effectiveness.

Website

If you have internet access, you can learn more about the package and how it works on: **www.steppingstonesfeedback.org**

This site also has links to many related materials on participatory approaches to gender, sexual and reproductive health and well-being, and rights, and monitoring and evaluation of all these.

Vimeo: There are now several films about the use of *Stepping Stones* available online or on your smartphone Vimeo app: https://vimeo.com/salamandertrust

Adaptations

If you want to adapt this programme you must contact us for information, advice and permissions, in order to comply with our requirements. This programme has been adapted and translated widely across Africa, Asia, Latin America, Eastern Europe, Central Asia and the Pacific, where many similar results from diverse Muslim, Christian, Hindu and other communities have been reported. There may already be a local translation and/or adaptation of *Stepping Stones* **relevant to your needs, and we can help you find** out about these and how to get hold of them. There is an excellent resource available on request from us, entitled *Implementing Stepping Stones* (ACORD 2007), which can help you to adapt it. We also offer our own advice and support services, to ensure that any adaptation maintains the original principles of the manual. **Please read and observe the permissions paragraph at the start of this volume.**

Monitoring and evaluation

See Annex 4.

Contact

enquiries@steppingstonesfeedback.org
Postal Address:
Stepping Stones Coordinator
Salamander Trust
Positively UK
345 City Road
London EC1V 1LR, UK